Introduction to Health Care in a
FLASH!

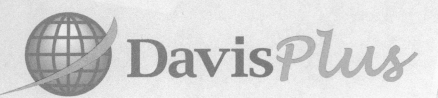
 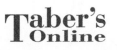

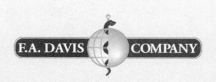

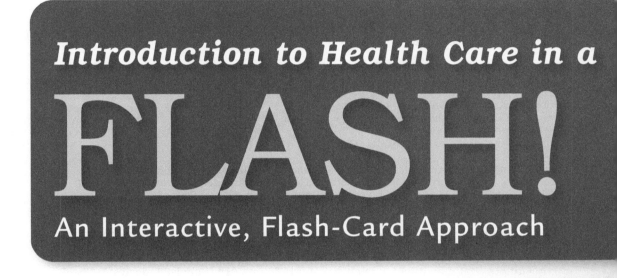

Introduction to Health Care in a
FLASH!

An Interactive, Flash-Card Approach

Marilyn Turner, RN, CMA (AAMA)
Medical Assisting Program Director
Ogeechee Technical College
Statesboro, Georgia

 F.A. Davis Company • Philadelphia

F. A. Davis Company
1915 Arch Street
Philadelphia, PA 19103
www.fadavis.com

Printed in the United States of America

Last digit indicates print number: 10 9 8 7 6

Senior Acquisitions Editor: Andy McPhee
Manager of Content Development: George W. Lang
Developmental Editor: Grace Caputo
Manager of Art and Design: Carolyn O'Brien

As new scientific information becomes available through basic and clinical research, recommended treatments and drug therapies undergo changes. The author(s) and publisher have done everything possible to make this book accurate, up to date, and in accord with accepted standards at the time of publication. The author(s), editors, and publisher are not responsible for errors or omissions or for consequences from application of the book, and make no warranty, expressed or implied, in regard to the contents of the book. Any practice described in this book should be applied by the reader in accordance with professional standards of care used in regard to the unique circumstances that may apply in each situation. The reader is advised always to check product information (package inserts) for changes and new information regarding dose and contraindications before administering any drug. Caution is especially urged when using new or infrequently ordered drugs.

Library of Congress Cataloging-in-Publication Data
Turner, Marilyn (Marilyn M.)
  Introduction to health care in a flash! : an interactive, flash-card approach / Marilyn Turner.
      p. ; cm.
  Includes index.
  ISBN 978-0-8036-2586-0 (pbk. : alk. paper)
  I. Title.
  [DNLM: 1. Allied Health Personnel. 2. Infection Control. 3. Patient Care. 4. Vocational Guidance. W 21.5]

362.1—dc23   2012002501

DEDICATION

To my family—Barry, Brooks, Whitney, and Andrew—who has tolerated my hills and valleys on this journey of accomplishment. Also, to Mama, Robert, and Jan. Thank you all for knowing when to ask and when to be quiet.

PREFACE

Health care is a challenging yet rewarding career. There are many levels of direct patient care jobs and administrative jobs, all working together for the patient's benefit. Regardless of the type of healthcare career you choose, *Introduction to Health Care in a Flash!* will give you insight.

Health care is one of the most rapidly changing fields in today's society. Advances in technology allow physicians to treat patients more rapidly and with greater precision, and research and development of new treatments and medications provide management for previously untreatable diseases. Advances in health care are expensive, and insurance companies are striving to cover the costs. With increasing costs, we must look at ways to provide quality health care in the most economical manner. But regardless of the costs involved, the personal touch of health care cannot be ignored.

This text will take you back to the early institutions of healing and through the development of today's healthcare facilities and technologies. You will learn the fundamental skills of teamwork, medical terminology, infection control, patient assessment, and vital signs.

Cultural sensitivity has become a concern in health care as the population grows and changes. Learning to work with those who may think differently is essential to the quality care that we seek to deliver.

Protecting yourself and your patients from infectious diseases is paramount in today's healthcare environment. This text will focus on what you can do at work and at home to protect yourself, your patients, and your family.

Every industry has standards that must be met, and health care is no exception. Learning the legal issues that surround patient information is an important part of this text. There are specific federal regulations that govern the release of this information. Understanding and abiding by these rules will help you document successfully and maintain confidentiality.

This text will take you from the classroom through job interviews to your final goal of working in the healthcare discipline of your choice. After you are employed, you will want to stay challenged and continue your learning process. This text ends with tips for maintaining your career.

Throughout the text, you will be prompted to *Stop, Think, and Learn*, with real-world situations in health care. These activities will help develop your critical thinking skills that are essential for working with patients and other members of the healthcare team. Chapters will provide Internet resources for additional information and helpful tips. Flashpoints appear throughout each chapter to give additional facts about the information in the text. Practice exercises are designed to help you understand the material in each chapter.

Software

At the back of this book there is a CD-ROM with interactive learning activities to help reinforce the information you learn in each chapter. There are several types of activities to benefit multiple styles of learning. Additional activities are available online at http://davisplus.fadavis.com, keyword Turner.

Flash Cards

This text has a printable set of flash cards available online at http://davisplus.fadavis.com, keyword: Turner. These can be helpful for reviewing the key terms in each chapter. Reviewing flash cards on your own or with a partner is a great way to prepare for tests.

REVIEWERS

ACKNOWLEDGMENTS

Thank you, F.A. Davis Company, for allowing me to combine my creative spirit with my passion for health care in a book that I hope will inspire future healthcare professionals.

A very special thank you to Andy McPhee. You believed in me more than I believed in myself and never gave up on me. We did it!

Thanks to Grace Caputo at Dovetail Content Solutions for your firm yet gentle nudging and the occasional swift kick when I needed it.

Many thanks to my colleagues at Ogeechee Technical College. Our healthcare partners are fortunate to have such a committed group of teachers preparing the next generation of healthcare professionals. A special thanks to Michelle, Jan, and Michele for giving me the courage to keep pushing through.

And thanks to all of my friends for understanding when I couldn't come out to play.

The secret of teaching is to appear to have known all of your life what you just learned this morning.
—ANONYMOUS

CONTENTS IN BRIEF

CONTENTS

INTRODUCTION

Learning Styles

Individuals learn information in different ways according to unique abilities and traits. The ways in which individuals perceive, understand, and remember information will be somewhat different from the styles of others.

In truth, everyone possesses a combination of styles. You may be especially strong in one style and less so in others. You may be strong in two or three areas or may be equally strong in all areas. No style is inherently good or bad. It simply indicates how you perceive and process new information most effectively. As you learn about the styles described here and come to identify your own, you will be able to modify your study activities accordingly. This will help you make the most of your valuable study time, enhance your learning, and support you in doing your very best in future classes.

Visual Learners

Most people are strongly visual learners. To grasp new information most accurately and quickly, these people need to see it represented visually. The more complex the data, the truer this is. Visual learners especially like content that is colorful and visually striking.

If you are a visual learner, you may have already noticed that you are drawn to visual information. Unless you are also an auditory learner, you may have some difficulty remembering information that is shared only verbally. Consequently, you may ask others to repeat themselves or, better yet, to write down their information. When looking through books, magazines, or instruction manuals, you are especially drawn to photos and illustrations because they help you "see" more accurately what is being discussed. In the classroom, you may prefer instructors who use written outlines and many visual aids.

You generally have a good sense of direction, rarely get lost, and can interpret and use maps easily. Your office and home may be littered with lists and notes that you have written to organize yourself and to remember things. You love self-adhesive note pads. You find listening to a lecture without stimulating visuals to be boring and tedious. You need to take notes, draw, or doodle to prevent falling asleep. In fact, you may appear to other people as if you are distracted or daydreaming. However, you know that doodling actually helps you listen better. Your work and hobbies include activities that make use of color, shapes, and design or visual art. Just a few examples include drawing, painting, quilting, photography, and keeping a scrap book.

Study Strategies for Visual Learners

If you are a visual learner, try using study or memory techniques that aid you in being able to visualize and recall information. You may find **mnemonics** (memory aids) especially helpful for remembering lists or sequenced pieces of information. Generally, the more creative, whimsical, funny, or absurd the aids, the better you will remember the information. There are many types of mnemonics. For example, children use the well-known alphabet song, a musical mnemonic, to learn their ABCs. Students in anatomy class use one of several mnemonic variations to remember the 12 cranial nerves (Olfactory, Optic, Oculomotor, Trochlear, Trigeminal, Abducens, Facial, Acoustic, Glossopharyngeal, Vagus, Spinal Accessory, and Hypoglossal). The mnemonic is: *"On Old Olympus' Tower Tops, A Finn And German Viewed Some Hops."* The first letter of each word is the same as the first letter of each of the cranial nerves. Similarly, many people use a spelling mnemonic: "I before E, except after C."

Another form of common mnemonic is the **acronym.** An acronym is an abbreviation created by using the first letters or word parts to create names or readable words. Examples of acronyms include LASER (Light Amplification by Stimulated Emission of Radiation), FAQ (Frequently Asked Questions), and PIN (Personal Identification Number). In addition, the seven warning signs of cancer can be represented in the acronym CAUTION (Change in bowel or bladder habits, A sore throat that does not heal, Unusual bleeding or discharge, Thickening or a lump in the breast or other area, Indigestion or difficulty swallowing, Obvious change in a mole or wart, and Nagging cough or hoarseness).

Auditory Learners

Many people are auditory (or aural) learners. In order to grasp new information, these people need to hear it spoken. The more complex the information, the more they need to hear it. The most common example of auditory information is a classroom lecture. Other auditory sources of information are audiotapes, videotapes, computer tutorials (with audio content), and discussion groups.

If you are an auditory learner, you may have already noticed that you are drawn to information presented aloud. Unless you are also a visual learner, you may have some difficulty remembering written information without some verbal discussion or review. You may often ask others to elaborate on details or ask them to repeat themselves so you can hear the content again. When recalling events, you can sometimes "hear" how someone else speaks. You notice subtle inflections that convey meaning.

Study Strategies for Auditory Learners

If you are an auditory learner, try using study or memory techniques that allow you to hear information aloud, whether it is the spoken word or data set to music or any other auditory format. Auditory learners are also usually verbal learners as well. If this is true for you, then you learn best when you have the chance for a verbal exchange. This allows you to speak to and listen to others. You find mnemonics helpful, especially if they include rhyming or are catchy and fun to say out loud. A common example is the following mnemonic used to help people remember the number of days in each month:

30 days hath September,
April, June, and November;
All the rest have 31,
Excepting February:
Which has 28, that's fine;
'Til leap year gives it 29.

Verbal Learners

It is sometimes said that some people must think (first) in order to speak. For verbal learners, the reverse may be true. They feel compelled to speak in order to think. Speaking aloud helps them to process information and think things through. This is especially true when the information is complex or the situation feels stressful. These people often "talk to themselves." Such individuals may state that doing so helps slow their brain down in order to help them focus and think more clearly.

If you are a verbal learner, you may seek a friend to act as a "sounding board." You do not expect this person to solve your problem; rather, you need someone to listen as you "think out loud" and "bounce things around." Most likely, you love to read and enjoy some type of writing. This could take a professional form such as becoming an author or writing poetry for your own enjoyment or writing in a private journal. You enjoy learning new words and incorporating them into your vocabulary. You find rhymes and tongue-twisters entertaining. You may enjoy reading poetry aloud because speaking it is more enjoyable than reading it silently.

Study Strategies for Verbal Learners

If you are a verbal learner, try using study or memory techniques that allow you to recite data or explain concepts aloud. Like auditory learners, you find mnemonics helpful, especially if they are fun to say or include rhyming. You may also find writing to be very helpful. Writing important data into outlines, summaries, or vocabulary helps you remember the content. You are very likely a social learner who benefits from studying with a partner or in a study group. This provides ample opportunity for discussion. You especially benefit from explaining challenging concepts or "teaching" your study partners about a given topic.

For example, the members of your study group may decide to teach one another about the four major joint types in the body: hinge, ball and socket, pivot, and gliding. Each person describes the appearance and function of the assigned joint and gives an example. For instance, one person may compare a hinge joint, such as those found in the knee and elbow, with a door hinge. The person describes how the joint moves back and forth like a door that swings open and shut. The next person may compare a pivot joint, such as the one in the neck, with a chair that turns back and forth in a 180-degree half circle. Other students go on to teach about their assigned joints and give examples. To maximize the value of this exercise, have all members of the group repeat key information or phrases after the "teacher" states it.

Kinesthetic Learners

Most people have some kinesthetic (tactile) aspects to their learning style, even though it may not be their most dominant style. People who are strong kinesthetic learners need to use their bodies as they learn. They like to touch and manipulate objects. This is especially important when learning physical skills. When assembling things, they may skip reading the instructions and just assemble the product based on inclination. They are usually successful, but if not, then they may check the instructions, which will make much more sense to them after they have become physically acquainted with the parts.

If you are a kinesthetic learner, you may have already noticed that you are eager to get your hands on objects to do things yourself. When the information being learned is theoretical, you are still eager to move your body somehow, even if it is to draw a diagram or fidget in your chair. Sitting through lengthy lectures feels tedious and almost painful to you. You like to touch things, and you very likely have hobbies that include manipulating objects or making things. You notice textures and like how they feel. Your most productive thinking time occurs when you are on the move in activities such as biking, hiking, walking, or running on a treadmill. You get restless if you sit around too long and feel eager to "do" something. You are very physical when communicating and may use big hand and arm gestures. You may enjoy dancing, sports, and other physical activities.

Study Strategies for Kinesthetic Learners

If you are a kinesthetic learner, try using study or memory techniques that allow you to move your body or touch objects. When learning skills or procedures, your best strategy is to get your hands on the needed supplies and practice the procedure. For example, consider again the study group in which you and your friends are each describing major body joints. In addition to describing the joints and giving examples, each person must act out or physically mimic the joint movement. The person describing the hinge joint now must stand up and find a door to open and shut while describing its function or might even play the part of the door and move back and forth in an open-door way. The next person compares a pivot joint, such as the one in the neck, with a chair that turns back and forth in a 180-degree half circle, demonstrating by turning the head back and forth and then turning the chair back and forth in a 180-degree half circle. After each person performs, other members of the group must perform the same physical movement. This gives everyone full kinesthetic value from the activity.

When actual physical practice of a skill is not possible, visualization is a great alternative. Play learning games, use flash cards, complete activities included in your textbook, use the student activity disk that accompanies many textbooks (including this one), and interact with a study partner or group.

Social Learners

Many people are social learners. They learn most effectively when they are able to interact with other people. They enjoy the group **synergy** (enhanced action of two or more agents working together cooperatively) and are able to think things through with the verbal exchange that occurs during a lively discussion.

If you are a social learner, you may have already noticed that you are drawn to social situations and do not like to study alone. You communicate and interact well with others. You enjoy listening to and helping others. You may also be a verbal-auditory learner and may enjoy discussions and "bouncing ideas" off other people. You are drawn to social situations and may stay after class to talk with others. If you are athletic, you may prefer group sports to solo activities. You also enjoy social activities such as dancing and board games. You like working through problems with a partner or a group. Work activities may include teaching, coaching, or working in a people-oriented setting such as a restaurant or retail store.

Study Strategies for Social Learners

If you are a social learner, you may find that you feel restless and have difficulty staying focused when you try to study alone. You need to study with other people. Consider starting a study group. Group activities can include discussion, learning games, role playing, and creating mnemonics together.

Solitary Learners

Many people are solitary learners. They learn most effectively when they are able to study alone without distraction from others. They are often somewhat private and enjoy time alone so they can reflect. They are strongly independent and know what works for them. Trying to conform to the group can be a source of frustration.

If you are a solitary learner, you may feel frustrated trying to study with a partner or a group. You may feel like they are wasting your time and believe you would do better by yourself. You focus and concentrate best when alone. You are analytical and goal-oriented. You are also a self-starter and do not need anyone to prompt you or to provide structure. You have learned to enjoy your own company and enjoy solitude. Many people, especially work colleagues, may find this difficult to understand because they may not like being alone. You may be known to travel alone, dine out alone, and go to movies or concerts alone because you do not have to negotiate with anyone else about what to do or where to go.

Study Strategies for Solitary learners

There are many ways that solitary learners study. The important thing is that they do it alone. They may read, review notes, and listen to taped lectures (if they are also auditory), or incorporate other strategies noted in this chapter, and they do so alone.

Global Learners

Global learners, sometimes called *holistic learners,* generally see the big picture first and pay more attention to details later. For example, when studying the human body, global learners first see it as a whole, complete organism. With that picture in mind, they are then able to begin studying the parts. This is true even when studying individual body systems, such as the cardiovascular system. Global learners first grasp the big picture of the entire system as it circulates blood throughout the body. With further study and thought, they appreciate how the system delivers oxygen and nutrients and eliminates wastes through a complex network of vessels including veins, arteries, and capillaries.

If you are a global learner, you may often respond based on intuition or emotion and are able to grasp symbolism. You may be able to accept rules, such as a math equation, without necessarily understanding how the steps work. You are probably good at recognizing relationships and "reading between the lines." You are flexible and do well with multitasking. When studying new concepts, you usually compare them with concepts you already understand. For example, when first learning about the lymphatic system, you may think, "This is very similar to what I know about the vascular system. They both have a complex network of vessels that convey fluid through the body." As you study the lymphatic system in detail, you then begin to distinguish the important differences.

Study Strategies for Global Learners

If you are a global learner, you are probably also a visual/auditory learner, so try the study and memory techniques previously described. If you find studying details to be tedious and boring, try to find other, more creative and fun ways to learn the same material. For example, you may prefer drawing your own colorful diagrams or may enjoy using audio/visual tutorials or other activities that are often on the student disks that accompany textbooks or are online.

Use your strengths. You are flexible. You are a multitasker. Do not be afraid to make your study efforts more lively and enjoyable. You are good at seeing the big picture and recognizing relationships. Therefore, begin each study session by identifying the relationship between what you are currently studying and your future career ambitions. While reading, make note of terms, concepts, or sections that you skipped over or did not understand. You can do this by highlighting these areas in a specific color or by writing notes in the margins. After your initial read-through, force yourself to return to each of these areas, and investigate them further.

Analytical Learners

Analytical learners, sometimes called *logical, linear, sequential, or mathematical* learners, generally need to see the parts before fully comprehending the whole. For example, when studying the human body, analytical learners prefer to study in a methodical fashion, beginning with the smallest parts and working up to the whole. Such people will prefer to take classes such as chemistry and cellular biology before taking classes like anatomy and physiology. As they continue learning about each of the body systems, they begin to appreciate how each relates to the other and comprises the whole organism. Analytical learners readily identify patterns and like to group data into categories for further study. They love to create and follow agendas, make lists with items ranked by priority, and approach problem solving in a methodical manner. They like to create and follow procedures and may grow impatient with others who do not. Analytical learners are often linear and orderly in their thinking and seek to quantify things whenever possible. They often pursue careers in accounting, sciences, computer technology, engineering, law enforcement, and mathematics.

Study Strategies for Analytical Learners

Put your organizational talent to work to make your study efforts productive. Make an agenda, or create a list of topics to be studied. Prioritize topics to ensure that you address the most important ones first. This is your *need to know* list. Set and follow time limits. It is most important to get busy studying. Rather than get sidetracked with interesting but low-priority items, make another list of topics as you go along titled *nice to know*. Come back to this list later if, and only if, time permits.

Use your gift for identifying patterns by noting patterns within the material you are studying. This can be useful when you prepare for exams because test questions often focus on features that are similar and those that are different. For example, a myocardial infarction (MI, also known as a heart attack) and angina both cause chest pain. In both cases, the pain is caused by inadequate blood supply to the heart. These are two important and similar features when comparing these disorders (chest pain and lack of oxygen). On the other hand, an MI causes actual death of heart muscle tissue, but angina does not. This is an important difference.

To make the most of some study strategies, give yourself permission to be illogical or even silly. If a technically "inaccurate" mnemonic or silly song will help you remember something, use it.

As you continue through this book you will find study tips included in every chapter. These tips suggest study techniques for all learning styles. Keep an open mind as you move forward, and be willing to try any that you believe may be helpful. Make notes as you do so about what did and did not work well and anything you might do differently next time.

Resources

Visit http://davisplus.fadavis.com and search for keyword "Turner" for pertinent resources to aid in your studies.

THE EVOLUTION OF MODERN HEALTH CARE

Learning Outcomes

1.1 Identify early healthcare delivery systems

1.2 Contrast early healthcare facilities with current facilities

1.3 Describe early physicians and their contributions to current health care

1.4 Discuss various types of healthcare facilities and the patients they treat

1.5 Contrast healthcare professionals and their roles in patient care

1.6 Identify technological advances in health care

Competencies

CAAHEP

• Discuss principles of using electronic medical record. (CAAHEP V.C.11)
• Discuss legal scope of practice for medical assistants. (CAAHEP IX.C.1)
• Discuss licensure and certification as it applies to healthcare providers. (CAAHEP IX.C.5)
• Compare and contrast physician and medical assistant roles in terms of standard of care. (CAAHEP IX.C.7)

ABHES

• Compare and contrast the allied health professions and understand their relation to medical assisting. (ABHES 1.b)

Key Terms

algorithm Detailed treatment scenarios that can be used to tailor a patient's care regardless of where he or she is being treated

asclepeion An ancient Greek healing temple

avatar A virtual reality coach that one day may replace health call centers

electronic medical record (EMR)

electronic health record (EHR) A computerized record of a patient's healthcare encounters

Elizabeth Blackwell The first female to qualify as a physician in the United States

emergency medical services Healthcare professionals that provide pre-hospital care to victims of sudden illnesses, accidents, or injuries at the scene of the accident or illness and during transport to a healthcare facility

Continued

Health care is one of the fastest changing fields in today's society. Advances in technology allow physicians to treat patients more rapidly and with greater precision, while research and development of new treatments and medications provide management for previous untreatable diseases. Developments in health care are important because our life expectancy has increased 30 years over the last century. As life expectancy increases, so do the healthcare needs of the increasingly elderly population.

Flashpoint

Modern society uses the spa experience to relax and de-stress, which may contribute to a person's good health.

The History of Health Care

It is interesting to look back to see how modern health care has evolved over the centuries and to try to imagine life without the sophisticated treatment modalities that are available to us today. For instance, in the pre-Christian era (4000–3000 BC) illness and disease were viewed as a punishment from the gods for which healers used herbs to restore patients to health. Many cultures contributed to early health care in the pre-Christian era, including the ancient Egyptians, Greeks, Romans, and Chinese.

The early Christian era (1–500), medieval era (500–1500), and modern era (1500–1800) saw advances in healthcare technology and medical practices that have shaped health care as we know it today.

The Egyptians

From 3000 to 300 BC, ancient Egyptian priests also served as physicians and used bloodletting or leeches as medical treatment. A system of community planning that involved hygiene, sanitation, embalming, and dentistry existed. Medical records were preserved in papyrus, and women assisted the priest-physicians as midwives and wet nurses. Because human dissection was a forbidden practice, future progress of health care was stalled.

The Greeks

Most references to early health care begin in ancient Greece (1200–200 BC). The Greeks actively participated in behaviors that benefited their health, including a daily exercise routine and a diet that included the use of herbs and vitamins. Some ancient Greeks believed that illness was a curse from the supernatural or that they had angered one of the gods in some way; others believed a chemical imbalance within the sick person was the cause for illness. Those who believed in the supernatural would trek miles in search of a healing temple, called an **asclepeion,** named for Asclepius, the Greek god of healing. Treatment was often sought in these temples after conventional medicine had failed.

Services provided in the temple included healthy foods, hydrotherapy, music therapy, and psychotherapy. Once the temple therapists felt that a person was ready for healing, the patient went into a small room to sleep in hopes of a visit from Asclepius in their dreams. Such a dream was thought to start the healing process. Treatments such as this gained popularity in Greece and eventually spread throughout other areas of Europe and the Middle East. It is possible to find care similar to that given in the asclepeions in modern-day spas, where treatments may include massage, hydrotherapy, aromatherapy, and botanical aesthetic skin care, services that pamper the consumer and lead to an overall feeling of well-being.

The early Greek physician **Hippocrates** (circa 460–377 BC; Fig. 1-1) was opposed to the belief that illness was the result of a curse or supernatural causes. He believed that for healing to occur the body should be treated as a whole. He taught the healing process consisted of fresh air, good food, rest, and above all, cleanliness. This was the beginning of the philosophy known as **holistic medicine.** Hippocrates began to train other scholars and today is

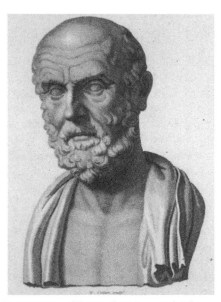

FIGURE 1-1 **Hippocrates.** (From the National Library of Medicine.)

revered as the "father of Western medicine." He is also credited with writing the ***Hippocratic Oath,*** a pledge in which a new physician swears to uphold a number of professional ethical standards, a promise that can be boiled down to "harm not." A modernized version of the Hippocratic Oath (Box 1-1) is a part of every medical school graduation.

Several centuries later, the Greek physician ***Galen*** (circa 130–200) began to study disease through dissection of deceased patients as well as dead

---

Box 1-1 The Modern Hippocratic Oath

I swear to fulfill, to the best of my ability and judgment, this covenant:

I will respect the hard-won scientific gains of those physicians in whose steps I walk, and gladly share such knowledge as is mine with those who are to follow.

I will apply, for the benefit of the sick, all measures [that] are required, avoiding those twin traps of overtreatment and therapeutic nihilism.

I will remember that there is art to medicine as well as science, and that warmth, sympathy, and understanding may outweigh the surgeon's knife or the chemist's drug.

I will not be ashamed to say "I know not," nor will I fail to call in my colleagues when the skills of another are needed for a patient's recovery.

I will respect the privacy of my patients, for their problems are not disclosed to me that the world may know. Most especially must I tread with care in matters of life and death. If it is given me to save a life, all thanks. But it may also be within my power to take a life; this awesome responsibility must be faced with great humbleness and awareness of my own frailty. Above all, I must not play at God.

I will remember that I do not treat a fever chart, a cancerous growth, but a sick human being, whose illness may affect the person's family and economic stability. My responsibility includes these related problems, if I am to care adequately for the sick.

I will prevent disease whenever I can, for prevention is preferable to cure.

Continued

Key Terms—cont'd

"if/then" A plan of care based on the patient's symptoms; for example, *if* the patient has a fever, *then* the patient should take an antipyretic

nurse practitioner A registered nurse with an advanced degree (master's) who takes health histories, performs basic physical examinations, helps establish treatment plans, orders medical procedures and laboratory tests, refers patients to physicians, treats common illnesses, and teaches patients to promote optimal health

physician's assistant A master's degree–prepared healthcare professional who works under the supervision of physicians to take medical histories and perform physical examinations, order laboratory and diagnostic tests, make preliminary diagnoses, prescribe and administer medications and treatments, and treat minor injuries

trauma center A hospital, designated by the state, which houses a unit that specializes in the care of catastrophic physical events.

Box 1-1 The Modern Hippocratic Oath—cont'd

I will remember that I remain a member of society, with special obligations to all my fellow human beings, those sound of mind and body as well as the infirm.

If I do not violate this oath, may I enjoy life and art, respected while I live and remembered with affection thereafter. May I always act so as to preserve the finest traditions of my calling and may I long experience the joy of healing those who seek my help.

This version of the Hippocratic Oath was written in 1964 by Louis Lasagna, Academic Dean of the School of Medicine at Tufts University. It is used in many medical schools today.

---

animals. Galen was one of the first experimental physiologists, using controlled experiments to research the function of the kidneys and spinal cord. Specifically, Galen's theory that the brain controls all the motions of the muscles by means of the cranial and peripheral nervous systems is still believed today. As he studied, he recorded all of his findings in journals. Galen's message that observation and investigation are the cornerstones of medical research began to take hold, and his research findings were studied for centuries to come.

Table 1-1 summarizes early physicians and researchers and their contributions to health care.

TABLE 1-1

EARLY PHYSICIANS, RESEARCHERS, AND NURSES AND THEIR CONTRIBUTIONS TO HEALTH

Physician/Researcher	Date	Accomplishment/Contribution
Hippocrates	460-370 BC	The "Father of Medicine" established one of the first medical schools in ancient Greece.
Galen of Pergamon	130-200	Recorded very early discoveries in anatomy and research in the function of the kidneys and spinal cord. Galen's theory of observation and investigation in medicine led to today's modern research practices.
Ignaz Philipp Semmelweiss	1818-1865	Semmelweiss discovered the relationship of improperly washed hands to puerperal (childbed fever) infections. He observed medical students performing dissections on cadavers just prior to examining pregnant women. The mortality rate of these women was extremely high, and Semmelweiss is credited with decreasing the mortality in these women by requiring all of the healthcare workers to wash their hands in chlorinated lime water.
Louis Pasteur	1822-1885	Pasteur is known for his work in the development of vaccines against deadly diseases. He also discovered the process of pasteurization that is still used today as a method of preservation of foods. Pasteurization prevents spoilage of products such as milk by heating to just under the boiling point.

TABLE 1-1

EARLY PHYSICIANS, RESEARCHERS, AND NURSES AND THEIR CONTRIBUTIONS TO HEALTH—cont'd

Physician/Researcher	Date	Accomplishment/Contribution
Sir Alexander Fleming	1881–1955	During his research on the influenza virus, Fleming noted that mold growing on a culture plate of staphylococcus germs had created a bacteria-free area. He continued to work with this mold and discovered that it would kill the staphylococcus even when diluted. Fleming called this mold penicillin.
Elizabeth Blackwell	1821–1910	The first female recognized as a graduate of medical school who went on to become the first female physician in the United States. She pioneered the medical education of women as well as many other women's rights.
Wilhelm Roentgen	1845–1923	While conducting studies on cathode rays, this German physicist accidentally discovered a different type of emission ray. Because he did not know what to call this new discovery, he called them x-rays although they were often referred to as Roentgen rays. After the discovery and explanation of the rays, Roentgen left the further research to other physicists.
Robert Gallo and Luc Montagnier	1937–present 1932–present	These physicians are credited with the discovery of the HIV retrovirus that causes AIDS. Each of the physicians had worked tirelessly to identify the virus that was causing the devastating disease. Each claimed victory in their discovery when actually it was the same organism. When the battle became political, there was a joint announcement from both the French and American governments about the discovery.
Nurses		
Florence Nightingale	1820–1910	One of the best-known early nurses, Florence Nightingale's parents were totally against her career choice. Florence was extremely intelligent and excelled in nursing. She helped to improve the care of soldiers in the Crimean War and decrease the mortality rate from infection.
Walt Whitman	1818–1892	Little known as a nurse, the great American poet Walt Whitman served for several years as a volunteer nurse during the Civil War. He used his experience caring for the soldiers as inspiration for his poetry collection *Drumtaps*.
Mary Ezra Mahoney	1845–1926	The first African American nurse who graduated from the New England Hospital for Women and Children Training School for Nurses, Mary had a long and rewarding career in nursing.
Clara Barton	1821–1912	Clara Barton is best known for establishing the American Red Cross. The Baltimore Riots left many soldiers wounded, and Clara found that these soldiers were not suffering from lack of attention, but lack of supplies to care for their medical needs. She was very successful in soliciting donations to provide necessary medical supplies. After a stint as the superintendent of nurses in the Civil War, Clara focused her efforts on establishing the Red Cross organization.

Continued

TABLE 1-1		
EARLY PHYSICIANS, RESEARCHERS, AND NURSES AND THEIR CONTRIBUTIONS TO HEALTH—cont'd		
Physician/Researcher	**Date**	**Accomplishment/Contribution**
Mary Breckenridge	1881-1965	Mary Breckenridge realized a need for rural care for women and founded the Frontier Nursing Service in southeastern Kentucky in 1925. This network of nurse midwives provided care for some of the country's poorest and most isolated families. The nurse midwives visited homes on horseback and set up small healthcare facilities in the rural areas.

The Romans

The Romans, as well as the Greeks, had a powerful impact on the development of health care. During the Roman Empire (753 BC to AD 410), the military recognized the need for the development of organized health care for the citizens of ancient Rome. While the military attempted to organize health care by training soldiers to become physicians, there were untrained individuals who surfaced and called themselves physicians. Many of these self-proclaimed physicians offered treatments, such as bloodletting, that were in fact deadly. If you were ill, you had "bad blood," and draining your blood was the treatment offered. Practicing physicians knew how to control the treatment, but the self-proclaimed physicians often continued the bloodletting until the patient died. Treatment with herbs was also popular during these times, but not knowing the difference between helpful and poisonous herbs led to the deaths of many people. Other treatments that resulted in patient death included treatment with arsenic and excessive doses of belladonna and opium.

Roman society continued to investigate Hippocrates's theory of cleanliness in relation to disease. One of the most important inventions of the Roman Empire was the aqueduct system of water and waste management, which made it possible for clean water to be available in all public areas, including the public baths.

Flashpoint

The ancient Roman baths were used as a gathering place after a long day's work for bathing, exercise, and socialization and were segregated for men and women.

These baths were an incredible engineering achievement in their day. The baths were built over natural hot springs, and the water was pumped through elaborate systems into the pools. Interestingly, these baths were sometimes surrounded by exercise equipment, similar to today's health spas. Some of these baths were large enough to accommodate 3000 people at one time.

Romans instituted public toilets that were flushed clean by running water and that were supported by an effective drainage system. Seven rivers flowed through the city's sewers to keep the septic system functioning.

The Romans built what many consider to be civilization's first hospitals. The hospitals were built for the military because the Romans felt that these hygienic institutions would restore their soldiers to the battlefield sooner than if the soldiers were cared for in private homes. The hospitals had specialized rooms for different tasks and even isolation areas to prevent the spread of disease among patients. Even though the Romans did not fully understand how germs related to disease, they did boil their tools in the hospitals before use and would not reuse a soiled tool on a new patient without boiling it first.

The Chinese

The ancient Chinese (1700 BC to AD 220) used therapies such as acupuncture and believed in the *yin* (passive female) and *yang* (active male) forces. The ancient Chinese implemented the rule of the physical exam: look, listen, ask, and feel. Baths to reduce fever, bloodletting to free evil spirits, and the use of vaccinations and physiotherapy were part of Chinese medical practices. It was the ancient Greeks and Romans, however, who had the most influence on health care as we know it today.

The Early Christian Era

The early Christian era, from 1 to 500, follows the pre-Christian era. The first Christian community was centered in Jerusalem, and its leaders included James, Peter, and John. During the early Christian era, people were encouraged to feed the hungry and care for the sick. As religion became an important part of people's lives, caring for others became a priority. Rituals, chants, and prayers were offered up as a measure of healing the sick. In the ensuing years, science joined the healthcare effort and universities emerged across Europe to train physicians. Medical knowledge expanded and provided much needed information to allow the field of organized medicine to progress. The research that started hundreds of years ago continues to this day, with new discoveries and treatment modalities seemingly daily.

Throughout history, inventors have developed implements, medications, and procedures that changed the course of medical history (Table 1-2). With the exception of ether anesthesia, the inventions listed in Table 1-2 are still in use today. Many of these discoveries have been refined over the last several decades, such as lasers and kidney dialysis machines, and others, such as bleach and the compound microscope, have remained very close to their original form.

The Medieval Era

In the medieval era (500–1500), there was a poor understanding of the human body despite the earlier efforts of the Greeks and Romans. A population explosion and the unsanitary conditions of many medieval cities led to the Black Death (or bubonic plague), a pandemic illness that killed nearly half of the population of Europe.

Infectious disease was not understood, and antibiotics had not yet been invented. Illness was thought to occur due to some weakness of the soul, with prayer being the main action of treatment. The body was thought to be governed by four systems of "humors": earth, water, air, and fire. Health was maintained when the humors were balanced. To restore balance during illness, bloodletting, in which blood was drained to return the body to balance, was an unsuccessful practice. Herbal remedies, another treatment option, sometimes included poisons, urine, or feces.

Physicians would examine a patient's blood, urine, or stool to diagnose illness. Barbers were considered the first surgeons, although the concept of anesthesia was unknown. In order to balance the humors, brain surgery and cataract removal were often performed. Folk healers, monks, and saints also served as medical practitioners.

TABLE 1-2

HISTORICAL HEALTHCARE DISCOVERIES

Year	Application	Inventor	Use
1564	Condom	Gabriele Falloppio	Protects user from sexually transmitted diseases
1660	Compound microscope	Robert Hooke	Allows identification of microorganisms
1785	Chlorine bleach	Claude Louis Bertholett	Serves as disinfectant
1816	Stethoscope	Rene Laennec	Allows the healthcare worker to listen to internal body sounds including the heart, lungs, and bowels
1842	Ether anesthesia	Crawford Long	Allows patients to undergo surgery without pain or knowledge of the procedure
1847	Ophthalmoscope	Hermann Ludwig Ferdinand von Helmholtz	Allows view of the internal structures of the eye
1867	Antiseptic surgery	Joseph Lister	Reduces the number of deaths after surgical procedures
1870	Vaccines	Louis Pasteur	Prevents deadly diseases
1895	x-rays	Wilhelm Roentgen	Views bones and other radiopaque structures within the body
1899	Aspirin	Felix Hoffman	Serves as pain reliever, blood thinner
1922	Insulin	Frederick Sanger	Treats patients with diabetes and uncontrolled blood sugar levels
1923	Hearing aids	Marconi Company	Allows patients with decreased hearing the gift of sound
1933	Electron microscope	Ernst Ruska	Allows identification of smaller organisms with much more detail than the compound microscope
1939	Streptomycin	Selman Waksman	Treats bacterial infections
1952	Cardiac pacemaker	Paul Zoll	Stimulates a diseased heart to beat in a regular rhythm
1954	Kidney dialysis	Willem Kolff, Karl Walter, and George Thorn	Provides patients in kidney failure with a regular means of purifying the blood
1958	Laser (light amplification by stimulated emission of radiation)	Theodore Merriman	Serves as a surgical tool to cut or disintegrate body structures through a powerful light beam.
1960	Oral contraceptives	Gregory Pincus	Provides birth control through hormones
1967	Heart transplant	Christian Barnard	Was the beginning of organ donation to save lives

The medieval era was generally not a time for great advancements in medical science, although some researchers such as Leonardo da Vinci, who studied the mechanical functions of the skeleton and muscular system, did make an impact that was accepted many years later.

The Modern Era

The modern era (1500–1800) includes the Renaissance (1300–1600), when the *scientific method* came into use. The scientific method used information based on observation and careful note taking to acquire medical knowledge instead of guesswork. Dissection of the human body led to an increased knowledge of anatomy and physiology, and the invention of the microscope by Anton van Leeuwenhoek and improved upon by Robert Hooke allowed physicians to see disease-causing microorganisms. The invention of the printing press allowed medical knowledge to be shared, and apothecaries led to the development of pharmacies.

The Industrial Revolution (1700–1899) occurred in the modern era, and it is at this time when populations moved from rural to urban areas and machines were introduced to help facilitate labor and production. Noteworthy discoveries during this period include the invention of the stethoscope and the ophthalmoscope. Capillaries were discovered, along with the understanding that blood is carried through the body by vessels, which led the way to the development of techniques for measuring blood pressure as well as body temperature. One of the most exciting findings of the time was Louis Pasteur's discovery that bacteria are the cause of specific diseases in humans as well as animals, followed by Sir Alexander Fleming's discovery of the mold penicillin as a treatment for the staphylococcus germ, which was thought to cause the influenza virus. Edward Jenner pioneered the smallpox vaccine and was referred to as the "father of immunology." Along with the discovery of pathogens and vaccines, during this time came the development of the modern concept of medical asepsis, in which medical equipment was sterilized prior to use to avoid the spread of infection among patients.

From the 1900s to the present, advances in engineering, chemistry, physics, and research and technology, specifically computers, have affected the evolution of health care. These advances have brought about the invention of antibiotics, x-rays, ultrasound, chemotherapy, and pacemakers, to name just a few. The specialization of medicine in the 20th century has included genetic research, which looks for the causes of certain diseases and disorders, as well as the development of the polio vaccine, in vitro fertilization, artificial organs and organ transplantation, and the identification of the human genome. Healthcare concepts such as medical insurance, access to care, and patient rights have evolved in step with these technological and genetic advances.

The Beginning of Nursing

With the evolution of health care through the centuries came the development of the role of the nurse. Nursing began as a job for working-class women and those considered unfit to live in society. In the early 1800s, a well-to-do woman named **Florence Nightingale** (1820–1910; Fig. 1-2) opted to study nursing instead of following her parents' wishes to marry someone of their choosing. Nightingale met **Elizabeth Blackwell** (1821–1910), the first female to qualify as

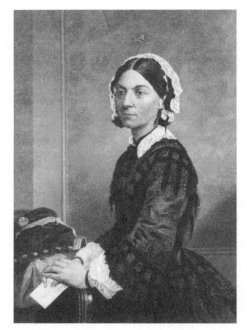

FIGURE 1-2 **Florence Nightingale.** (From the National Library of Medicine.)

a physician in the United States, at a hospital in London, England, and was encouraged by her to continue her quest to become a nurse. After studying in Germany, Nightingale returned to her native England as the leader of a hospital for invalid women.

During the Crimean War (1853–1856), many English soldiers at the front fell victim to diseases such as cholera and malaria. A contingency of nurses, including Nightingale, traveled from England to the war zone only to find deplorable conditions in the military hospitals. Military-trained physicians were offended by Florence Nightingale's suggestion that the environment contributed to the high mortality rate of the wounded soldiers. After much bad press in England, the physicians relented and allowed her to reorganize and sanitize the facilities. Because of her work in decreasing the mortality of the soldiers, she was regarded as a hero in her native country. Her work also earned her an audience with Queen Victoria to explain her views on sanitation and the care of soldiers in the military hospitals. The royal endorsement prompted Nightingale to author two books on nursing: *Notes on Nursing; What It is, and What It Is Not* and *Florence Nightingale–To Her Nurses.* The proceeds from these books allowed her to open a school of nursing in England that taught students both the necessary clinical skills and nursing ideologies. Nightingale was the inspiration for the Nightingale Pledge, which is a variation of the Hippocratic Oath for nurses. Most nursing schools use this pledge during pinning or graduation ceremonies: "I solemnly pledge myself before God and in the presence of this assembly, to pass my life in purity and to practice my profession faithfully. I will abstain from whatever is deleterious and mischievous, and will not take or knowingly administer any harmful drug. I will do all in my power to maintain and elevate the standard of my profession, and will hold in confidence all personal matters committed to my keeping and all family affairs coming to my knowledge in the practice of my calling. With loyalty will I endeavor to aid the physician, in his work, and devote myself to the welfare of those committed to my care."

Modern Careers in Nursing

Due to Florence Nightingale's efforts in founding the practice of nursing, several careers in the profession of nursing are now available (Table 1-3). A career in nursing focuses on the mental, emotional, and physical needs of the patient as directed by physicians. Nurses work closely with other members of the health-care team, such as medical assistants, pharmacists, rehabilitation specialists, and laboratory disciplines to name a few.

TABLE 1-3
NURSING CAREERS

Nursing Career	Duties	Education	Certification	Career Outlook	Average Annual Salary
Nurse practitioner (CRNP)	• Take health histories/physical examinations • Order laboratory tests/procedures • Refer patients to physicians • Treat common illnesses	• Registered Nurse • Masters degree in nursing • Additional educational and clinical practice requirements	• National certification exam • Licensure by state	Above average growth	• $36,500–$84,600 • $60,300–$108,900 with advanced specialties
Registered nurse (RN)	• Assesses patient needs • Administers prescribed medications and treatments • Reports to other health-care personnel • Supervises other health-care personnel • Teaches health care	• 2- to 3-year diploma program in hospital school of nursing, or 2-year associate's college degree, or 4-year bachelor college degree • Master's or doctoral degree for some educational/administrative/advanced practice positions	• Graduate from approved program • National Council Licensure Examination for Registered Nurses (NCLEX-RN) • Licensure by state	Above average growth	
Licensed practical/vocational nurse (LPN/LVN)	• Provide technical patient care under physician/RN supervision • Duties determined by work environment and state laws	• 1- to 2-year state-approved certificate or diploma program (HSTE practical/vocational nurse program)	• Graduate from approved program • National Council Licensure Examination for Licensed Practical/Vocational Nurses (NCLEX-PN) • Licensure by state	Above average growth	

Continued

TABLE 1-3

NURSING CAREERS—cont'd

Nursing Career	Duties	Education	Certification	Career Outlook	Average Annual Salary
Certified nursing assistant (CNA)	• Work under the supervision of RNs or LPNs/LVNs • Take vital signs • Provide baths, bed making, feeding • Assist in transfer and ambulation • Administer basic treatments	75- to 120-hour state-approved training program (HSTE program) for long-term care facilities	Omnibus Budget Reconciliation Act of 1987 (OBRA) requires all states have certification for work in long-term care facilities	Above average growth, especially in geriatric or home care	
Patient care technician (PCT)/patient care assistant (PCA)	• Work under the supervision of RNs or LPNs/LVNs • Take vital signs • Provide baths, bed making, feeding • Assist in transfer and ambulation • Administer basic treatments	75- to 120-hour state-approved training program (HSTE program) for long-term care facilities	Certification required if nursing assistant duties are included	Above average growth, especially in geriatric or home care	
Home health aide/ geriatric aide/ medication aide	• Trained to perform certain tasks such as medication administration • Provide care for specific patient population such as elderly or terminally ill • Trained to work in patients' homes	75- to 120-hour state-approved training program (HSTE program) for long-term care facilities	Approval requirements vary by state according to OBRA	Above average growth, especially in geriatric or home care	

Nurses work within the framework of a structured process to assess the patient's needs, develop a plan of care based on the patient's individual needs, implement this plan, and then evaluate the effectiveness of the plan. A key element of the nursing role is to advocate for the patient and family while providing ongoing education to promote self-care and health maintenance in the patient.

Levels of nursing include the advanced practice nurse, registered nurse, licensed practical/vocational nurse, and nurse assistant/technician.

Nurse Practitioner

Registered nurses with an advanced education can specialize. Examples of advanced practice nurses and their duties include the following:

Nurse practitioners: Take health histories, perform basic physical examinations, help establish treatment plans, order medical procedures and laboratory tests, refer patients to physicians, treat common illnesses, and teach patients to promote optimal health. Nurse practitioners typically work in clinics and physician offices.

Clinical nurse specialists: Specialize in specific nursing areas such as intensive care, trauma or emergency care, psychiatry, pediatrics, neonatology (premature infants), and gerontology (older adults). Clinical nurse specialists work in clinics and hospitals.

Nurse midwives: Provide total care for normal pregnancies, examine the pregnant woman at regular intervals, perform routine tests, teach childbirth and childcare classes, monitor the mother and infant during childbirth, deliver the infant, teach the mother and partner, and refer any problems to the physician. Nurse midwives typically work in clinics and physician offices with practicing rights at hospitals and birthing centers.

Nurse anesthetists: Administer anesthesia during surgical procedures, monitor patients during surgery, and assist anesthesiologists. Nurse anesthetists work in hospitals and surgery centers.

Nurse educators: Provide education to students and community members and teach in health science technology education (HSTE) programs, schools of nursing, colleges and universities, wellness centers, healthcare facilities, and community programs.

Registered Nurse

Registered nurses (RNs) work under the direction of physicians to provide total care to patients. The RN observes and assesses the patients' needs, administers prescribed medications and treatments, teaches health care, and reports to and supervises other healthcare personnel. RNs work in hospitals, clinics, physician offices, long-term care facilities, surgery centers, wellness centers, schools, correctional facilities, psychiatric hospitals, hospices, and cancer centers, to name a few.

Licensed Practical/Vocational Nurse

Licensed practical/vocational nurses (LPNs/LVNs) work under the supervision of physicians or RNs to provide patient care requiring technical knowledge but not the level of knowledge that is required of RNs. Duties are determined by work environment and state laws. LPNs/LVNs work in hospitals, patients' homes, long-term care facilities, adult day-care centers, physician offices, clinics, wellness centers, and health maintenance organizations.

Certified Nursing Assistant

Certified nursing assistants work under the supervision of nurses and the mandate of state laws to take vital signs, assist patients with hygiene and feeding, provide comfort measures, change bedding, and help transport patients. Nursing assistants work in patients' homes, hospice centers, and long-term care facilities.

Additional Healthcare Careers

Nursing is not the only healthcare career available to those who wish to enter a profession that focuses on the mental, emotional, and physical needs of the patient. The hundreds of job titles in health care (Table 1-4) require different amounts of education and training. It is important that learners interested in pursuing occupations in health care discover as much as possible about the responsibilities, requirements, and work conditions of their areas of interest. Learners should focus on choosing a career that interests them and matches their preferences and abilities.

TABLE 1-4

HEALTH SCIENCE CAREERS
PLANNING, MANAGING, AND PROVIDING THERAPEUTIC SERVICES, DIAGNOSTIC SERVICES, HEALTH INFORMATICS, SUPPORT SERVICES, AND BIOTECHNOLOGY RESEARCH, AND DEVELOPMENT

Sample Career Specialties/Occupations

Acupuncturist	Audiologist	Admitting clerk	Animal behavioralist	Biochemist
Anesthesiologist/ assistant	Blood bank technology specialist	Applied researcher	Biomedical/clinical engineer	Bioinformatics Scientist
Anesthesia technologist/technician	Cardiovascular technologist	Clinical account manager	Biomedical/clinical technician	Biomedical chemist
Art/music/dance therapist(s)	Clinical lab technician	Clinical account technician	Clinical simulator technician	Biomedical manufacturing technician
Athletic trainer	Clinical laboratory technologist	Clinical data specialist	Central service manager	Biostatistician
Audiologist	Computer tomography (CT) technologist	Community services specialists	Central service technician	Cancer registrar
Certified nursing assistant	Cytogenetic technologist	Compliance technician	Community health worker	Cell biologist
Chiropractor	Cytotechnologist	Data quality manager	Dietary manager	Clinical data management specialist
Chiropractic assistant	Dentist	Epidemiologist	Dietetic technician	Clinical pharmacologist
Dental assistant/ hygienist	Diagnostic medical sonographer	Ethicist	Environmental health advocate	Clinical trials monitor
Dental lab technician	Electrocardiographic (ECG) technician	Health educator	Environmental health practitioner	Clinical trials research coordinator
Dietitian/nutritionist	Electroneurodiagnostic technologist	Health information management administrator	Environmental services/specialist	Crime scene investigator
Dosimetrist	Electronic diagnostic (EEG) technologist	Health information management technician	Facilities manager	Diagnostic molecular scientist
EMT/paramedic	Exercise physiologist	Healthcare access manager	Food safety specialist	Forensic biologist
Endodontist	Geneticist	Healthcare administrator	Health advocate	Forensic chemist
Exercise physiologist	Geriatrician	Healthcare finance information	Hospital maintenance engineer	Forensic odontologist
Home health aide	Histotechnician	Information privacy officer	Industrial hygienist	Forensic pathologist
Kinesiotherapist	Histotechnologist	Managed care contract analyst	Interpreter	Genetic counselor
Licensed practical nurse	Magnetic resonance technologist	Medical coder	Marital, couple, family counselor/therapist	Geneticist/lab assistant
Massage therapist	Mammographer	Medical historian	Materials manager	Lab technician
Medical assistant	Medical technologist/clinical laboratory scientist	Medical illustrator	Medical health counselor	Medical editor/writer
Mental health counselor				Microbiologist
Naturopathic doctor				Molecular biologist
Nurse anesthetist				Nurse researcher
Nurse midwife				Packaging technician
Nurse practitioner				Patent lawyer
Occupational therapist/assistant				Pharmaceutical/clinical project manager
Oral surgeon				

TABLE 1-4

HEALTH SCIENCE CAREERS
PLANNING, MANAGING, AND PROVIDING THERAPEUTIC SERVICES, DIAGNOSTIC SERVICES, HEALTH INFORMATICS, SUPPORT SERVICES, AND BIOTECHNOLOGY RESEARCH, AND DEVELOPMENT—cont'd

Orientation/mobility specialist
Orthodontist
Orthoptist
Orthotist/prosthetist/technician
Pedorthist
Perfusionist
Pharmacist
Pharmacy Technician
Physical therapist/assistant
Physician (MD/DO)
Physician Assistant
Podiatrist
Psychologist
Psychiatrist
Radiation therapist
Recreation therapist
Registered nurse
Rehabilitation counselor
Respiratory therapist
Speech-language therapist
Surgical technician
Veterinarian
Veterinarian assistant/technician
Vision rehabilitation therapist
Wellness coach

Nuclear medicine technologist
Optician
Ophthalmologist
Ophthalmic assistant/technologist
Optometrist
Pathologist
Pathologist's assistant
Phlebotomist
Polysomnographic technologist
Positron emission tomography (PET) technologist
Radiologic technologist
Radiologist
Speech-language pathologist

Medical information technologist
Medical librarian
Medical transcriptionist
Patient account manager
Patient account technician
Patient advocate
Patient information coordinator
Project manager
Public health educator
Quality data analyst
Quality management specialist
Research and decision support specialist
Reimbursement specialist
Risk manager
Unit coordinator
Utilization manager
Utilization review manager

Mortician/funeral director
Nurse educator
Occupational health nurse
Occupational health and safety Expert
Social Worker
Transport Technician

Pharmaceutical sales representative
Pharmaceutical scientist
Pharmacokineticist
Pharmacologist
Product safety scientist
Process development scientist
Processing technician
Quality assurance technician
Quality control technician
Regulatory affairs specialist
Research assistant
Research scientist
Toxicologist

Cluster Knowledge and Skills

Cluster K & S

♦ Academic Foundation ♦ Communications ♦ Systems ♦ Employability Skills ♦ Legal Responsibilities ♦ Ethics
♦ Safety Practices ♦ Teamwork ♦ Health Maintenance Practices ♦ Technical Skills ♦ Information Technology Applications
Revised July 2009

From the National Consortium for Health Science Education. "Career Specialties Chart." 2009. Accessed January 17, 2011 from http://www.healthscienceconsortium.org/health_science_careers.php. Used with permission.

Therapeutic and Treatment Services Careers

Therapeutic and treatment careers focus on regaining and improving the wellness of patients who are physically, mentally, or emotionally injured or disabled. The goal of treatment is to restore patient function to maximum capacity. The majority of healthcare occupations fall into this category.

Dental Careers

Dental professionals focus on the health of the patient's teeth and soft tissues of the mouth. They prevent dental disease, repair or replace damaged or diseased teeth, diagnose and treat diseases of the gums, perform cosmetic dentistry, and provide patient education. Dental professionals include dentists (doctors of dental medicine [DMDs] or doctors of dental surgery [DDSs]), dental hygienists (DHs), dental laboratory technicians (DLTs), and dental assistants (DAs) who work in private dental offices, laboratories, and clinics or in dental departments in hospitals, schools, health departments, or government agencies (Table 1-5).

Emergency Medical Services Careers

Emergency medical services workers, called emergency medical technicians (EMTs), provide emergency, pre-hospital care to victims of sudden illnesses, accidents, or injuries at the scene of the accident or illness and during transport to a healthcare facility. EMTs provide life support care including managing shock, restoring breathing, controlling bleeding, administering oxygen and medications, bandaging wounds, and operating complex medical equipment. These healthcare technicians are also responsible for collaborating with other healthcare team members at the emergency and trauma center locations to ensure increased quality of care for the patient. EMTs work for fire and police departments, rescue squads, ambulance services, hospital or private emergency rooms, urgent care centers, industry, emergency helicopter services, and the military. See Table 1-6 for a list of emergency medical services careers.

Medical Careers

Medical career professionals include physicians and those who work under the supervision of physicians, such as physician assistants and medical assistants, with the focus on diagnosing, treating, and preventing illness in patients. These healthcare personnel work in private practices, clinics, hospitals, public health agencies, research facilities, health maintenance organizations (HMOs), government agencies, and colleges or universities.

Physicians

It is important to learn some historical background on the evolution of the physician's role to better understand how physicians practice today. In the beginning of the 20th century, physicians made house calls for patients who did not have transportation to the office or who were too ill to travel to the

TABLE 1-5

DENTAL CAREERS

Dental Career	Duties	Education	Certification	Career Outlook	Average Annual Salary
Dentist (DMD, DDS)	• Diagnose and treat diseases of teeth and mouth tissues • Perform surgery • Provide preventive care and teaching	• 2–4 years college preprofessional education • 4 years dental school • 2–4 years additional education if seeking specialty	• Graduate from accredited dental school • Certification exam • Licensure by state	Below average growth	$84,000–$200,000
Dental hygienist (DH)	• Perform preliminary examinations of teeth and mouth tissues • Clean teeth Provide dental treatments • Expose and develop x-rays	• 2-year associate's college degree, or 4-year bachelor's college degree, or master's college degree	• Graduate from accredited dental hygiene school • National board exams by American Dental Association Joint Commission on National Dental Examinations • Licensure by state	Above average growth	$39,300–$83,200
Dental laboratory technician (DLT)/ certified dental laboratory technician (CDLT)	• Make and repair dental prostheses	2-year associate's college degree, or 3–4 years on-the-job training, or 1–2 years HSTE program	Optional certification by National Board for Certification in Dental Technology	Average growth	$23,200–$53,600
Dental assistant (DA)/certified dental assistant (CDA)	• Prepare patients for examination • Pass instruments to dentist • Take and develop x-rays • Sterilize instruments • Teach preventive dental care	2-year associate's college degree, or 1–3 years on-the-job training, or 1–2 years HSTE program	• Licensure or registration required in most states • Voluntary certifications through Dental Assisting National Board	Above average growth	$19,900–$38,700

physician's office or the hospital. Physicians were often paid with produce or other products raised or grown by the patient, although not always in accordance with the services rendered. As transportation became less of an issue, house calls decreased and the modern physician's office concept became the location to seek and receive health care.

Physicians obtain medical histories, perform physical examinations, order laboratory and diagnostic tests, perform surgery and medical procedures, treat

TABLE 1-6

EMERGENCY MEDICAL SERVICES CAREERS

Emergency Medical Service Career	Duties	Education	Certification	Career Outlook	Average Annual Salary
Emergency medical technician paramedic (EMT-P) (EMT-4)	• Perform basic EMT duties • Perform in-depth patient assessment • Provide advanced cardiac life support (ACLS) • Interpret electro-cardiograms (ECGs) • Perform endotracheal intubation • Administer medications • Operate complex equipment	2-year associate's college degree, or 6–9 months to 2 years (over 1000 hours) approved EMT-intermediate training	• 6 months' experience as paramedic • State certification • Registration by the National Registry of EMTs (NREMT) in most states • Other states identify as EMT-4 and administer own certification examination	Above average growth	$28,400–$52,600
Emergency medical technician intermediate (EMT-1) (EMT-2) (EMT-3)	• Assess patients • Interpret electro-cardiograms (ECGs) • Administer defibrillation • Manage shock • Insert intra-venous lines and esophageal airways	• EMT-Basic • Additional approved training (at least 35–55 hours with clinical experience)	• State certification • Registration by NREMT in some states • Other states identify as EMT-2 and EMT-3 and administer their own certification exam	Above average growth	$21,200–$44,300
Emergency medical technician basic (EMT-B) (EMT-1)	Care for wide range of illnesses and injuries, including medical emergencies	• 110 hours approved EMT program • 10-hour internship in emergency room	• State certification • Registration by NREMT in some states • Other states identify as EMT-1 and administer own certification exam	Above average growth	$19,200–$35,700
First responder	• First to arrive at scene of accident or illness • Interviews and examines victim • Calls for emergency medical assistance • Maintains safety and infection control at scene • Provides basic emergency medical care	Minimum 40 hours approved training program	Certification can be obtained by NREMT	Above average growth	Salary depends on regular job

diseases and disorders, and teach preventative health. Levels of physicians include doctor of medicine (MD), doctor of osteopathic medicine (DO), doctor of podiatric medicine (DPM), doctor of chiropractic (DC), and hospitalist.

There are more than 145 specialties and subspecialties available for physicians today (Table 1-7). Some concentrate on specific body systems, such as cardiologists, or on disease processes like diabetes, and others concentrate on a specific age group such as pediatrics or geriatrics. Some physicians may choose a career in research, education, and prevention of diseases.

Doctor of medicine (MD): Assesses, diagnoses, treats, and prevents diseases, disorders, and illnesses.

TABLE 1-7
MEDICAL SPECIALTIES

Physician Title	Specialty
Anesthesiologist	Administration of medication to cause loss of feeling during surgery or treatments
Cardiologist	Heart and blood vessels
Dermatologist	Skin
Emergency Physician	Acute illness and injury
Endocrinologist	Endocrine glands
Family Practice Physician	Treatment and promotion of wellness in all age groups
Gastroenterologist	Stomach and intestine
Gerontologist	Treatment and promotion of wellness in elderly individuals
Gynecologist	Female reproductive organs
Internist	Internal organs (heart, lungs, kidneys, intestines, glands)
Nephrologist	Kidneys
Neurologist	Brain and nervous system
Obstetrician	Pregnancy and childbirth
Oncologist	Diagnosis and treatment of tumors (cancer)
Ophthalmologist	Eye
Orthopedist	Muscles and bones
Otolaryngologist	Ear, nose, throat
Pathologist	Diagnosis of disease by studying changes in cells, tissues, and organs
Pediatrician	Treatment and promotion of wellness in children
Physiatrist	Physical medicine and rehabilitation
Plastic surgeon	Corrective surgery to repair injured or malformed body parts
Proctologist	Lower part of large intestine
Psychiatrist	Mind
Radiologist	Use of x-rays and radiation to diagnose and treat diseases
Sports medicine physician	Prevention and treatment of injuries sustained in athletic events
Surgeon	Surgery to correct deformities or treat injuries or disease
Thoracic surgeon	Surgery of the lungs, heart, and chest cavity
Urologist	Kidney, bladder, urinary system

Doctor of osteopathic medicine (DO): Treats diseases and disorders of the nervous, muscular, and skeletal systems while focusing on the balance of the body, mind, and emotions.

Doctor of podiatric medicine (DPM): Assesses, diagnoses, and treats diseases and disorders of the feet or leg below the knee.

Doctor of chiropractic (DC): Focuses on maintaining the alignment of the spine and the balance of the nervous and muscular systems to optimize health.

Hospitalist: A physician who chooses to practice exclusively in the hospital treating the patients of local physicians. Many physicians are choosing to admit their patients to the **hospitalist,** leaving physicians to provide committed care to the patients in the office. There is a constant line of communication open between the hospitalist and the primary physician to ensure that the hospitalized patient receives the best possible care. All reports from the patient's hospitalization are forwarded to the primary care physician to be included in the patient's permanent record. This arrangement has become popular in recent years in the United States prompting medical schools to initiate an educational track for students who wish to practice hospital medicine.

Physician assistants (PAs) work under the supervision of physicians to take medical histories and perform physical examinations, order laboratory and diagnostic tests, make preliminary diagnoses, prescribe and administer medications and treatments, and treat minor injuries.

Medical assistants (MAs) work under the supervision of physicians to prepare patients for examination, take vital signs, assist the physician or physician assistant with examinations and procedures, perform basic procedures and laboratory tests on patients, prepare and maintain equipment and supplies, and perform receptionist duties. See Table 1-8 for a discussion on medical careers.

Mental Health and Social Services Careers

Mental health professionals provide care, treatment, counseling, and activities for patients with mental or emotional disorders or those who are developmentally delayed or mentally impaired. Social workers assist patients with illness, employment, family, and community issues. Mental health and social workers may be employed in the following settings: psychiatric hospitals and clinics, home healthcare agencies, halfway houses, group homes, hospitals, public health departments, government agencies, crisis counseling centers, drug and alcohol treatment facilities, prisons, educational institutions, and long-term care facilities.

The levels of employment include psychiatrists, psychologists, psychiatric/mental health technicians, social workers/sociologists, and genetic counselors with educational requirements and duties that vary based on the occupation (Table 1-9).

Vision Services Careers

Vision care workers correct vision problems, diagnose and treat diseases of the eye, provide education to maintain good vision and eye health, and make eyeglasses and contact lenses. Vision professionals work in offices, clinics,

TABLE 1-8

MEDICAL CAREERS

Medical Career	Duties	Education	Certification	Career Outlook	Average Annual Salary
Physician	• Treat diseases and disorders • Examine patients • Obtain medical histories • Make diagnoses • Order tests and treatments • Teach preventive health	• Doctoral degree • 3–8 years additional postgraduate training of residency or internship	• State licensure • Board certification in specialty area	Above average growth	$120,000–$425,500
Physician assistant (PA)/certified physician assistant (PAC)	• Take medical histories • Perform physical examinations • Make preliminary diagnoses • Prescribe and administer medications and treatments	• 4-year bachelor's college degree • 2 or more years accredited physician assistant program	• Registration, certification, or licensure required in all states • Certification from National Commission on Certification of Physician's Assistants	Above average growth	$49,800–$104,600
Medical assistant (MA)/certified medical assistant (CMA)/registered medical assistant (RMA)	• Prepare patients for examination • Take vital signs • Perform medical histories • Assist with procedures and treatments • Perform basic laboratory tests • Prepare and maintain equipment and supplies • Perform receptionist duties	Associate's college degree, or 1–2 year HSTE program	• Graduate of CAAHEP- or ABHES-accredited medical assistant program • Certification from American Association of Medical Assistants (AAMA) • Registration from American Medical Technologists (AMT)	Above average growth	$18,400–$46,700

optical shops and laboratories, department stores, hospitals, schools, health maintenance organizations (HMOs), and government agencies.

Career levels include ophthalmologist, optometrist, ophthalmic medical technologist, ophthalmic technician, ophthalmic assistant, optician, and ophthalmic laboratory technician (Table 1-10).

Ophthalmologist: Specializes in diseases, injuries, and disorders of the eyes by diagnosing and treating disease, performing surgery, and correcting vision defects. Ophthalmologists are medical doctors.

TABLE 1-9

MENTAL HEALTH AND SOCIAL SERVICES CAREERS

Mental Health and Social Services Career	Duties	Education	Certification	Career Outlook	Average Annual Salary
Psychiatrist	Diagnose and treat mental illness	Doctoral degree 2-7 years post-graduate specialty training	• State licensure • Certification in psychiatry	Average growth	$95,500–$297,000
Psychologist PsyD (Doctor of Psychology)	Assist patients with mental and emotional aspects of every-day living	• Bachelor's or master's college degree • Doctor of psychology required for many positions	• Licensure or certification in all states • Certification in specialty areas from American Board of Professional Psychology	Above average growth	$34,900–$97,800 or $45,900–$136,500 with doctorate
Psychiatric/ mental health technician	• Assist patients with treatment and rehabilitation plans • Assist with physical care • Teach constructive social behavior	Associate's college degree	• Licensure required in some states • Some states require nursing degree	Average growth	$28,500–$52,600
Social worker/ sociologist	Refer patients to community resources	Bachelor's degree, or master's degree, or doctor of philosophy of social work (DSW)	• Licensure, certification, registration required in all states • Credentials available from National Association of Social Workers	Above average growth	$33,500–$76,800
Genetic counselor (GC)	Teach patients about genetic diseases and inherited conditions	Master's degree	Certification from American Board on Genetic Counseling	Above average growth	$38,900–$97,600

Optometrist (DO): Examines the eyes for vision defects, prescribes corrective lenses, and in some states, uses drugs for diagnosis and treatment. A doctor of optometry, or optometrist, refers a patient to an ophthalmologist for eye disease treatment or eye surgery.

Ophthalmic medical technologist (OMT): Works under the supervision of ophthalmologists and may perform any tasks that ophthalmic technicians or assistants perform. Other duties include obtaining patient histories, performing routine eye tests, measurements, and advanced diagnostic tests,

TABLE 1-10

VISION SERVICES CAREERS

Vision Services Career	Duties	Education	Certification	Career Outlook	Average Annual Salary
Ophthalmologist (MD)	• Diagnose and treat diseases of the eye • Perform surgery • Correct vision problems	Doctoral degree 2-7 years post-graduate special-ty training	• State licensure • Certification in ophthalmology	Average growth	$108,000–$248,500
Optometrist (OD)	• Examine eyes for vision defects • Prescribe corrective lenses	• 3-4 years pre-optometric college • 4 years college of optometry for doctor of optometry degree	State licensure	Average growth	$62,300–$125,300
Ophthalmic medical technologist COMT (certified)	• Obtain patient histories • Perform routine eye tests and measurements • Fit patients for glasses and contacts • Perform advanced diagnostic tests • Assist with surgery	Associate's or bachelor's college degree	Certification from the Joint Commission on Allied Health Personnel in Ophthalmology (JCAHPO)	Average growth	$28,600–$68,500
Ophthalmic technician COT (certified)	• Prepare patients for examinations • Obtain medical histories • Take ocular measurements • Administer basic vision tests	Associate's college degree	Certification from JCAHPO	Average growth	$27,500–$50,200
Ophthalmic assistant COA (certified)	• Prepare patients for examinations • Measure visual acuity • Help patients with eyeglass frame selection and fit • Assist with receptionist duties	• 1-month to 1-year HSTE program • Some on-the-job training	Certification from JCAHPO	Average growth	$14,900–$31,500

Continued

TABLE 1-10

VISION SERVICES CAREERS—cont'd

Vision Services Career	Duties	Education	Certification	Career Outlook	Average Annual Salary
Optician	Make and fit eyeglasses or lenses	Associate's college degree, or HSTE program, or 2- to 4-year apprenticeship, or 2–4 years on the job	• Licensure or certification in some states • Certification from American Board of Opticianry and National Contact Lens Examiners	Average growth	$19,400–$46,500
Ophthalmic laboratory technician	Cut, grind, finish, polish, and mount lenses used in eyeglasses, contact lenses, telescopes, and binoculars	1-year HSTE certificate program, or 2–3 years on-the-job training	Certification in some states	Below average growth	$15,400–$35,600

administering prescribed medications and treatments, fitting patients for contacts, assisting with eye surgery, and performing advanced microbiological procedures.

Ophthalmic technician (OT): Works under the supervision of ophthalmologists and optometrists to prepare patients for examinations, obtain medical histories, take ocular measurements, administer basic vision tests, maintain ophthalmic and surgical instruments, adjust glasses and measure for contacts, teach care and use of glasses and contacts, and perform receptionist duties.

Ophthalmic assistant (OA): Works under the supervision of ophthalmologists, optometrists, and ophthalmic medical technologists to prepare patients for examinations, measure visual acuity, assist patients with frame selections and fittings, order lenses, perform minor adjustments and repairs of glasses, teach proper care and use of glasses and contacts, and perform receptionist duties.

Optician: Makes and fits lenses and eyeglasses prescribed by ophthalmologists and optometrists.

Ophthalmic laboratory technician: Cuts, grinds, finishes, polishes, and mounts the lenses used in eyeglasses, contact lenses, and optical instruments such as telescopes and binoculars.

Nutrition and Dietary Services Careers

Nutrition and dietary service personnel support patients by providing dietary guidelines, nutritious foods, and nutrition counseling and teaching to facilitate health. Places of employment include hospitals, clinics, offices, long-term care facilities, child and adult day-care facilities, schools, wellness centers, home health agencies, public health agencies, community agencies, and industry.

Nutrition and dietary services careers include registered dietician (RD), dietetic technician (DT), and dietetic assistant, with educational requirements and duties that vary depending on the job title (Table 1-11).

Additional Therapeutic Services Careers

There are many additional therapeutic services careers that require varied educational levels and skills to restore or maintain a patient's health. Most of these occupations include levels of therapist, technician, and assistant/aide and may be found in healthcare settings ranging from hospitals and long-term care facilities to home health agencies and beyond.

Table 1-12 discusses these most common therapeutic services careers.

Diagnostic Services Careers

Diagnostic services personnel help determine the causes of diseases and extent of injuries to help guide treatment. Duties include performing tests, collecting

(text continues on page 29)

TABLE 1-11

NUTRITION AND DIETARY SERVICES CAREERS

Nutrition and Dietary Service Career	Duties	Education	Certification	Career Outlook	Average Annual Salary
Dietitian, registered (RD)	• Manage food service systems • Assess patients' nutritional needs • Plan menus • Teach nutrition	Bachelor's or master's college degree	• Licensure, certification, or registration required in many states • Registration from Commission on Dietetic Registration of the American Dietetic Association	Average growth	$32,700–$68,300
Dietetic technician, registered (DTR)	• Plan menus • Order food • Test recipes • Provide basic dietary teaching	Associate's college degree	• Licensure, certification, or registration in many states • Registration from Commission on Dietetic Registration	Average growth	$24,200–$49,200
Dietetic assistant	• Assist with food preparation • Help patients select menus • Clean work areas • Assist other dietary workers	• 1 or more years HSTE or food service career/technical program • 6–12 months on-the-job training	No certification required	Average growth	$13,600–$24,900

TABLE 1-12

ADDITIONAL THERAPEUTIC SERVICES CAREERS

Additional Therapeutic Services Career	Duties	Education	Certification	Career Outlook	Average Annual Salary
Pharmacist (PharmD)	• Dispense medications • Provide information on and use of drugs • Ensure patient safety	5- to 6-year college program with doctor of pharmacy degree and internship	Licensure required in all states	Above average growth	$56,800–$103,500
Pharmacy technician	• Label medications • Perform inventory • Order supplies • Maintain records	Associate's college degree, or 1- to 2-year HSTE program, or 1 or more years on the job	• Licensure required in many states • Certification from Pharmacy Technician Certification Board	Above average growth	$17,300–$36,400
Registered occupational therapist (OTR)	• Help patients overcome disabilities • Assist with activities of daily living • Prepare patients to return to home or work	Master's college degree and internship	• Licensure required in all states • Certification from American Occupational Therapy Association	Above average growth	$43,900–$93,600
Certified occupational therapy assistant (COTA)	• Direct patients in arts and crafts projects • Provide recreation and social events • Teach rehabilitation exercises	Associate's college degree, or certificate and internship	• Licensure or certification required in most states • Certification from American Occupational Therapy Association	Above average growth	$32,500–$56,600
Physical therapist (PT)	• Improve mobility • Prevent disability • Apply treatments • Develop exercise programs	Master's or doctoral college degree	Licensure required in all states	Above average growth	$48,400–$108,300
Physical therapist assistant (PTA)	• Perform exercises and massage • Administer treatments • Ambulate patients	Associate's college degree and internship	Licensure required in most states	Above average growth	$23,500–$54,900

TABLE 1-12

ADDITIONAL THERAPEUTIC SERVICES CAREERS—cont'd

Additional Therapeutic Services Career	Duties	Education	Certification	Career Outlook	Average Annual Salary
Massage therapist	• Provide pain relief for injuries and chronic conditions • Improve lymphatic circulation • Relieve stress and tension			Above average growth	$22,400–$46,500
Recreational therapist (TR) Certified therapeutic recreation specialist (CTRS)	• Use recreation and leisure as a form of treatment • Organize activities	Bachelor's college degree plus internship	• Licensure or certification required in few states • Certification from National Council for Therapeutic Recreation Certification (NCTRC) • Registration from Association for Rehabilitation Therapy	Average growth	$26,800–$54,500
Recreational therapist assistant (activity director)	• Carry out planned activities • Arrange activities and events	Associate's college degree, or 1- to 2-year HSTE certificate program	• Certification from National Council for Therapeutic Recreation Certification	Average growth	$14,700–$32,800
Registered respiratory therapist (RRT)	• Treat patients with heart and lung disease • Administer oxygen and medications • Monitor ventilators • Perform respiratory function tests	Associate's or bachelor's college degree	• Licensure required in most states • Registration from National Board for Respiratory Care	Above average growth	$32,800–$66,300
Respiratory therapy technician (RTT) Certified respiratory therapy technician (CRTT)	• Administer respiratory treatments • Perform basic diagnostic tests • Clean and maintain equipment	Associate's college degree, or 1- to 2-year HSTE program	• Licensure or certification required for most states • Certification from National Board for Respiratory Care	Above average growth	$23,400–$49,800

Continued

TABLE 1-12

ADDITIONAL THERAPEUTIC SERVICES CAREERS—cont'd

Additional Therapeutic Services Career	Duties	Education	Certification	Career Outlook	Average Annual Salary
Speech-language therapist/ pathologist/ audiologist	• Treat patients with speech and language problems • Help patients communicate • Test hearing • Prescribe hearing treatments	• Master's college degree with 9 months postgraduate clinical experience • Clinical doctoral degree for audiologists	• Licensure required in most states • Audiologists obtain certification from American Board of Audiology Certificate of Clinical Competence in Speech-Language Pathology (CCC-SLP) or Audiology (CCC-A) obtained from American Speech-Language-Hearing Association (ASHA)	Above average growth	$40,100–$82,500
Certified surgical technician/ technologist (CST)	• Prepare patients for surgery • Set up surgical instruments • Maintain surgical equipment • Assist surgeons during surgery	Associate's college degree, certificate, or diploma, or 1- to 2-year HSTE program	Certification from Liaison Council on Certification for Surgical Technologists	Above average growth	$24,800–$48,500
Art therapist (ATR), dance (DTR) therapist, music therapist	Use the arts to help patients deal with physical, emotional, and social problems	Bachelor's or master's college degree	• Certification for art therapist from American Art Therapy Association • Registration for music therapist from National Association of Music Therapy and American Association for Music Therapy • Registration for dance therapist from American Dance Therapy Association • Registration for art therapist from Art Therapy Credentials Board	Average growth	$25,700–$64,500

TABLE 1-12

ADDITIONAL THERAPEUTIC SERVICES CAREERS—cont'd

Additional Therapeutic Services Career	Duties	Education	Certification	Career Outlook	Average Annual Salary
Certified athletic trainer (ATC)	• Prevent and treat athletic injuries • Apply treatments including first aid	Bachelor's or master's college degree	• Licensure required in some states • Most states require certification from National Athletic Trainers Association	Above average growth	$35,000–$73,800
Dialysis technician	• Operate kidney hemodialysis machines • Monitor patients during dialysis	Associate's college degree, or 1- to 2-year HSTE state-approved dialysis program	• Some states require RN or LPN license and state-approved dialysis training • Certification from National Association of Nephrology Technicians/Technologists	Average growth	$18,700–$56,800
Certified clinical perfusionist (CCP) Extracorporeal circulation technologist	• Operate heart-lung machines used in coronary bypass surgery • Monitor patients during surgery	• Bachelor's college degree • Specialized extracorporeal circulation training and supervised clinical experience	• Licensure required in some states • Certification from American Board of Cardiovascular Perfusion	Above average growth	$51,600–$112,800

specimens, and operating complex equipment in hospital and private laboratories, outpatient centers, physician offices, clinics, public health agencies, pharmaceutical (drug) companies, research companies and agencies, and government agencies (Table 1-13).

The more common diagnostic services careers are discussed in Table 1-13.

Health Informatics Careers

People in the health informatics profession gather, analyze, organize, store, and document patient information. Those who work with medical information must maintain patient confidentiality while adhering to regulatory compliance. Health informatics careers are among the fastest growing in the healthcare industry and include health information administrators or technicians, health educators, medical transcriptionists, epidemiologists, medical illustrators and photographers, medical writers, librarians, and admitting office personnel.

TABLE 1-13

DIAGNOSTIC SERVICES CAREERS

Diagnostic Services Careers	Duties	Education	Certification	Career Outlook	Average Annual Salary
Cardiovascular technologist Registered diagnostic vascular technologist (RDVT)	• Assist with cardiac catheterization procedures and angioplasty • Monitor patients during open heart surgery • Perform circulation tests	Associate's or bachelor's college degree	• Certification or registration from Cardiovascular Credentialing International • Registration from American Registry of Diagnostic Medical Sonographers	Above average growth	$27,500–$58,600
Electrocardiograph (ECG) technician Certified cardiographic technician (CCT)	Operate electrocardiograph machines that record electrical impulses in the heart	6- to 12-month HSTE program, or 1–12 months on the job	Certification from Cardiovascular Credentialing International	Below average growth	$17,300–$32,800
Electroencephalographic (EEG) technologist	Operate electroencephalograph that records electrical activity of brain	Associate's college degree, or 1- to 2-year HSTE certification program, or 1–2 years on the job	Registration from American Board of Registration of Electroencephalographic and Evoked Potential Technologists	Below average growth	$22,300–$46,200
Electroneurodiagnostic technologist (END)	• Perform nerve conduction tests • Measure sensory responses to stimuli • Operate monitoring devices	1- to 2-year program usually leading to associate's college degree	• Registration from American Board of Electroencephalographic and Evoked Potential Technologists • Polysomnographic technologists obtain registration from Association of Polysomnographic Technologists	Above average growth	$35,800–$56,200
Medical clinical laboratory technologist (MT) Certified medical clinical laboratory technologist (CMT) Registered medical clinical laboratory technologist (RMT)	Perform chemical, microscopic, and computer tests to study tissues, fluids, and cells of the human body	Bachelor's or master's college degree	• Licensure or registration required in some states • Certification from American Medical Technologists Association and the National Credentialing Agency for Laboratory Personnel	Average growth	$35,800–$66,900
Medical clinical laboratory technician (MLT) Certified laboratory technician (CLT)	Perform routine tests that do not require advanced knowledge of medical technologist	Associate's college degree, or 2-year HSTE certification program	• Licensure or registration required in some states • Certification from American Medical Technologists Association and the National Credentialing Agency for Laboratory Personnel	Average growth	$26,300–$48,900

TABLE 1-13

DIAGNOSTIC SERVICES CAREERS—cont'd

Diagnostic Services Careers	Duties	Education	Certification	Career Outlook	Average Annual Salary
Medical clinical laboratory assistant	• Perform basic laboratory tests • Prepare specimens for testing • Maintain equipment	1- to 2-year HSTE program, or on-the-job training	Certification from Board of Certified Laboratory Assistants	Below average growth	$14,500–$26,300
Phlebotomist	Collect blood and prepare it for testing	1- to 2-year HSTE program, or 1–2 years on-the-job training, or 100- to 300-hour certification program	Certification from National Credentialing Agency for Laboratory Personnel and the American Society of Phlebotomy Technicians	Average growth	$14,600–$28,300
Registered radiologic technologist RT(R)	Use scanners to produce images of body parts to diagnose disease	Associate's or bachelor's college degree	Licensure in most states Registration from American Registry of Radiologic Technologies (ARRT)	Above average growth	$28,900–$68,600

These personnel work in hospitals, clinics, health departments, research centers, long-term care facilities, colleges, law firms, and insurance companies. Table 1-14 discusses the more common health informatics careers.

Research and Development Careers

Research and development professionals use living cells and their molecules to help produce new diagnostic tests, forms of treatment, medications, vaccines to prevent disease, food products, and methods to detect and clean up environmental contamination.

Career paths include biological or medical scientists, biotechnological engineers, biological technicians, process technicians, and forensic science technicians. The professionals work in research laboratories, hospitals, colleges or universities, pharmaceutical companies, chemical companies, forensic laboratories, agricultural facilities, government facilities, and industry. The more common research and development careers are discussed in Table 1-15.

EARLY HEALTHCARE FACILITIES

The word **hospital** is a derivative of the Latin word *hospes* or *host*. Interestingly, this is also the root of the English word *hotel*. The Greek

TABLE 1-14

HEALTH INFORMATICS CAREERS

Health Informatics Career	Duties	Education	Certification	Career Outlook	Annual Average Salary
Registered health information (medical records) administrator (RHIA)	• Develop and manage systems for storing and obtaining medical records • Prepare information for legal claims • Compile statistics Manage medical records departments • Ensure patient confidentiality	Bachelor's or master's college degree	Registration from American Health Information Management Association (AHIMA)	Above average growth	$41,400–$88,700
Registered health information (medical records) technician (RHIT)	• Organize and code patient records • Gather statistical and research data • Monitor information to ensure confidentiality	Associate's college degree	Registration from American Health Information Management Association (AHIMA)	Above average growth	$22,700–$52,300
Medical transcriptionist/ certified medical transcriptionist (CMT)	• Enter data into computer from recording device used by healthcare professionals to create or add to medical record	Associate's college degree, or 1 or more years career or technical education program, or on-the-job training	Certification from American Association for Medical Transcription	Above average growth	$18,700–$37,400
Admitting officer or clerk	• Admit patient to facility • Maintain records • Process patient discharge paperwork	Bachelor's college degree for admitting manager, 1- to 2-year HSTE program, or business, career, technical education	No certification required	Average growth	$15,300–$36,800
Unit secretary ward clerk Health unit coordinator Medical records clerk	• Add information to patient records • Schedule procedures and tests • Answer telephones • Order supplies	1 or more years career or technical education program	No certification required	Average growth	$14,200–$34,300

TABLE 1-14

HEALTH INFORMATICS CAREERS—cont'd

Health Informatics Career	Duties	Education	Certification	Career Outlook	Annual Average Salary
Epidemiologist	• Identify and track diseases • Determine risk factors for disease • Evaluate statistical data	Master's or doctoral degree in environmental health, public health, or health management sciences	No certification required	Above average growth	$55,000–$96,500
Medical interpreter/translator	• Assist cross-cultural communication by converting one language to another Interpreters convert the spoken word. • Translators convert the written word.	Associate's, bachelor's, or master's college degree	Certification from American Translators Association Certification for sign language interpreters from National Association of the Deaf and the Registry of Interpreters for the Deaf	Above average growth	$31,800–$76,300
Medical illustrator	Produce illustrations, charts, graphs, and diagrams for medical publications	Bachelor's or master's college degree	Certification from Association of Medical Illustrators	Average growth	$43,700–$132,500
Medical librarian	• Organize reading materials for healthcare professionals • Research information	Master's college degree in library science	No certification required	Average growth	$41,600–$136,300

temples were the first examples of facilities dedicated to caring for the sick. During the height of the Roman Empire and the rise of Christianity, the temples became not only healthcare facilities but also a place for weary travelers and the homeless to stay. Hospitals founded as early as the fifth century in India and Southeast Asia began as private institutions, and government-sponsored hospitals began to surface in the early part of the sixth century. European hotels served as hospital facilities staffed by nuns and clergy. The Hotel Dieu Paris (Fig. 1-3), one of the earliest recorded hospitals in France, remains open today with a reputation for excellent care. There are also hotel rooms available within the hospital, which is located next to the Cathedral of Notre Dame.

The first American hospitals originated in the mid 1700s. The Pennsylvania Hospital in Philadelphia was established in 1752, followed by New York City's

TABLE 1-15

RESEARCH AND DEVELOPMENT CAREERS

Research and Development Career	Duties	Education	Certification	Career Outlook	Annual Average Salary
Biological or medical scientist	• Study viruses, bacteria, protozoa • Assist in development of vaccines, medicines, treatments • Administer programs for testing food and drugs	Bachelor's, master's, or doctoral college degree	Licensure required in some states	Average growth	$52,600–$110,500
Biotechnological engineers (bioengineers)	• Develop medical devices • Research materials for use in human body • Design artificial organs • Research injury and wound healing	Bachelor's or master's college degree	Licensure required in some states	Average growth	$48,600–$82,700
Biological technicians	• Perform laboratory experiments • Assist in development of medications	Associate's or bachelor's college degree	Certification from National Credentialing Agency for Laboratory Personnel	Average growth	$32,300–$62,500
Process technicians	Operate and monitor biotechnical machinery	Associate's or bachelor's college degree	No certification required	Average growth	$32,300–$59,400
Forensic science technicians	• Investigate crimes • Collect physical evidence • Reconstruct crime scenes	Associate's, bachelor's, or master's college degree	• Certification from American Society for Clinical Pathology • Must meet proficiency levels established by national accreditation associations for criminal laboratories	Above average growth	$38,600–$67,300

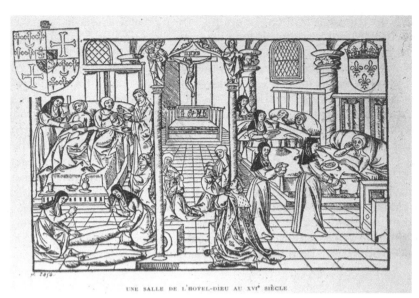

UNE SALLE DE L'HOTEL-DIEU AU XVI⁰ SIÈCLE

FIGURE 1-3 **Hotel Dieu Paris in Lyons, France.** (From the National Library of Medicine.)

New York Hospital in 1771. Very few of the five million Americans at that time had access to these facilities because these areas of the new world were sparsely populated; however, after the beginning of World War I, the number of hospitals soared to more than 5000, a surge necessitated by the need to care for those fighting in the war.

Hospitals were originally set up as general or full-service hospitals, and all patients were housed in multibed wards without regard to diagnosis, segregated only by sex and race. As hospitals progressed, rooming changed to semiprivate and private accommodations for patients with insurance coverage or those with enough money to cover the extra expense. Wards remained an option for the uninsured. An emergency room provided immediate attention to stabilize patients before admission. Inpatient services included laboratories, operating rooms, and maternity wards. Patients in need of continuous or specialized care were admitted to the hospital for around-the-clock care. Nurses and trained nurses' aides provided bedside care on the orders of the attending physician.

Because health care was expensive and not affordable to most during the Great Depression, in 1929 a group of teachers in Dallas, Texas, offered Baylor Hospital a small "premium" or fee, about 50 cents per month, in exchange for a maximum of 21 days of hospitalization per year. Known as the "Baylor Plan," this was the first prepaid hospital insurance plan in the United States and helped many area citizens afford hospital care. The Baylor Plan evolved and thus became the predecessor of the Blue Cross insurance company.

As technology advanced, healthcare costs increased and insurance companies became less eager to cover these rising costs. Some physicians ordered unnecessary laboratory testing to protect themselves from litigation and to meet the demands of patients. This led to a major change in the way insurance companies reimbursed healthcare facilities. These practices eventually led to the demise of small, rural hospitals. With these closures, hospitals in larger urban areas expanded their services to handle the increase in the number of patients served. Urban hospitals also increased in size and capabilities to become more than just larger general hospitals. These larger, more profitable facilities began

Flashpoint

The Bureau of Labor Statistics (www.bls.gov) estimates that there are 580,000 healthcare facilities and 14 million healthcare jobs in our country.

to capitalize on the lack of local hospital care in rural areas by constructing outpatient and urgent care facilities closer to the smaller communities. We continue to see the expansion of healthcare services beyond the hospital as patients or healthcare consumers become more aware and selective about healthcare facility options. For example, some physicians have chosen the route of "boutique" or "concierge" medicine, also called *direct care medicine*, which is a relationship between the patient and a primary care physician in which the patient pays an annual fee or retainer for medical services. In exchange for the retainer, the physician provides special services above and beyond the normal care a patient may receive from a non-concierge physician. Special services may include 24-hour cell phone and e-mail access to the physician, annual comprehensive physicals that include extensive diagnostic and laboratory testing, and longer physician-patient appointment visits. Concierge physicians are able to offer these more personalized services because they care for fewer patients than in a conventional practice, ranging from 100 patients per physician to 1000, instead of the 3000–4000 that the average physician now sees every year.

TODAY'S HEALTHCARE FACILITIES

Healthcare facilities today are much different from the early asclepeions and even the early 19th century hospitals. Hospitals and physicians have expanded their facilities and services to provide expert care to those in need of health care.

General Hospitals

A general acute care hospital, found in rural and urban areas, provides all of the necessary services to care for patients and is similar to the first hospitals established in this country. Today's **general hospital** encompasses services to meet the healthcare needs of the community, including emergency services, intensive care, surgery, maternity and newborn care, and some basic psychiatric care. General hospitals have an association with emergency medical services for transferring patients to larger facilities when adequate care is not available there. You will find all types of healthcare professionals dedicated to providing high-quality patient care in a general hospital.

Hospitals may be identified as for-profit, nonprofit, or government-owned facilities. Profit is usually determined by the patient mix. For-profit hospitals are found in areas where the population is typically well covered by insurance. Approximately two-thirds of urban hospitals are nonprofit, with for-profit and governmental facilities making up the remaining one-third.

Flashpoint

The future of health care may see an increase in free-market competition and consumer choice for healthcare services.

General Hospitals With Specialty Services

Some general hospitals may provide specialized care for a certain type of illness, such as tuberculosis, while continuing to offer general services to other patients. A physician on staff at a general hospital may be an expert in the care of certain diseases, and the hospital would provide accommodations to care for patients suffering from these conditions. The staff assigned to this area would be given all of the training necessary to care for these patients.

Teaching Hospitals

A teaching hospital is associated with a university medical school and provides hands-on training for all medical students, interns, and residents. A patient seeking care at a teaching hospital should expect to be seen and treated by all levels of practitioners, ranging from medical and allied health students to attending physicians. There is never a compromise in the quality of care in a teaching hospital. Some patients may choose not to participate in such care, but many others value the extended care provided by the students, interns, residents, and attending physicians. Public university medical schools use the teaching hospitals to care for many of the state's medically indigent population.

Veterans Affairs Hospitals

Veterans Affairs (VA) hospitals are government-sponsored, nationwide hospitals that offer care to all veterans. Eligibility for hospitalization and other benefits is based on "a person having served in any branch of the military and having been discharged under other than dishonorable conditions" (www.va.gov). Eligibility is also extended to Reservists and National Guard members who were called into active duty by an Executive Order. Benefits are not limited to those who served in combat situations or to injuries and illnesses acquired during service. Health care at VA facilities include any and all veterans. VA hospitals also serve as teaching facilities for nearby medical schools, giving the patients access to many levels of care. As with other teaching hospitals, there is a staff of attending physicians who oversee the practice of the medical students, interns, and residents who provide care for the veterans.

Specialty Hospitals

There are times when patients need very specialized care. This care is provided by hospitals dedicated to providing special services to a particular group of patients or diagnoses.

Trauma Center

A hospital that houses a unit that specializes in the care of catastrophic physical events is designated by the state as a **trauma center.** States choose these trauma centers in large medical centers based on the employment of highly specialized physicians, nurses, and other healthcare professionals who are trained to provide care for the critically injured patients. The goal of the trauma center is to prevent further damage to the patient and increase his or her chance of survival. Trauma centers contain the most technologically advanced equipment and supplies to care for patients at any time. Trauma centers are accessible by air or ground ambulances.

Children's Hospitals

Children are not little adults and should not be treated as such. Likewise, not all healthcare providers are suited to care for children. Children's hospitals provide dedicated facilities staffed by trained physicians, nurses, and other healthcare professionals to care specifically for the needs of children from

Flashpoint

The definition of a medically indigent patient is someone who cannot afford private health insurance but who does not qualify for national or state healthcare assistance.

birth through age 19. Often, a neonatal intensive care unit (NICU) may be a part of a children's hospital so that premature and sick newborns can be transferred in to receive the best possible care. Facilities such as St. Jude's Children's Research Hospital and the Shriner's Hospital for Children provide care for specific diseases and disorders without regard to the family's ability to pay for care. Because facilities like these specialize in certain illnesses and disorders, the research done on site provides more rapid treatment to the patients.

Burn Centers

Burn centers provide care for patients suffering moderate to severe burns. Because infection is one of the primary causes of death in burn victims, the burn centers strive to maintain the cleanest possible environment and a highly trained staff to care for the patient from injury to return to society. The staff of a burn center is committed to care for the physical and psychological needs of the patient and the family with a goal of returning the patient to the highest level of function through physical, emotional, and vocational care.

Flashpoint

The skin is the largest organ of the body and the body's first line of defense against infections and trauma. Burns disrupt the protective functions of the skin.

Psychiatric Hospitals

A psychiatric hospital cares for patients with documented mental diseases and disorders that prevent them from living independently. The facilities promote a nonthreatening environment for short-term or long-term care. In early days, these facilities were known as asylums, but as physicians came to better understand psychiatric illnesses, the facilities changed to provide more than just custodial care for patients who needed assistance with activities of daily living. Today, psychiatric hospitals treat patients with eating disorders, acute emotional crises, and other debilitating mental illnesses.

Branches of psychiatric facilities provide care for patients with alcohol and drug abuse or addiction. These settings, which can be inpatient or outpatient, provide detoxification and rehabilitation for patients who want to become clean and sober. Support groups for patients of all psychiatric hospitals offer an immeasurable service for long-term care.

Cancer Centers

Another specialty facility that may be a freestanding building or one located within the confines of a general or teaching hospital is a cancer center. These facilities are known for their extensive research and comprehensive care of patients with cancer. Some facilities specialize in a specific cancers, and others treat most types of primary and secondary cancers. Among the cancer centers in the United States are those that use holistic methods of treating the mind, body, and spirit of the patients they serve. The extensive research at these centers helps not only with treatment of the disease but also with prevention and education as well. The National Cancer Institute, which is a part of the U.S. government, has facilities around the country dedicated to research, treatment, and education for patients and healthcare providers. There are also many private cancer centers that are operated with private funds or donations.

Rehabilitation Centers

Patients who undergo orthopedic surgery or suffer the effects of a stroke and other debilitating illnesses and injuries often find themselves in need of daily rehabilitation exercises to return to a normal or near-normal state of health. Rehabilitation centers provide physician-directed care by physical therapists, occupational therapists, and speech therapists. The physician, therapist, and patient develop a plan of care jointly. Families are encouraged to participate in this care to promote continuity of care at home. Rehabilitation centers focus on the patient's abilities and not their disabilities. Services that are used in a rehabilitation center include aquatic therapy, sports medicine, range-of-motion therapy, and activities of daily living. Some rehabilitation centers have mock-ups of stores, homes, and outside spaces to allow patients to refamiliarize themselves with the environment in which they live.

Birthing Centers

Birthing centers provide a home-like atmosphere where low-risk mothers can safely deliver their babies. The staff of the birthing center, which creates family-centered care, includes nurse midwives, nurse practitioners, and registered nurses. Patients receive prenatal care at the center, which familiarizes the mother-to-be with the facility and the staff. Most birthing centers provide total women's health care as well as newborn and pediatric care. Insurance typically covers the costs of a birthing center delivery as it is less than that for conventional hospitalization. The size of the facility determines the number of patients accepted for care. This keeps the average number of births per month low, and there is usually only one patient in the facility at any given time. Families are welcomed and encouraged to interact with the mother during the entire labor and delivery process. Women can use the facility showers and whirlpool tubs to assist with relaxation. After delivery, the mother and newborn may go home as soon as the mother is stable and feels that she is ready, usually within 12 hours of birth. Birthing centers are equipped with the latest technology, but they must also have an agreement with a nearby hospital and emergency service contacts to transfer any mother who becomes high risk during labor or delivery.

Outpatient Facilities

As inpatient hospitalizations have declined, outpatient facilities have emerged as the new wave in health care. Gone are the days of entering the hospital on the day before surgery and having several days of recuperation afterward. More procedures are done on an outpatient basis in the ambulatory care unit of the hospital or in freestanding outpatient centers, or surgicenters, staffed with physicians, nurses, and other allied health professionals with access to the latest technology and equipment. These centers provide preoperative assessment as well as recovery after the procedure. Patients have the benefit of being able to recuperate at home once they are awake and alert and are discharged. It is believed that patients recover more quickly and are more comfortable in their own surroundings. Insurance companies often offer incentives for physicians and patients who choose the outpatient setting for minor surgeries.

Clinics

The term *clinic* describes many different types of outpatient healthcare settings. Often, people think of a clinic as a "free clinic," a place that offers reduced or no-charge healthcare services. This is not always the case. Clinics can be privately owned and provide a specific type of care or be government sponsored to provide more general services. An example of a private clinic may be a weight loss clinic or an orthotic fittings and service clinic. Both types of clinics offer a specific service to a specific audience. A government-sponsored clinic may be a public or free clinic within the confines of a public health department. Services you may find in the public health department clinic include limited physical exams, immunizations, administration of the Women, Infants and Children Program (WIC), and documentation of birth and death certificates. If not totally free, services are offered on an income-based scale. A hospital or private investor may sponsor urgent or emergent care clinics. The original intent of these clinics was to offer walk-in care for patients who cannot get in to their regular physician for an acute illness or non–life-threatening injury. This clinic offers some relief to overcrowded emergency rooms and allows all patients to be seen in a more timely manner.

Flashpoint

WIC provides nutritional support, healthcare referrals, and information on healthy eating for low-income mothers, infants, and children up to age 5 years.

Physician Offices

Patients visit their family physician for both routine care and when sick or injured in a nonemergent way. Routine care may be an annual physical, medication evaluation, or care related to a specific condition such as asthma or diabetes. Some patients choose to see their family physician for routine care and a specialist for other conditions or they may see one physician for all of their healthcare needs. A patient's insurance may also dictate which physician the patient may see. In the managed care environment, an insurance company may negotiate a contract with a particular physician to treat all patients covered by their plan at a reduced rate.

Physicians practice in either a solo practice or a group practice. A solo practice requires that the physician be on call 24 hours per day, seven days per week and see all of the patients in the practice. They must also care for their hospitalized patients. Some solo physicians hire a **physician's assistant** (PA) or a **nurse practitioner** (NP) to assist with the daily patient load, but after-hours call and weekend calls are the responsibility of the physician.

A group practice includes more than one physician in the same specialty. In larger cities, there may be as many as 10 physicians in one practice. This type of practice allows each physician guaranteed time off. A group practice may also employ a PA or NP for daily patient visits and routine care. Patients who use physicians in a group practice must be willing to see any of the physicians in the group if they need care and their usual physician is not scheduled to be in the office that day. Each multi-physician practice maintains the patient medical record so that it is available to all physicians when the patient visits the office.

Physician offices employ nurses, medical assistants, medical receptionists, billers, and coders. Specialty offices may employ healthcare professionals specific to the practice, such as an electroencephalogram (EEG) technician in a neurology practice, a radiologic technologist in an orthopedic practice, or a sonographer for ultrasounds in an obstetrical practice. Having allied health professionals in a medical office provides onsite services for patients who would otherwise have to leave the office to have testing completed.

Emergency Medical Services

Today, very few communities in our nation lack access to some type of healthcare facility, whether it is a community hospital, urgent care facility, physician office, or government-sponsored clinic. When a hospital is not available in a community, **emergency medical services** (EMSs) are available in small communities and townships for the transfer of patients to neighboring towns where healthcare facilities are available. EMSs provide treatment to those in need of urgent medical care, with the goal of treating the presenting illness at the scene and during transport as well as transferring the patient to a location where further medical services are provided. This location is typically the emergency department at a local or regional hospital.

Looking Forward

We have seen quite a progression of health care through the ages and the current trends in health care available for patients today. As technology advances, we will continue to see the growth of specialized health care, but we must remember that with expanding technology come increased costs and the need for additional training for healthcare professionals.

In an attempt to follow the lead of other nations around the world, the United States is slowly adopting a nationwide **electronic health record** (EHR), or electronic medical record (EMR), in an attempt to move away from a paper record-keeping system. A government mandate will require that all physicians employ the EHR/EMR technology by 2014. The Centers for Medicare and Medicaid Services currently offers eligible professionals and hospitals that adopt and demonstrate meaningful use of EHR technology financial incentives. The hope is that the electronic format will be available through the Internet for access by all healthcare professionals caring for a patient. Although the concept may be ideal, the confidentiality of the record must take top priority when a patient's health information is available in such an open format as the Internet. Digital storage of records and greater security controls must be engaged to protect all personally identifiable health information.

In addition to computerized records, standard **algorithms,** or detailed treatment scenarios, can be used to tailor a patient's care regardless of where he or she is being treated. These algorithms would be developed nationally based on best practices and used with the patient's profile to determine an **"if/then"** plan of care. Virtual reality **avatars** are emerging as one of the newest technologies in health "coaching" and may one day replace medical call centers or become a realistic outlet for both general and disease-specific information. These new technologies may increase access to health care for all people, which should continue to be one of the major goals of future generations.

Future trends in health care must not only focus on technology but also on research opportunities for the reduction of morbidity and mortality worldwide, especially in underserved populations. Each of these efforts, combined with the common goal of providing care to those in need, makes health care an exciting and dynamic career choice.

Summary

Health care has changed significantly from the early ages and continues to change on an almost daily basis. New technologies provide patients with more rapid diagnoses and treatments. As a healthcare professional, it is imperative that you stay up-to-date with developments in the world of medicine.

Practice Exercises

Multiple Choice

1. Which of the early civilizations thought illness was the result of a curse from the supernatural?

    a. Egyptians

    b. Greek

    c. Romans

    d. Chinese

2. The physician who began to study disease through dissection of deceased patients and dead animals is:

    a. Galen

    b. Hippocrates

    c. Blackwell

    d. Fleming

3. All of the following early inventions are still in use today, except:

    a. Ophthalmoscope

    b. Kidney dialysis

    c. Compound microscope

    d. Ether anesthesia

4. Nursing began as a job for:

    a. Well-to-do women

    b. Working-class women

    c. Unemployed men

    d. Upper-class women

5. Florence Nightingale was considered a hero after her work with soldiers in:

    a. The Crimean War

    b. World War I

    c. The Korean War

    d. World War II

6. The first hospital in the United States was built in which city?

    a. New York

    b. Atlanta

    c. Philadelphia

    d. Boston

Fill in the Blank

1. Advances in technology allow physicians to treat patients more
   _____ and with greater _____.

2. Detailed treatment scenarios, known as _____, can be
   used to tailor a patient's care regardless of where he or she is being
   treated.

3. The early Greeks followed a diet rich in _____ and
   _____.

Short Answer

1. **What qualifies a person as "medically indigent"?**

2. **What is an advantage of having a hospitalist? What is a disadvantage
   of a hospitalist?**

3. **What are some similarities in the ancient asclepeion temples and
   today's spas?**

INTERNET RESOURCES

Organization	Web Address	Resources
U.S. Bureau of Labor Statistics	www.bls.gov	Healthcare career information including job descriptions, salary ranges, and job outlook
U.S. Department of Veterans Affairs	www.va.gov	Information for veterans' healthcare initiatives, coverage, and benefits
Centers for Medicare and Medicaid Services	www.cms.gov	Medicare and Medicaid regulations, coverage, and benefits
Blue Cross/Blue Shield	www.bcbs.com	Proprietary site for health insurance coverage
Healthcare Reform	www.healthreform.gov	Information concerning the healthcare reform legislation
Women, Infants, and Children (WIC)	www.fns.usda.gov	Eligibility for inclusion in the WIC program to promote healthy women and children
Hotel Dieu	www.hotel-hospitel.com	Site for the oldest hospital still in operation today
National Association of Emergency Medical Technicians	www.naemt.org	Information related to the EMT profession
American Nurses Association	www.nursingworld.org	Information related to the nursing profession
U.S. Department of Veteran Affairs	www.va.org	Site for veteran services
Centers for Medicare and Medicaid Services	www.cms.gov	Site for Medicare and Medicaid services
American Academy of Physician Assistants	www.aapa.org	Information related to the physician assistant profession
American Medical Association	www.ama-assn.org	Professional organization for physicians
American Association of Medical Assistants	www.aama-ntl.org	Information related to the medical assistant profession
American Psychiatric Association	www.psych.org	Information related to the mental health profession
National Association of Social Workers	www.naswdc.org	Information related to the social work profession
Joint Commission on Allied Health Personnel in Ophthalmology	www.jcahpo.org	Information related to the ophthalmology profession
Opticians Association of America	www.oaa.org	Professional organization for opticians
American Dietetic Association	www.eatright.org	Information related to the nutrition and dietary services career
American College of Radiology	www.acr.org	Information related to the radiology profession
American Medical Technologists	www.amt1.com	Information related to the medical technologist profession

INTERNET RESOURCES—cont'd

Organization	Web Address	Resources
American Society for Clinical Laboratory Science	www.ascls.org	Professional organization for laboratory scientists and technologists
Association of Schools of Allied Health Professions	www.asahp.org	Information related to allied health professions
American Association for Medical Transcription	www.ahdionline.org	Professional organization for medical transcriptionists
American Health Information Management Association	www.ahima.org	Professional organization for health information managers
American Academy of Forensic Sciences	www.aafs.org	Professional organization for forensic scientists
American Institute of Biological Sciences	www.aibs.org	Professional organization for biological scientists
Pharmaceutical Research and Manufacturers of America	www.phrma.org	Information related to the pharmaceutical industry
American Dental Association	www.ada.org	Professional organization for dentists
American Dental Hygienists' Association	www.adha.org	Professional organization for dental hygienists
American Academy of Audiology	www.audiology.org	Professional association for audiologists
American Association of Colleges of Pharmacy	www.aacp.org	Professional association for pharmacists
American Physical Therapy Association	www.apta.org	Professional association for physical therapists
American Occupational Therapy Association	www.aota.org	Professional association for occupational therapists
Association of Surgical Technologists	www.ast.org	Professional association for surgical technologists

2 WORKING AS A TEAM

Key Terms

administrative Those who manage or direct the business side of health care. Administrative information includes the patient's demographics and insurance information.

certification Validation of education through an examination that grants an individual permission to work in a profession.

clinical Those roles that are involved in the direct observation and care of the patient and are diverse and categorized by the level of education and responsibility within the healthcare environment.

communication Verbal exchange, written messages, active listening, and nonverbal behavior, such as facial expressions, body language, and touch used to share information.

credentialed Healthcare workers who have been granted the evidence of their authority of their title or profession

defensiveness Excessive sensitivity to criticism that can destroy a conversation.

group A collection of workers in which everyone has an individual task and goal.

Learning Outcomes

2.1 Discuss the significance of teamwork in health care

2.2 Differentiate between teams and groups

2.3 Compare the different pathways to becoming a physician

2.4 Define administrative and clinical professions within health care

2.5 Describe the healthcare information collection process

Competencies

CAAHEP

- Identify styles and types of verbal communication. (CAAHEP IV.C.1)
- Identify nonverbal communication. (CAAHEP IV.C.2)
- Recognize communication barriers. (CAAHEP IV.C.3)
- Identify techniques for overcoming communication barriers. (CAAHEP IV.C.4)

ABHES

- Compare and contrast the allied health professions and understand their relation to medical assisting. (ABHES 1.b)

By nature, we are born with the desire to make our own decisions and choose our own path. This independence is a necessary skill to survive in today's world, and we all share specific needs for personal gain, reward, and control. There are, however, times and places when this independence is a hindrance. Certain situations require that people work together for the good of a mission. **Teamwork** is a concept that requires each person involved to relinquish some of his or her individual traits to become a part of a group that works together for overall gain, rewards, and control. A team shares the accomplishments as well as the responsibility for the outcomes.

The first thing that usually comes to mind when you think of teamwork is a sports environment. Games are not won by an individual but rather by all of the team members working together. Certain members of the team may have specific skills that contribute to the win, but without the contributions of the other team members, winning is not likely. The team begins with an overall plan, and each member must buy into the plan and follow through with the execution. True teamwork requires that all members of the team listen, discuss, participate, respect, and, above all, communicate.

There is a well-known saying that a chain is only as strong as its weakest link. The same is true in health care. Within the healthcare environment, individual care providers compose loose or well-defined teams of physicians, nurses, assistants, technicians, and so forth, and many of these smaller teams merge into one large team—a department, a practice, a hospital—to provide quality patient care. One person in a healthcare facility who does not perform to his or her best ability can cause an interruption in providing high-quality patient care.

Healthcare Teams

Healthcare workers who are involved in the actual face-to-face care of patients, such as physicians and nurses, are often thought of as the backbone of health care; however, there are many people interested in working in health care who prefer not to work in the clinical aspect of the facility. Health care requires both administrative and clinical teams, and neither can survive without the other. A *team,* whether in health care or other industries, is a group of people with a full set of complementary skills required to complete a task, job, or project. *Team building* occurs when the members of the team work together to improve the team and reach its goals.

Clinical teams may be made up of physicians, nurses, nursing assistants, medical assistants, therapists (respiratory, occupational, physical), dietitians, and psychologists. Administrative teams may consist of healthcare administrators, medical records administrators, office clerks, unit secretaries, health insurance personnel, and billing specialists.

Administrative Members

It is necessary to collect patient information before treatment can begin, a task that often falls to *administrative* workers. Administrative workers are those who manage or direct an institution. Both the health and demographic information belongs to the patient, but the physical record becomes the property of the facility and is protected by the Health Insurance Portability and Accountability Act (HIPAA) of 1996. Along with basic demographics, insurance information is collected and used to authorize benefits and initiate payment for services. Once administrative employees create the physical record, it is passed to the clinical staff to proceed with the encounter.

The rule strikes a balance that permits important uses of information while protecting the privacy of people who seek care and healing.

Other administrative entities that participate in a healthcare visit may seem less involved, but they are important just the same. These entities may include the patient's insurance company, ancillary physicians such as radiologists or pathologists, government-sponsored agencies such as Medicare and Medicaid, independent billing services, and related healthcare service industries, such as rehabilitation facilities. Collecting the correct demographics at the patient's first encounter is important to all of these groups. Not sharing this information would require that the patient contact each entity individually and repeat the same information multiple times. Working as a team relieves the patient of this burden.

Let's follow a patient's medical information through a physician's office visit to learn a bit more about the administrative personnel involved and their roles in processing the patient's information.

- The patient calls the physician's office and schedules an appointment with the receptionist. The receptionist collects some basic demographic and

Key Terms—cont'd

licensure Another method of validation of education through an examination that grants an individual permission to work in a profession.

recertification Renewing credentials through continuing education or examination.

team A group of people with a full set of complementary skills required to complete a task, job, or project.

team building The members of the team work together to improve the team and reach its goals.

teamwork A concept that requires each person involved to relinquish some of his or her own individual traits to become a part of a group that works together for overall gain, rewards, and control. A team shares the accomplishments as well as the responsibility for the outcomes.

Flashpoint

A major goal of the privacy rule under HIPAA is to ensure that an individual's health information is properly protected while allowing the flow of health information needed to provide and promote high-quality health care and to protect the public's health and well being.

health insurance information from the patient and schedules the appointment.

- The patient arrives at the physician's office for the scheduled appointment, at which time several forms are completed, including a demographic profile (address, telephone number, birth date), a medical history, a payment form (medical insurance information), and a HIPAA form. The receptionist collects the paperwork and makes a copy of the patient's insurance card.
- The receptionist enters the patient's information into the computer system and may also create a paper medical record for the patient.
- The patient meets with the clinical team (medical assistant, nurse, physician), and the details of this meeting are transcribed as notes into the patient's chart.
- Upon leaving the physician's office, the patient pays for the visit (either pays an insurance copayment or pays for the visit in full) and possibly schedules an appointment for a follow-up visit.
- The receptionist completes the patient's medical record and forwards any billing information to the accounts payable department. Someone in accounts payable then files the patient's insurance paperwork with the patient's insurance company and ensures that the patient's account is in good standing. If the insurance company does not cover part or all of the office visit and the patient owes the physician payment, the accounts payable person works with the patient's insurance company and the patient to receive payment.
- The receptionist forwards the patient's medical record to the physician to complete notes and review the patient's care. The physician may dictate patient notes into a recorder that a medical transcriptionist transcribes into print form and places in the patient's medical record for future reference.
- If the physician wishes to refer the patient to another healthcare provider, this is done while the physician reviews the patient's medical record after the patient's visit. If a referral is required, the medical assistant or nurse completes the referral paperwork and assists the patient in making the referral appointment.
- When the physician is finished with the patient's medical record, the receptionist files the record until the patient comes to the office for another visit.

Administrative personnel in hospitals, specialty clinics, nursing homes, rehabilitation facilities, and laboratories fulfill these same functions, regardless of the facility size. Administrative personnel have the additional responsibilities of managing other administrative personnel, creating and maintaining staff schedules, maintaining equipment and ordering supplies, facilitating the organization's marketing and public relations efforts, facilitating payroll for employees, maintaining safety for the patients and staff, protecting patient privacy, and ensuring the organization adheres to clinical and administrative regulatory guidelines.

Clinical Members

All healthcare entities require a myriad of hands-on providers to deliver high-quality patient care. **Clinical** roles are those that are involved in the direct observation and care of the patient, and these roles are diverse and categorized by the level of education and responsibility within the healthcare environment.

Within the clinical functions, physicians act as the leaders and provide guidance for the healthcare team to provide patient care. The team includes the following members:

- **Professional healthcare workers,** who typically have a minimum of a bachelor's degree with additional advanced education in their chosen field. Examples are physicians, advanced practice nurses, registered nurses, physician's assistants, physical therapists, occupational therapists, and pharmacists.
- **Allied health professionals,** who have postsecondary education specific to their career. Examples are paramedics, respiratory therapists, surgical technologists, laboratory technologists, and medical assistants.
- **Service technicians,** who provide valuable skills that contribute to the overall care of the patient. Examples are nursing assistants, phlebotomy technicians, and dietary aides.

There are two pathways to becoming a physician. The more common of the two is the medical doctor (MD) degree, but there is also the doctor of osteopathy (DO) pathway. Both professions are similar in that a person must obtain an undergraduate degree in a scientific field plus 4 years of medical school, followed by varying lengths of internships and residencies. Those who choose the DO pathway receive additional training in the interconnection of the musculoskeletal systems and in manipulative medicine to provide "whole person" medicine. For more information on the physician pathway, see the section on medical careers in Chapter 1, including corresponding Tables 1-7 and 1-8.

A "nurse" is a healthcare professional who cares for the patient's most basic needs in a hospital, outpatient setting, or long-term care facility. There are several levels of nurses that are part of the healthcare team. A practical nurse is trained for a minimum of 1 year in nursing theory and practice. After successful completion of a licensing examination, the licensed practical nurse (LPN) or licensed vocational nurse (LVN) can practice in most types of healthcare facilities, according to guidelines set by the state governing board. A registered nurse has completed a minimum of 2 years in training for an associate's degree in nursing. This training provides more intense training than the practical nursing programs for patient care. Graduates of these programs sit for the registered professional nursing licensing examination, and upon successful completion, they are awarded the registered nurse (RN) title. State boards of nursing regulate the scope and practice of RNs. Although there are only a few programs left in the United States, a diploma in nursing is a 3-year, hospital-based program that offers not only nursing theory but also additional clinical training. Graduates also sit for the registered professional nursing examination. Most nursing schools today offer the Bachelor of Science in nursing degree. These students receive advanced training in nursing theory and management. Graduates will sit for the registered professional nursing examination and are also awarded the title of RN. These nurses may also use the BSN credential. The recent development of bridge programs at many universities offer LPNs and associate and diploma RNs the option to advance their education to the bachelor's level by offering credit based on licensure and experiential learning.

Many nurses choose to continue their education beyond the RN level. Master's-level nurses can choose from different specialty tracks, including family nurse practitioner (FNP), pediatric nurse practitioner (PNP), nurse midwife (CNM), or nursing educator. Each state licensing board develops scope of practice guidelines for these advanced practice nurses. For more information on the nursing pathway, see the section on modern careers in nursing in Chapter 1 and Table 1-3.

A common thread among all healthcare professionals and allied health personnel is the **certification** or **licensure** requirement that grants an individual permission to work in a profession. These exams allow graduates to validate their education and obtain the recognized credentials of their chosen field. The education process does not end with obtaining the credentials. All agencies require that those who become **credentialed,** or granted the evidence of their authority of their title or profession, continue to update their knowledge and skills through the **recertification** or license-renewal process of the licensing board. The length of initial licensure or certification varies, but it allows individuals enough time to prepare for the recredentialing process. Each organization sets standards for maintenance of credentials either through documented continuing education or retesting at specified intervals. These requirements allow us to stay current regarding changes and updates not only in our field but also with health care as a whole. See the Internet Resources section at the end of this chapter for a list of several professional associations that offer credentialing and continuing education resources.

Service technicians are also a valuable part of the healthcare team. Although the education process is shorter, these occupations can act as stepping stones to higher-level professions in health care. Many people enter these fields to evaluate their own interest in a healthcare setting and as a bonus receive valuable hands-on experience while attending school for an advanced career. The service technicians, such as nursing assistants, work at the patient's bedside to provide assistance with the activities of daily living. In doing so, they act as a liaison between the patient and the nurses, physicians, and administrative members of the healthcare team. Together, the team provides complete care for the patient.

For information on additional healthcare pathways, please see the Additional Healthcare Careers section in Chapter 1 and Tables 1-4 to 1-15.

STOP, THINK, AND LEARN.

Think about the last time you visited a healthcare facility. How many employees contributed to your visit? What were their jobs? Could any of those jobs been eliminated and left you with the same level of care? How would a hospital or physician survive without the team of dedicated employees to manage the flow of patients?

Teams Versus Groups

How do all of these occupations work together to provide high-quality patient care? Healthcare facilities promote an atmosphere of teamwork throughout the disciplines, with some describing their employees as team leaders and team members. Within a facility, there may be more than one team, but in the big picture, all of the teams combine to form one complete team dedicated to patient care. In an office or clinic, you may find an administrative team and a clinical team working both independently and together as neither can function without the other.

There is a significant difference between working as a **group** and working as a team. In groups, everyone has an individual task and goal, whereas teams may have individual tasks that jointly work toward the same goal. Team members know they are all working together and do not hesitate to ask other team members for help or to offer help.

Healthcare facilities strive to develop a culture of teamwork in an effort to ensure that patients feel they have received the best care possible. In extremely large hospitals, it is impossible for all employees to know each other, but they can still successfully form an effective team willing to work with other departments. On the other end of the spectrum, small hospitals develop more of a family environment in which every employee knows everybody else, and they all work together as one team. Healthcare facility administrators have the responsibility to develop a teamwork approach in a way that stimulates all employees. An example would be offering facility-wide meetings or recreational activities in which all employees from all departments are invited to participate equally. For example, when nursing assistants are given the opportunity to interact with the director of health information, they begin to feel more like a part of the larger team. A facility that promotes career retreats, educational opportunities, and special gatherings for all employees is successful in promoting teamwork within the institution that leads to optimal patient outcomes.

Team building is a daily process that helps to solve real work issues and improve the work flow. Once a project has been identified, it is most important that progress be reviewed on a regular basis to ensure the team members feel secure in their duties, they are getting along, and results are forthcoming. Teams must feel a sense of empowerment before they begin and must be reassured during the process. It is also necessary to keep all employees informed of the project so even though they may not be a part of this smaller team, they are involved in the process and will be responsible for the outcomes. A vital facet of team building is creating a feeling in employees that they are a part of something larger.

Health care has a culturally diverse population in both patients and employees. When working as a team, we must remember to respect the importance of each person's beliefs as they relate to the situation. We will discuss cultural diversity in Chapter 3.

Teamwork can be very effective in solving problems or improving processes. We should be interdependent on those in our work environment. By letting everyone contribute his or her strengths to the process, we find that the task is easier to accomplish. See Box 2-1 for an example of how we can work together for a common cause—just as geese do!

Communication

Without the ability to communicate, or exchange information, teamwork is impossible. It follows that **communication** can make or break a team or a group project. Verbal exchange, written messages, active listening, and nonverbal behavior such as facial expressions, body language, and touch are all components of communication. When communicating with team members, you should always start with a communication goal so that your communication and the actions that follow your communication will produce positive results.

Flashpoint
The load is always lighter when everybody lifts.

Box 2-1 Teamwork Lessons From Geese

Geese are known to fly in a V formation. As each goose flaps its wings, it creates "uplift" for the birds that follow it. By flying in formation, the whole flock adds 71% greater flying range than if each bird were flying alone.

- People who share a common direction and sense of community can get where they are going quicker and easier because they are traveling on the thrust of others.
- This helps us understand the concept of teamwork and cooperation. Things are easier if we cooperate and work as a team.

When a goose falls out of formation, it suddenly feels the drag and resistance of flying alone. It quickly moves back into formation to take advantage of the bird immediately in front of it.

- It makes sense to stay in formation with those who share our goals. We are willing to accept their help and give our help to others.
- Staying organized and focused really does make the job a lot easier.
- The geese flying in the back of the formation honk to encourage those up front to keep up their speed.
- Team members positively reinforce one another to ensure they keep progressing to reach the common goal.
- When the lead goose gets tired, it rotates back into the formation and another goose flies up to the point position.
- It may make sense to take turns doing the hard tasks and sharing leadership responsibilities. As with geese, people are interdependent on each other's skills, capabilities, and unique arrangement of gifts, talents, and resources.

When a goose gets sick or is shot down, two geese drop out of formation and follow it down to help and protect it. They stay with it until it dies or is able to fly again. Then they launch out with another formation or catch up to their flock.

- Team members stick by each other in both the good times and the bad. If someone in the office is having a bad day, don't let that person feel alone. Help him or her out; you may need help one day. Use good communication skills to let that person know that you are willing to provide support.
- Don't get pulled down by someone else's attitude. Both good attitudes and bad attitudes can be contagious. Use your best verbal and nonverbal communication skills to keep your team in top-notch shape.

Prior to communicating, know what you are talking about by being informed on your subject matter and what you hope to accomplish in the communication exchange.

Listening involves showing interest in what the other person is saying, avoiding interrupting the speaker, and watching the speaker closely to observe actions that may contradict what the person is saying. Conversation, a form of verbal communication that is used frequently in health care, may be formal, such as in a meeting, or informal, such as when you have a new idea that you wish to informally bounce off someone during a lunch break. Nonverbal communication may involve the use of facial expressions, body language, gestures, eye contact, and touch to convey a message. Examples of nonverbal communication are feet-tapping, shrugging the shoulders, smiling, nodding the head, a handshake, and a wink of an eye.

STOP, THINK, AND LEARN.
Think about the last time you worked on a team project. What communication skills were used within the group? Did everyone always agree on everything? List at least five verbal communication skills and five nonverbal skills or behaviors. For each of these traits, decide if they were helpful or disadvantageous to the team's goal.

When you ask a question, make sure that you listen to what others may say and respect their opinion regardless of whether you share that opinion. Once you ask a question or make a contribution, be quiet and let others respond. It may be necessary to rephrase your question, but you should not try to help your team members formulate their response with your own comments or suggestions. Relax as much as possible during a conversation to allow for purposeful interaction. Nonverbal communication, such as a frown on the face, and body language, such as crossing your arms, may indicate your disapproval without saying anything. Because you want conversations to be productive, it is important to keep emotions out of the way as much as possible. Many people are passionate about a topic one way or the other, and some will express that emotion to the point of exhaustion, damaging not only the conversation but the group dynamics as well, shifting the conversation from productivity to personal agenda.

Flashpoint
We have two ears and only one mouth, which tell us that we should listen twice as much as we talk.

All team members should feel that they are important to the goal and that their input is valued. The word "why" can be very threatening to some people, and we should try to avoid using it whenever possible. Rephrase "why" questions into a less intimidating format, such as "Can you tell me what makes you feel that way?," in order to keep the other person from becoming defensive. **Defensiveness** is excessive sensitivity to criticism and can destroy a conversation, sometimes changing the focus of the group and hurting feelings.

We have all heard clichés used in conversations. A *cliché* is an expression that has been overused to the point of losing its original meaning. Remember when you were growing up and relatives or family friends would say, "She is growing like a weed?" After hearing that repeatedly, you got tired of hearing it. The same is true for using clichés in teams. Members want to hear thoughts and ideas, not tired sayings that have been used to fill a conversation and serve no useful purpose. Leave clichés for times when conversations are personal and light-hearted.

To produce effective communications, we can follow a list of suggestions called the C's of communication found in Box 2-2.

Effective communication will always enhance teamwork and improve the quality and quantity of the work. We can learn effective communication skills through understanding our own style and by observing others. We are comfortable with our own communication style, but how others perceive our communication is very important. For example, those who communicate aggressively may seem angry or rude to those with a more passive style, whereas the passive may appear timid and weak to those with the aggressive style. Those with a very technical style of communication that is devoid of examples and emotions may have difficulty connecting with more emotional communicators who rely on details and feelings to express themselves.

Box 2-2 The Cs of Communication

- Be **clear**. You want to make sure that everyone understands you when you speak or ask a question. Have you ever had to stand up and talk in front of a group? Did you feel nervous? Most people do feel somewhat anxious when they become the focus of a crowd's attention. We tend to talk faster, which sometimes causes our listeners to lose interest and become distracted. Speaking clearly and slowly will help you remain in control and will give your audience the information that they need.

- Be **concise**. Be specific with your information. If you are communicating with a group of coworkers or team members, be careful that you do not digress from your topic. Information should be to the point and delivered in an appropriate manner. Communicating with patients must also be concise. Instructions for tests or information about treatment should be delivered both verbally and in written form to patients to prevent misunderstanding and a delay in treatment. When giving the instructions to patients, review the written instructions verbally and always include a telephone number so the patient or family may call if they have questions once they get home.

- Be **confident**. Have confidence in yourself as a communicator. For others to believe what you say, you must believe in what you say. Nonverbal communication such as not making eye contact or speaking in a faint voice may decrease your effectiveness in getting your point across. Do your research ahead of time and make sure you understand and believe what you say. When addressing a group or talking with team members, stand tall and make eye contact with everyone in the group. Use notes if necessary, but do not rely on them totally to communicate. It is acceptable to refer to written materials if everyone has access to those written materials.

- Be **complete**. It is not a good idea to begin a team meeting or project without having complete information. Conversations tend to lose focus when members interrupt to retrieve information that is important to the task. Handouts or presentations may help when members of the group are expected to retain information and report later. Regardless of whether your information is presented orally, in writing, or both, it is a good idea to have it proofread for completeness and grammar.

- Be **considerate**. Everyone comes to a meeting with his or her own ideas and interests. If you are the team leader, give all members an equal opportunity to express their ideas. Imagine how you would feel if after giving your ideas someone in the group immediately said, "That will never work!" It is likely that you would not speak up in future meetings and possibly prevent the group from being cohesive. Show a true interest in everyone that you work with. Respect is earned by treating people the way that you would like to be treated.

- Give **compliments**. When given in earnest, compliments may improve a person's self-esteem. Most people do not appreciate compliments that are empty or shallow and given as a consolation, but true compliments will give some team members the confidence to become more active in conversations, discussions, and projects. Inappropriate compliments may be construed as sexual harassment, so it is important to remember that giving compliments on clothing or personal appearance should be saved for those people with whom you have a personal relationship.

STOP, THINK, AND LEARN.
Personality traits may affect a person's ability to work with others, whether it is someone's shyness or outspokenness. The team leader will likely be the one to harmonize the group's dynamics. What other qualities should a team leader possess?

Communication is necessary for teamwork. Without both communication and teamwork working hand-in-hand in the healthcare environment, decisions would be impossible, tasks could not be accomplished, and patients would suffer.

Summary

Regardless of the healthcare occupation that you choose, working together as a team will provide better patient care and lessen the stress in the fast-paced healthcare field. Being a part of a team means giving and taking to accomplish a single goal.

Practice Exercises

Multiple Choice

1. Team members must do all of the following, except:
   a. Listen to everyone
   b. Discuss all suggestions
   c. Participate in discussions
   d. Insist on their way

2. Which of the following professionals is a part of the administrative healthcare team?
   a. Physician
   b. Office manager
   c. Nurse
   d. Certified nursing assistant

3. The minimum education for a registered nurse is:

   a. Diploma

   b. Associate's degree

   c. Bachelor's degree

   d. Master's degree

4. Recredentialing for a license or certification may be done through:

   a. Retesting

   b. Continuing education

   c. Payment of fees

   d. All of the above

5. Teamwork is most effective in:

   a. Setting the work schedule

   b. Solving problems and improving work flow

   c. Determining current pay scales

   d. Providing discipline for employees

Fill in the Blank

1. A team shares the _____ as well as the _____ for the outcomes.

2. When a physician chooses to send a patient to another provider, _____ paperwork must be completed by the clinical staff.

3. When working with a team, you must remember to _____ each member's _____.

4. _____ involves showing interest in what another person is saying.

Short Answer

1. **The patient's demographic and health information is protected by what statute?**

2. **What is an example of nonverbal communication?**

INTERNET RESOURCES

Career	Professional Organization	Web Address
Medical doctor (MD)	American Medical Association	www.ama-assn.org
Doctor of osteopathy (DO)	American Osteopathic Association	www.osteopathic.org
Dentist (DMD, DDS)	American Dental Association	www.ada.org
Optometrist (OD)	American Optometric Association	www.aoa.org
Podiatrist (DPM)	National Podiatric Medical Association	www.npmaonline.org
Pharmacist (PharmD)	American Pharmacists Association	www.pharmacist.com
Physician's assistant (PA)	National Commission on the Certification of Physician's Assistants	www.nccpa.net
Nurse practitioner (NP)	American Academy of Nurse Practitioners	www.aanp.org
Certified registered nurse anesthetist (CRNA)	American Association of Nurse Anesthetists	www.aana.com
Nurse midwife (CNM)	American College of Nurse Midwives	www.midwife.org
Registered nurse (RN)	American Nurses Association	www.ana.org
Social worker (ACSW) (DCSW) (QCSW)	National Association of Social Workers	www.socialworkers.org
Occupational therapist (OTR)	The American Occupational Therapy Association	www.aota.org
Physical therapist (PT)	American Physical Therapy Association	www.apta.org
Respiratory therapist (CRT) (RRT)	American Association for Respiratory Care	www.aarc.org
Medical laboratory technologist (MT) (MLT)	American Medical Technologists	www.amt1.com
Dental hygienist (RDH)	American Dental Hygienists' Association	www.adha.org
Dietitian (RD)	American Dietetic Association	www.eatright.org
Dental assistant (CDA), Registered dental assistant (RDA)	American Dental Assistants Association American Medical Technologists	www.dentalassistant.org www.amt1.com
Medical assistant (CMA), Registered medical assistant (RMA)	American Association of Medical Assistants American Medical Technologists	www.aama-ntl.org www.amt1.com
Radiologic technologist (RT-R)	American Society of Radiologic Technologists	www.asrt.org
Diagnostic medical sonographer	American Registry for Diagnostic Medical Sonography	www.ardms.org
Echocardiographer	American Society of Echocardiography	www.asecho.org
Licensed practical nurse (LPN) Licensed vocational nurse (LVN)	National Association for Practical Nurse Education and Service	www.napnes.org
Certified pharmacy technician (CPhT)	National Pharmacy Technician Association	www.pharmacytechnician.org

Continued

INTERNET RESOURCES—cont'd

Career	Professional Organization	Web Address
Surgical technologist (CST)	Association of Surgical Technologists National Board of Surgical Technology and Surgical Assisting	www.ast.org www.nbstsa.org
Emergency medical technician (NREMT-I) Paramedic (NREMT-P)	National Registry of Emergency Medical Technicians	www.nremt.org
Optician (ABOC) (ABOC-AC) (NCLE) (NCLE-AC)	American Board of Opticianry/National Contact Lens Examiners	www.abo-ncle.org
Certified nursing assistant (CNA)	National Association of Career Nursing Assistants	www.cna-network.org
Medical transcriptionist (CMT)	Association for Healthcare Documentation Integrity	www.ahdionline.org
Medical coder (CCS), (CCS-P) (CPC)	American Health Information Management Association American Academy of Professional Coders	www.ahima.org www.aapc.com

CULTURAL SENSITIVITY

Learning Outcomes

3.1 Define cultural sensitivity

3.2 Identify reasons that cultural sensitivity is important in health care

3.3 List barriers to transcultural health care

3.4 Distinguish between personal sensitivity and cultural sensitivity

Competencies

CAAHEP

- Demonstrate respect for diversity in approaching patients and family. (CAAHEP I.A.3)
- Demonstrate respect for individual diversity, incorporating one's own biases, in areas including gender, race, religion, age, and economic status. (CAAHEP IV.A.10)
- Demonstrate awareness of diversity in providing patient care. (CAAHEP X.A.3)

ABHES

- Analyze the effect of hereditary, cultural, and environmental influences. (ABHES 5.g)
- Demonstrate professionalism by being cognizant of ethical boundaries. (ABHES 11.b.4)

Key Terms

conscientious objection A personal disagreement on moral or ethical grounds voiced by a healthcare worker so that the worker may abstain from participation in a procedure as long as the patient's access to care is not adversely affected

cultural competency Healthcare workers successfully functioning within the framework of cultural needs, beliefs, and behaviors both as individuals and as a healthcare organization

cultural knowledge What a healthcare worker knows about other cultures and their beliefs, behaviors, and customs

culture Beliefs, values, practices, and social behavior of a particular nation or people

custom Something that people always do or always do in a particular way by tradition

diversity Having ethnic variety, as well as socioeconomic and gender variety, in a group, society, or institution

ethnicity The normal practices of a specific population that guide all decisions and actions; these practices are learned from elders and passed to younger generations
Continued

The Need for Transcultural Health Care

There are almost as many differences as there are people. There are differences in skin color, family structure, religious beliefs, and dietary preferences, just to name a few. Everyone can be identified by features as simple as one's clothing, actions, or address, or by more complex traits such as culture, customs, or beliefs. The world would be a boring place if people were identical.

Learning about and focusing on cultural diversity recognizes the fact that everyone has unique characteristics that make them who they are. Language, race, literacy level, and religion are a few more traits that divide people into cultures or ethnicities. Healthcare professionals must appreciate these differences and care for those in need without regard to whether they agree with their patients' beliefs. When caring for patients from a different culture, ask them what they would like you to know and understand about their care. This can ease patients' anxiety as well as that of the staff.

Transcultural health care is both a scientific and a humanistic approach to caring for the needs of society. According to the Culturally Competent Care Education Committee at Harvard Medical School, transcultural health care is defined as "the knowledge, skills, and attitudes required to provide quality clinical care to patients from different cultural, ethnic, and racial backgrounds."

It is important to focus not only on absolute healthcare needs but also on the similarities and differences among the many cultures of people that live in this country. A person's healthcare needs are based on a person's cultural values,

Key Terms—cont'd

generalization Broad statements about groups of people based on trends seen through specific examples

language barriers Inability to communicate due to not understanding another language

personal sensitivity An awareness of your personal feelings and reactions to situations

prejudice An unfavorable opinion or feeling formed beforehand or without knowledge, thought, or reason and having a negative effect on health care

religious beliefs Each person's belief in a supreme deity or specific religion and showing devotion or reverence to that higher power

stereotyping Labeling everyone from a certain culture as exactly the same

transcultural health care A scientific and a humanistic approach to caring for the needs of everyone in society

Flashpoint

The more familiar you are with other cultures, the more likely you are to provide culturally sensitive health care.

beliefs, and practices. Many cultures do not emphasize preventive healthcare services as the typical American does, so many times when treating someone of a different culture, it is a medical crisis. It is important to understand the concepts of transcultural health care to be able to provide more holistic and culturally sensitive health care.

Some individuals do not hesitate to discuss their customs or beliefs in an effort to help healthcare workers understand how to better care for them. Learning to communicate effectively with those from other cultures is an asset to working in health care. When working in a location that has a culturally diverse population, it is a good idea to research customs and beliefs that may affect health care for those people.

It is important not to stereotype people of another culture. A stereotype is a commonly held public belief about specific social groups or types of individuals or an assumption that "everyone" is a certain way. For example, you would be **stereotyping** if, when during a patient interview, you assume that all Mexican families are large and thus do not ask the patient about family size. **Generalizations,** broad statements about groups of people, are based on trends seen through specific examples. A generalization is that many Mexican families are large, so perhaps the patient has many brothers and sisters. You should ask the patient about her family, and record the correct information. Stereotyping assumes that all members of a particular culture believe and act on identical standards, whereas generalizations recognize trends within a culture.

Prejudice is an unfavorable opinion or feeling formed beforehand or without knowledge, thought, or reason and can have a negative impact on health care. Statements like "dizzy blond," "fat cow," and "lazy slob" are prejudicial. Prejudiced people regard their ideas and behavior as right and other ideas or behavior as wrong. Prejudice often stems from the fear of people or things that are different and that are not understood. To prevent prejudice, healthcare workers must treat all patients with respect and dignity, regardless of their appearance, lifestyle, and social or economic status.

Culture, or **ethnicity,** is the normal practices of a specific population that guides all decisions and actions; it is learned from elders and passed to younger generations. It is a way of life, and each member develops his or her values from living in society. To provide the best possible health care, it is important that you as healthcare workers allow each person to hold on to his or her cultural beliefs or practices and provide care that is sensitive to these needs, while remaining within the scope of safe and effective treatment. Lack of knowledge of cultural beliefs and languages can present barriers to providing patients with the best possible care. Even a simple misunderstanding of a belief or custom or a lack of thorough explanation could result in a missed diagnosis or unnecessary treatment. It is important that you become culturally competent healthcare providers.

Your **cultural knowledge** is what you know about other cultures and their beliefs, behaviors, and customs. **Cultural competency** means that you can successfully function within the framework of cultural needs, beliefs, and behaviors, both as an individual and within a healthcare organization. Knowledge of customs is very important when working with patients of a different cultural background. While many of those from different cultures are indoctrinated by American culture, they usually remain steadfast to their own culture in healthcare issues. When working in an area with a high population of culturally diverse people, it is important to learn about the various cultures to better provide care for these groups, regardless of their beliefs.

There may often be a lack of trust between patients and the healthcare team if they are not of the same background or ethnicity, so it is important to gain patients' trust through nonjudgmental discussions and explanations. Allaying apprehension and decreasing suspicions take compassion and a thorough knowledge of the treatment that is being proposed.

Knowledge of other customs is not enough, however. You must also be aware of those around you with cultural differences and not take them for granted when delivering health care. Always stop and consider how you would want to be treated if you found yourself in a culture different from your own. Arming yourself with both the knowledge and the awareness of cultural differences allows you to become a culturally competent healthcare professional and to deliver quality patient care to everyone.

Some people believe that anyone living in the United States should learn English and follow the customs. Is that compassionate or even practical? Imagine visiting another country and finding yourself in need of health care. Would you feel comfortable? Could you adapt?

STOP, THINK, AND LEARN.
Research finds that many Americans are traveling to foreign countries for procedures not covered by their insurance or because they do not have insurance and the cost savings are tremendous. What questions would you want answered before traveling to another country for medical treatment?

Flashpoint
The Centers for Disease Control and Prevention (CDC) offers information about traveling to other countries, including tips about diseases, vaccinations, and protecting yourself.

The Patient as an Individual

All patients have the right to be seen as and treated as an individual. Healthcare workers must use sensitivity when caring for patients and thus recognize and appreciate the personal characteristics of others. Individuals also have needs or a lack of something that is required or desired. Every human being has needs from the moment of birth until death. Needs motivate an individual's behavior in an attempt to meet these needs. Certain needs have a priority over other needs. For instance, the need for food, water, and shelter takes priority over the need to be invited to the school dance.

A noted psychologist named Abraham Maslow created a hierarchy of needs to show that basic needs, such as physiological and safety needs, must be met before attaining higher needs, such as self-esteem and self-confidence. Maslow's hierarchy of needs, which is discussed at length in Chapter 7, includes physiological needs, safety and security needs, love and affection needs, esteem needs, and self-actualization.

When the basic needs of both patients and healthcare workers are not met, anger, frustration, tension, and dissatisfaction can occur. The more intense a need, the greater the desire to meet it.

Barriers to Transcultural Health Care

The United States often looks at health care strictly as a biomedical or "by the book" process. Patients seeking medical care leave their homes and familiar surroundings to be treated in clinics, hospitals, and other healthcare settings. This can be a frightening experience for anyone and especially for someone who does not understand Western medicine. As healthcare professionals, you must be prepared to facilitate the care these people receive in a manner that is comforting and therapeutic. It is important to exercise compassion when you do not understand a language or a custom so that you do not appear to be frustrated or impatient. You should afford a patient from a different culture the same level of care and concern as you would a patient from your own culture. A few examples of cultural barriers follow.

Language

While some people may not think of language as a cultural barrier, it can present many challenges in health care. **Language barriers** are becoming more common as people emigrate from other countries. It is not possible for all healthcare workers to learn all languages, but you must be prepared to work with the patient and family to create a comfortable and knowledgeable conversation. Translators should be provided when detailed information must be given to the patient and family because many languages cannot be literally translated from the written word. Is a family member the best translator? Do you know for sure that the patient and other family members are getting the correct information? Likewise, is the healthcare team getting the correct information from the patient through the family translator?

 ### STOP, THINK, AND LEARN.
Mr. Hsu Son, a Chinese immigrant, must undergo a bone marrow transplant. His immediate family speaks no English. He calls for his brother to come to the hospital to translate. His brother is determined to be a viable donor; however, the extended family tries to convince him that donating bone marrow is harmful to his own health. The family members ask the brother to tell Mr. Son that he is not a donor. How do you think this scenario will end? Will Mr. Son get the needed transplant from his brother? Will the extended family accept the transplant option? What is the most appropriate way to educate all of the involved family members?

When complex procedures are necessary, it is always in the best interest of the healthcare facility to provide a neutral translator to ensure that the patient understands and provides the correct information. In a culturally diverse population, healthcare facilities must secure a network of translators to provide the necessary communication between patients and physicians. Informed consent for procedures is an example of the need for expert translation. There are software programs available, some at no cost, if your need for translation is not a daily occurrence. The Office of Minority Health of the U.S. Department of Health and Human Services has developed the *Patient-Centered Guide to Implementing Language Access Services in Healthcare Organizations* in an effort to give those with language difficulties the ability to increase their access to health care in the United States. These language access services (LASs), such as telephone language lines, local nonbiased interpreters, and written patient information packets, are helpful in preventing barriers to quality health care.

Research by the Institute of Medicine (IOM) found a true disparity in care and health status of racial and ethnic groups as compared with white counterparts. The IOM found that racial and ethnic groups received substandard care, resulting in poorer health, most likely due to language barriers and lack of equal access to health care. Language barriers can lead to reduced care or even the wrong treatment in some cases. Patients and healthcare workers often give up when communication or cultural boundaries become a burden. Patients may feel that they are expected to sacrifice their beliefs or customs and may become frustrated. This may cause patients to reject care and not seek further treatment. Healthcare workers may not understand the sacrifice and insist that the patient receive a treatment. Both situations require patience and compassion.

An important concept to remember is that when people have no knowledge of English, talking louder or slower does not help them understand. Hand gestures and basic demonstrations may be helpful in explaining procedures.

Religious Beliefs

Religious beliefs can play a significant role in health care. For example, Jehovah's Witnesses are unwilling to accept a blood transfusion, and Amish people may refuse preventive care such as immunizations. For many cultures, health care and religious or spiritual practices are intertwined. Some cultures believe in faith healing, evil spirits, nature as a spiritual healing force, and the spiritual balance of spirit, mind, and body. For instance, Native Americans combine folk medicine and spiritual natural elements with Western medicine to promote healing.

Studies have been conducted on the power of prayer in medicine with conflicting results. A study in the *New England Journal of Medicine* recently found that linking religion with medicine often oversimplifies these two major areas of patients' beliefs—prayer and modern medicine. Although religious beliefs and preferences are not a major portion of a patient assessment, it is important to understand that certain religions have very specific beliefs about healthcare practices. In some religious cultures, it is inappropriate for a female patient to be examined by a male physician or for a male baby to be circumcised before leaving the hospital. Many religions have ceremonial rights associated with health care and with end-of-life issues. These should always be addressed respectfully.

Flashpoint

Do not shout at a person whose language you do not speak. Use gestures, pictures, and other visual aids to help the patient understand you.

STOP, THINK, AND LEARN.
Using the earlier case of Mr. Son, make a "family" list and a "healthcare provider" list of the issues involved in this case. Prioritize your lists, and compare them. Are there common issues on both sides?

As a healthcare worker, there may be situations in which your own religious beliefs may be tested. When abortion was legalized in the United States, physicians and nurses with strong "right-to-life" beliefs were put into situations that required they participate in the procedures. The patients were often the ones who suffered when healthcare workers lashed out at them or failed to provide proper care and treatment. Was either party at fault for standing behind its beliefs? Another case of religious objection has surfaced since the approval of the "morning after" pill. Pharmacists have refused to provide the medication to women. Does this interfere with womens' ability to obtain the care they want? Eventually, the American Medical Association intervened to separate religion and medicine.

Healthcare workers with a **conscientious objection** to certain procedures or practices—that is, a personal disagreement on moral or ethical grounds—should be allowed to abstain from participation as long as the patient's access to care is not affected. If you, as a healthcare professional, have beliefs that do not allow you to participate in certain procedures, advise your employer of such so there are no awkward situations for you, the employer, or your patients. When this type of situation arises with a physician, it is his or her obligation to advise the patient to see another practitioner. If the patient is unable to make other arrangements, the physician must make sure that any necessary immediate care is provided while further care is arranged. If a physician does hold certain religious beliefs that affect his or her treatment options, it should be communicated to all patients who choose this provider for care. Practice brochures or information packets should include all of the necessary information to allow patients to make an informed decision about their healthcare provider.

When caring for patients with particular religious beliefs, you must remember that their beliefs may be fundamental to their well-being, and you must be sensitive to those beliefs without making the patient uncomfortable or angry. Physicians and other healthcare workers must be certain that patients have and fully understand all the information concerning their diagnosis and treatment options in order to make an informed decision about their health care.

Customs

The term **custom** indicates the way somebody or some group routinely behaves in a given situation. Social or ethnic groups may have customs that are viewed by their followers as laws. Because these customs are practiced from generation to generation, they become a part of the group's beliefs and foundations.

A person's culture may dictate the type of health care he or she seeks or treatment he or she allows. Asian people are known to be stoic, often refusing pain medication despite their suffering. Some cultures prevent eye contact with persons of authority such as physicians, healthcare providers, and teachers. This may interfere with proper communication in a healthcare setting but should never be viewed as a lack of concern from the patient. Table 3-1 outlines some differences in customs among cultures that may come into play in the healthcare context.

Pregnancy and childbirth customs differ among cultures with very strong beliefs about the safety of the mother and the child. Turkish culture requires that the mother and newborn be isolated for 20 days before they visit individual homes and celebrating with a special drink. Some German city governments have a list of approved baby names from which new parents must choose. The idea is to prevent the child from being ridiculed later in life by having an unusual name. Brazilian culture mandates that all women undergo a caesarean delivery, but the government is trying to impose other childbirth methods to reduce the costs associated with caesarean deliveries.

Americans tend to view these customs as odd, but these cultures may look at some American customs with the same curiosity. Being very careful with your conversations and even facial expressions can help put a patient at ease in the healthcare environment. Some children who come to this country early in life may even question their own family's customs after having grown up in the

TABLE 3-1

CULTURAL DIFFERENCES IN HEALTH CARE

Culture	Customs
Asian	Coining may be performed, in which a coin is heated or oiled and rubbed vigorously over the patient's back to "draw out the illness." The reddened areas are proof that the procedure has been successful.
Chinese/Japanese	The word for the number 4 sounds like the word for death. These patients do not want to be placed in a room with the number 4 in the room number. (Similar to the American belief that the number "13" is bad luck.)
Asian, Muslim, Navaho	Lack of eye contact with persons of authority is a sign of respect and not lack of interest, embarrassment, or depression. Navahos may be avoiding the loss of their soul through direct eye contact.
Orthodox Jew	Physical contact by someone of the opposite sex for hands-on care is prohibited.
Christian Scientist	Christian Scientists generally do not seek medical care in a hospital, but rather through a Christian Science hospital practitioner and prayer. When admission to a hospital after an accident is necessary, they wish to be treated totally drug free.
Jehovah's Witness	Taking blood, as in a transfusion, is morally wrong.
Russian culture	Bad news is not given directly to the patient but rather to the family, who decides whether or not to tell the patient.

host society. There will always be strong family ties that enable people to stay true to their cultural background, but they may also start adopting some newer customs relative to health care.

Personal Sensitivity

In addition to cultural sensitivity, you should be aware of your **personal sensitivity,** which is how you feel and react to situations. Your primary duty is to provide your patients with the care you are trained to give, in a nonjudgmental manner, being careful not to let facial expressions or other nonverbal expressions show. You should treat each patient equally, regardless of your personal reactions to or opinions about a patient's lifestyle choices. You may not agree with a patient's choice of hairstyles, tattoos, or body piercings, when in reality these have nothing to do with his or her need for health care. The patient's weight, sexual preference, personal hygiene, or socioeconomic status must not affect the type of care you provide.

These characteristics may not always be as obvious or seem as significant as the others listed in this chapter, but each patient is different and has a different level of sensitivity. Whereas one patient may be comfortable with what you consider a "harmless" comment or joke, another might be very offended or upset by the same comment. Moreover, a patient's presence in the sometimes high-stress environment of the hospital or physician's office may heighten sensitivities. Almost everyone is on edge when facing a health crisis, and each patient's reaction may be different, but most people will not react in the way they would normally. Always err on the safe side when conversing with a patient, steering clear of potentially offensive or inappropriate remarks. Use the patient's proper name to show respect and concern. In any healthcare facility, your job is to provide thoughtful, thorough care while making the patient as comfortable as possible.

Flashpoint

Sensitivity is easily accomplished by using the Golden Rule: Treat others as you want to be treated.

Diversity is everywhere in health care, both for patients and healthcare workers. Understanding that there will always be patients or even healthcare team members with ideas and beliefs different from your own will help you focus on the patient's healthcare needs. Teamwork is important in health care, and learning to work together with other healthcare professionals who do not share your values and beliefs will challenge you. Make the effort to put the patient first, and resolve to put personal differences with your team members aside to ensure the patient receives the best possible treatment.

Flashpoint

The culturally sensitive treatment plan may take a little longer to construct, but the patient's needs are the top priority.

Summary

As professionals, you should respect your patients' and coworkers' customs and beliefs. It is important that you do not let any personal biases get in the way of quality patient care. Practicing the Golden Rule will ensure that patients and family members will appreciate the care and respect that they receive.

Practice Exercises

Multiple Choice

1. Cultural differences include all of the following, except:
   a. race
   b. religion
   c. sex
   d. language

2. The best method of caring for patients from a different culture is to:
   a. tell them how our culture works
   b. ask them if they have any questions about your culture
   c. avoid talking about the subject
   d. ask them what they would like for you to know about their culture

3. Functioning within the framework of cultural needs, beliefs, and behaviors, both as an individual and as a healthcare organization, is the definition of:
   a. culture
   b. cultural competence
   c. cultural knowledge
   d. cultural experience

4. Believing that everyone of a certain culture is exactly the same is known as:

    a. stereotyping

    b. generalizing

    c. prejudice

    d. monotyping

5. Having a conscientious objection means that you:

    a. don't like the patient

    b. don't like the procedure

    c. have a personal disagreement based on moral and ethical grounds

    d. have a personal objection to the physician's practice

6. Many cultures do not emphasize which of the following aspects of health care?

    a. childbirth

    b. education

    d. medications

    e. prevention

Fill in the Blank

1. The term _____ indicates the way somebody or some group routinely behaves in a given situation.

2. An unfavorable opinion or feeling formed beforehand or without knowledge, thought, or reason about a person or group is known as _____.

3. _____ is the normal practices of a specific population that guides all decisions and actions of the group.

Short Answer

1. **Why is it important that you understand transcultural health care?**

2. **How can you communicate with someone who speaks a different language from your own?**

3. **What is one area of health care that varies greatly between cultures?**

INTERNET RESOURCES	
Organization/Service	**Web Address**
The Office of Minority Health of the U.S. Department of Health and Human Services	http://minorityhealth.hhs.gov
The National Institute on Minority Health and Health Disparities	http://nimhd.nih.gov
The National Coalition of Ethnic Minority Nurse Associations	www.ncemna.org
The Transcultural Nursing Society	www.tcns.org
Language translation	www.freetranslation.com http://babelfish.yahoo.com http://languageline.com

PREPARING FOR A CAREER IN HEALTH CARE

4

Learning Outcomes

4.1 Understand the importance of math in healthcare careers

4.2 Master the fundamentals of whole numbers, fractions, decimals, percentages, and ratios

4.3 Demonstrate an understanding of rounding and estimating

4.4 Differentiate between the metric and apothecary systems of measurement used in health care

4.5 Convert measurements, drug dosages, and temperatures using the appropriate system

Competencies

CAAHEP

- Demonstrate knowledge of basic math computations. (CAAHEP II.C.1)
- Apply mathematical computations to solve equations. (CAAHEP II.C.2)
- Identify measurement systems. (CAAHEP II.C.3)
- Define basic units of measurement in metric apothecary and household systems. (CAAHEP II.C.4)
- Convert among measurement systems. (CAAHEP II.C.5)

ABHES

- Demonstrate accurate occupational math and metric conversions for proper medication administration. (ABHES 6.a)

Importance of Math in Health Care

Preparing for a career in health care takes many forms: attending classes, studying, researching career options, and volunteering in a healthcare environment. However, there is one area of study that you must master to become proficient in health care, and this is math. Professionals working in health care use math skills to measure and perform various types of calculations. Math applications are used in all types of healthcare occupations, including:

- Taking height and weight readings
- Calculating medication dosages
- Performing laboratory tests
- Measuring the amount of intake (fluids consumed or infused) and output (e.g., urine, vomit)
- Developing dietary guidelines (food and liquid weights and measurements)
- Performing billing and bookkeeping tasks
- Mixing cleaning solutions

Key Terms

apothecary system Least used and oldest of the three drug calculation systems.

Arabic numerals Traditional numbering system that is used every day.

centigrade System of temperature measurement used in health care; also known as Celsius.

decimal Used to define parts of numbers expressed in units of ten. They represent the number of 10ths, 100ths, 1000ths, and so forth, that are available.

estimating Process used to approximate the result of a calculation to detect any possible errors.

Fahrenheit System of temperature measurement more familiar to people living in the United States.

fraction Method of expressing numbers that represent part of a whole. The numerator is the top number, which represents actual number of parts of a whole, and the denominator is the bottom number, which signifies how many parts it takes to make a whole.

Continued

Key Terms—cont'd

household system System of measurement commonly used in U.S. households that also has applications in health care, including volume, length, and weight.

improper fraction Fractions that have a numerator larger than the denominator.

math anxiety Situation in which learners react to math so strongly that their ability to memorize, concentrate, and pay attention is affected negatively.

metric system Measurement system based on units of 10.

military time Time based on a 24-hour day, meaning that the 12th hour represents 12 noon and the 24th hour represents 12 midnight.

Continued

Flashpoint

Instead of thinking negatively about math, tell yourself, "I can do this. I just have to take my time and think the problems through, but I don't have a problem with math."

Healthcare workers must be 100% accurate when performing math calculations. Mathematical errors can produce negative consequences in patients, so it is essential that healthcare workers double-check all calculations to enhance the quality of care and improve patient safety. This chapter covers several basic math concepts that are essential to understand when pursuing a career in health care.

Math Anxiety

Many healthcare professionals suffer from **math anxiety,** a situation in which learners react to math so strongly that their ability to memorize, concentrate, and pay attention is negatively affected. Many learners can overcome this fear. The first step is to recognize that the fear exists, followed by a willingness to correct the fear. Many learners believe common math myths that hinder learning. Some of these myths are that (a) math is not creative; (b) math requires a good memory; (c) men are better at math than women; (d) mathematicians do problems quickly in their heads; and (e) some people have a "math mind" and some do not. The following are some ways to improve math skills:

- Avoid procrastination, which increases anxiety.
- Employ a "can-do," positive approach to learning math.
- Be proactive about learning concepts and ideas, even those previously learned that may have been forgotten.
- Read and discuss some ideas several times to help them "stick" in your mind.
- Take a break when ideas feel like they are no longer clear and are creating confusion.

Basic Calculations

This section presents the basics needed to perform many medical math applications, including whole numbers, decimals, fractions, percentages, ratios, and proportions. The information presented should jog your memory regarding these basic skills, but do not hesitate to see if your campus has a resource center that offers assistance in reviewing math.

To work safely and proficiently in health care, you must know how to add, subtract, multiply, and divide whole numbers, decimals, fractions, and percentages. Although many healthcare workers use calculators, you should also know how to perform these basic functions "longhand," both in the workplace and when preparing to take licensure and certification examinations that may not allow the use of calculators.

Whole Numbers

Whole numbers are traditional numbers (1, 2, 3 . . .) that do not contain fractions or decimals and that are used in counting. For example, 25 is a whole number, but $25^1/_2$ and 25.5 are not. Healthcare professionals must be able to add, subtract, multiply, and divide whole numbers, such as the following:

- Add: 20 + 30 = 50
- Subtract: 85 − 25 = 60
- Multiply: 10 × 22 = 220
- Divide: 105 ÷ 5 = 21

 STOP, THINK, AND LEARN.
Add the following: 36 + 59; 25 + 98; 44 + 77; 18 +87
Subtract the following: 75 − 39; 93 − 21; 88 − 52; 69 − 27
Multiply the following: 31 × 22; 17 × 20; 23 × 9; 21 × 42
Divide the following: 36 ÷ 13; 48 ÷ 12; 57 ÷ 14; 89 ÷ 21

Fractions

Fractions are a method of expressing numbers that represent part of a whole. A fraction contains a numerator, the top number, which represents the actual number of parts of a whole, and a denominator, the bottom number, which signifies how many parts it takes to make a whole. One example of a fraction is $^7/_8$, where 7 is the numerator and 8 is the denominator.

Performing calculations with fractions is not difficult (Table 4-1). There are several considerations when performing these calculations, such as the following:

- When adding and subtracting fractions, convert the fractions, a process in which you change all the denominators to the same number. To do this, find a number that each denominator can divide into evenly and then adjust the numerators to maintain an equivalent fraction. For example, to add $^1/_2 + ^2/_5$, convert both fractions to tenths: $^5/_{10} + ^4/_{10} = ^9/_{10}$. The denominators 2 and 5 both divide into 10 evenly. Multiply the numerator by the number of times the old denominator divides into the new denominator.
- When multiplying fractions, first multiply the two numerators and then the two denominators, for example: $^2/_3 × ^2/_3 = ^4/_9$.
- When dividing fractions, the dividing fractions are inverted, or turned upside down (known as the ***reciprocal)***, and the numerators and denominators are then multiplied to get the answer. Here is one example: $^2/_4 ÷ ^1/_4 = ^2/_4 × ^4/_1 = ^8/_4$, or 2.

Also, fractions are reduced to their lowest common numbers, meaning that a number can be divided evenly into both the numerator and denominator. For example, the fraction $^3/_6$ can be reduced to $^1/_2$ by dividing both the numerator and denominator by 3 (3 ÷ 3 = 1, and 6 ÷ 3 = 2).

Improper fractions have numerators that are larger than the denominator and can easily be reduced by dividing the denominator into the numerator, which will yield a result of either a whole number or a mixed number (whole number and a fraction). Two examples of this are $^{18}/_3 = 6$ (18 ÷ 3) and $^{17}/_4 = 4^1/_4$ (17 ÷ 4).

Key Terms—cont'd

nomenclature Method of naming.

percentage Number that expresses either a whole (100%) or part of a whole (25%).

proportion Equality and relationship between two ratios.

ratio Relationship between one value and number as compared to another like value.

reciprocal Fractions that are inverted, or turned upside down.

Roman numerals Ancient numbering system consisting of seven key numbers represented by capital letters; still used in health care for medications, solutions, and ordering systems.

rounding numbers Changing a number to the nearest whole, 10th, 100th, or 1000th, depending on the original number and the final product.

whole numbers Traditional numbers that do not contain fractions or decimals and that are used in counting.

TABLE 4-1		
WORKING WITH FRACTIONS		
Function	**Example**	**Key Points**
Add (+):	$\frac{1}{4} + \frac{1}{5} = \frac{5}{20} + \frac{4}{20} = \frac{9}{20}$	1. If the denominators are not the same, find a number that both denominators divide into evenly. 2. Multiply the numerators by the number of times the old denominators divide into the new denominator. 3. Add the numerators. 4. Place the new numerator over the denominator. 5. Reduce the fraction, if necessary.
Subtract (−):	$\frac{1}{4} - \frac{1}{5} = \frac{5}{20} - \frac{4}{20} = \frac{1}{20}$	1. If the denominators are not the same, find a number that both denominators divide into evenly. 2. Multiply the numerators by the number of times the old denominators divide into the new denominators. 3. Subtract the numerators. 4. Place the new numerator over the denominator. 5. Reduce the fraction, if necessary.
Multiply (×)	$\frac{1}{4} \times \frac{1}{5} = \frac{1}{20}$	1. Multiply numerators. 2. Multiply denominators. 3. Reduce the fraction, if necessary.
Divide (÷)	$\frac{1}{4} \div \frac{1}{5} = \frac{1}{4} \times \frac{5}{1} = \frac{5}{4} = 1\frac{1}{4}$	1. Invert the dividing fraction. 2. Multiply numerators. 3. Multiply denominators. 4. Reduce the fraction, if necessary.

STOP, THINK, AND LEARN.

Add the following fractions: $1\frac{3}{4} + \frac{2}{8}$; $\frac{3}{5} + \frac{3}{10}$; $\frac{6}{8} + \frac{1}{4}$; $\frac{2}{3} + \frac{3}{4}$

Subtract the following fractions: $\frac{3}{4} - \frac{2}{3}$; $\frac{6}{8} - \frac{3}{4}$; $\frac{5}{9} - \frac{1}{3}$; $\frac{5}{8} - \frac{2}{3}$

Multiply the following fractions: $\frac{1}{2} \times \frac{2}{3}$; $\frac{3}{4} \times 1\frac{1}{2}$; $\frac{2}{3} \times \frac{3}{4}$; $\frac{5}{8} \times \frac{1}{2}$

Divide the following fractions: $\frac{3}{4} \div \frac{1}{3}$; $\frac{2}{3} \div \frac{1}{2}$; $\frac{5}{8} \div \frac{3}{8}$; $\frac{7}{8} \div \frac{2}{3}$

Decimals

Decimals are used to define parts of numbers and are expressed in units of 10. They represent the number of 10ths, 100ths, 1000ths, and so forth, that are available. For example, 0.9 represents 9 of the 10 parts into which something has been divided. Digits for placement values of decimals are placed to the right of the decimal point. A decimal point is verbally read as "and." Also, be aware that a zero is placed to the left of the decimal point if the number starts to the right of the decimal point. For example, learners would read the following numbers like this:

- 0.7 is read "seven-tenths"
- 2.3 is read "two and three-tenths"

Although decimals are added, subtracted, multiplied, and divided in the same manner as whole numbers, make sure that the decimal points are correctly placed throughout the calculation. An incorrect placement of a decimal point will yield an incorrect answer (Table 4-2) and could jeopardize patient care and patient safety.

STOP, THINK, AND LEARN.

Add the following decimals: 1.4 + 2.3; 1.47 + 3.19; 6.785 + 4.69; 2.389 + 5.124
Subtract the following decimals: 2.34 − 1.19; 3.07 − 1.897; 9.065 − 4.148; 5.009 − 2.762
Multiply the following decimals: 2.56 × 3.12; 3.461 × 8.23; 1.265 × 3.485; 2.445 × 1.995
Divide the following decimals: 5.23 ÷ 1.12; 12.34 ÷ 2.25; 25.873 ÷ 2.91; 9.1 ÷ 2.351

Percentages

Percentages express either a whole (100%) or part of a whole (25%) of something. If, for example, you had a cherry pie and sliced it into 10 slices, the 10 pieces

TABLE 4-2		
WORKING WITH DECIMALS		
Function	**Example**	**Key Points**
Add (+):	2.5 +1.75 4.25	1. Line up the decimal points. 2. Add the numbers. 3. Bring the decimal point straight down.
Subtract (−):	4.25 − 1.75 2.5	1. Line up the decimal points. 2. Subtract the numbers. 3. Bring the decimal point straight down.
Multiply (×)	1.5 × 1.5 75 + 15 2.25	1. Multiply the numbers. 2. Count the total number of digits to the right of the decimal points in the numbers you are multiplying. 3. Count the same number of places in your answer. Start to the right of the last digit in your answer and move that number of places to the left. This is where the decimal point is placed.
Divide (÷)	6.25⟌1.25 6.25 → 625 6.25⟌1.25 1.25 → 125 6.25⟌125.0 .2	1. Move the decimal point to the right in the number you are dividing by (to make it a whole number). 2. Move the decimal point the same number of places to the right in the number being divided. Add zeros, if necessary. 3. Divide the numbers. 4. Place the decimal point in the answer by moving it straight up from the number that was divided.

would equal the whole of 100%, one slice would equal 10%, and three slices would represent 30% of the pie (Fig. 4-1). Generally, it is easier to convert percentages into decimals and then calculate the addition, subtraction, multiplication, or division problem.

Ratios

Ratios show relationships between one value and number compared to another like value. The use of ratios to express the strength of a solution is commonly seen in healthcare settings. Solution strengths are frequently expressed as percentages. A 50% bleach solution, for example, is the same as a 1:2 ratio. A water and bleach solution with a 2:3 ratio means that two parts of water are added for every three parts of bleach (Fig. 4-2). This relationship is expressed the same regardless of the units used for example:

- 2 cups of water and 3 cups of bleach
- 2 quarts of water and 3 quarts of bleach
- ²/₃ cup of water and 1 cup of bleach

Converting Decimals, Fractions, Percentages, and Ratios

Decimals, fractions, and percentages all represent parts of a whole, and all are expressed differently. For example, the fraction ³/₄, the decimal 0.75, and the percentage 75% all represent the same calculation. The steps to convert these numerical forms from one application to another are shown in Table 4-3.

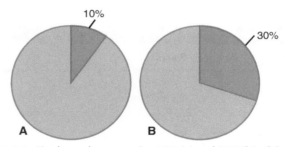

FIGURE 4-1 Pie charts demonstrating 10% (a) and 30% (b) of the whole.

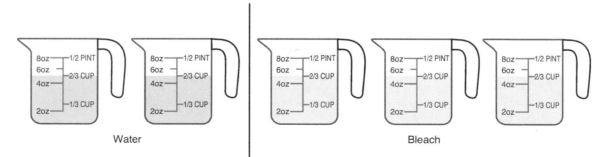

FIGURE 4-2 A visual representation of a 2:3 water-to-bleach solution strength.

TABLE 4-3		
CONVERTING FRACTIONS, DECIMALS, AND PERCENTAGES		
Conversion	**Example**	**Key Points**
Fractions to decimals	$^4/_{10} = 4 \div 10 = 0.4$	1. Divide numerator by denominator.
Fractions to percentages	$^5/_8 = 5 \div 8 = 0.625$ $0.625 \times 100 = 62.5$ 62.5%	1. Divide numerator by denominator. 2. Move the decimal point two places to the right because percentages are based on 100. This is the same as multiplying by 100. 3. Add percentage sign.
Decimals to fractions	$0.25 = {}^{25}/_{100} = {}^1/_4$	1. Drop the decimal point. 2. Position the number over its placement value. 3. If necessary, reduce the fraction.
Decimals to percentages	$3.155 = 3.155 \times 100 = 315.5$ 315.5%	1. Move the decimal point two places to the right because percentages are based on 100. This is the same as multiplying by 100. 2. Add percentage sign.
Percentages to ratios	75% = 75 75:100 3:4	1. Remove percentage sign. 2. Create a ratio using the former percentage and the number 100. 3. Insert a colon (:) between the numbers. 4. If appropriate, simplify ratio to lower numbers.
Ratios to percentages	$1:4 = {}^1/_4 = 0.25$ $0.25 \times 100 = 25$ 25%	1. Divide number on left of the colon by number on right of colon sign. 2. Move decimal point two places to the right. Add zero(s) if necessary. This is the same as multiplying by 100. 3. Add percentage sign.

STOP, THINK, AND LEARN.
Convert the following:
$^2/_3$ to decimal and to percentage
$^1/_2$ to decimal and to percentage

Rounding Numbers

When ***rounding a number*** (Table 4-4), you are changing it to the nearest 10th, 100th, or 1000th, depending on the original number and your final product. There will be times when you must calculate drug dosages, and your answer must be rounded to a measurable number.

You can round up or down, and this depends on the digits (numbers) located to the right of the value chosen for rounding. The following examples demonstrate how rounding is applied:

- **Example 1:** When your medication dosage is greater than 1 milliliter, the answer must be rounded to the 10ths place. Rounding rules state that if the number to the right of the 10th place is greater than 5, round up, and if the number is less than 5, round down.
    1.350 rounds up to 1.4
    1.421 rounds down to 1.4

TABLE 4-4

ROUNDING NUMBERS

Rounding the number 67.283 to the nearest:	Comments	Result
Whole number	The digit to the right of the whole number 67 is 2, so round down one number.	67
10s	The digit to the right of the 10s position is 7, so round up.	70
10ths	The digit to the right of the 10ths position is 8, so round up.	67.3
100ths	The digit to the right of the 100s position is 3, so round down.	67.28

- **Example 2:** When your answer is less than 1 milliliter, you must round to the 100ths.
  0.385 rounds up to 0.39
  0.323 rounds down to 0.32
- **Example 3:** When rounding to the nearest 10, look at the digit in the 1s place (which is to the right of the 10s place), and follow the same general rule found in example 1 above.
  72 rounds down to 70
  77 rounds up to 80

Proportions

A ***proportion*** shows the equality and relationship between two ratios. For example, the proportion 4:8 = 6:12 shows that 4 is related to 8 in the same manner that 6 is related to 12. When working with proportions, you can convert from one unit to another when three of the terms in the proportions are known. For example, you need $16.30, but only have dimes. How many dimes are needed? Three of the terms in the proportion are known:

1. $16.30
2. 10 (the number of dimes that are in $1.00)
3. $1.00

The proportion is set up as follows:

$$\frac{10 \text{ dimes}}{x \text{ dimes}} = \frac{\$1.00}{\$16.30}$$

The proportion above will answer the question: "If 10 dimes equal $1.00, how many dimes are there in $16.30?" Or put another way: "10 dimes is to $1.00 as *x* dimes are to $16.30." The *x* stands for the number of dimes to be calculated. The two unit measurements on each side of the equation are the same (dimes on the left and dollars on the right). Follow these steps to solve this problem:

1. Cross-multiply:

$$\frac{10 \text{ dimes}}{x \text{ dimes}} = \frac{\$1.00}{\$16.30}$$

$1 \times x = 10 \times \$16.30$

$1x = 163$

2. Divide each side by the number in front of *x*.

3. $1x \div 1 = 1$ and $163 \div 1 = 163$
4. 163 dimes are needed to make a payment of $16.30.
5. The completed proportion is presented as follows:
$$\frac{10 \text{ dimes}}{163 \text{ dimes}} = \frac{\$1.00}{\$16.30}$$

Converting units of measure is also commonly used in proportions. For example, you want to know how many feet are in 30 inches. Again, three of the terms in the proportion are known:

1. 30 inches
2. 12 (the number of inches in 1 foot)
3. 1 foot

The proportion is set up as follows:
$$\frac{1 \text{ foot}}{x \text{ feet}} = \frac{12 \text{ inches}}{30 \text{ inches}}$$
Follow these steps to solve this problem:

1. Cross-multiply:
$$\frac{1 \text{ foot}}{x \text{ feet}} = \frac{12 \text{ inches}}{30 \text{ inches}}$$
$12 \times x = 1 \times 30$
$12x = 30$
2. Divide each side by the number in front of "x."
$12x \div 12 = x$ and $30 \div 12 = 2.50$
$x = 2.50$
3. 2.5 feet = 30 inches.
4. The completed proportion is presented as follows:
$$\frac{1 \text{ foot}}{2.5 \text{ feet}} = \frac{12 \text{ inches}}{30 \text{ inches}}$$

Healthcare professionals use common applications for which they are required to find the value of an unknown when converting medications from one form to another. For example, a physician orders 30 grams of a medication be administered to a patient. When the nurse checks, he or she notes that the medication is available only in 10-gram tablets. How many tablets should the nurse give the patient? Follow these steps:

1. Set up your proportion:
$$\frac{1 \text{ tablet}}{x \text{ tablet}} = \frac{10 \text{ grams}}{30 \text{ grams}}$$
2. Solve this problem by taking the following steps:
   a. Cross-multiply:
   $$\frac{1 \text{ tablet}}{x \text{ tablet}} = \frac{10 \text{ grams}}{30 \text{ grams}}$$
   $10 \times x = 1 \times 30$
   $10x = 30$
   b. Divide each side by the number in front of x.
   $10x \div 10 = x$ and $30 \div 10 = 3$
   $x = 3$ tablets
   c. The completed proportion is presented as follows:
   $$\frac{1 \text{ tablet}}{3 \text{ tablets}} = \frac{10 \text{ grams}}{30 \text{ grams}}$$

STOP, THINK, AND LEARN.

1. Give 10 milligrams of valium. Your supply is 5-milligram tablets.
2. Give 500 milligrams of keflin. Your supply is 1000-milligram tablets.
3. Give 150 milligrams of gentamicin. Your supply is 100-milligram tablets.

Estimating Results

Healthcare professionals must check their work carefully for accurate results, and an important skill in helping professionals detect incorrect results is **estimating,** or anticipating the results. When checking your work, you can estimate (calculate the approximate answer) and judge if your results seem reasonable. This alerts healthcare professionals to results that don't make any sense and may be incorrect, and it provides a flag to go back and double-check the calculations involved. When you use it for its intended purpose, estimating can be a useful tool in detecting possible errors in healthcare calculations.

Here are some tips to help you perfect estimating techniques:

1. **Use rounding.** Rounding will help you reach numbers that are easier to mentally compute. For example, when multiplying 28 × 62, round 28 up to 30 and 62 down to 60. You can easily see how computing 30 × 60 is much easier!
2. **Does the answer make sense?** Look at the size of the answer and determine if it makes sense. Try multiplying whole numbers for a quick answer. Your answer should either be larger or smaller than either of the numbers in the problem.
3. **Watch your decimal point.** Be careful about placing decimal points. Remember that everything to the right of the point is a fraction.

Remember that estimating is just that—an anticipation of the results.

Flashpoint

One of the most common conversions in health care is a patient's weight. Many medications and treatments are based on a patient's kilogram weight. Because 1 kilogram equals 2.2 pounds, a quick estimation of kilogram weight is approximately half of the pound weight.

Roman Numerals

The traditional numbering system we use every day is referred to as **Arabic numerals** (1, 2, 3, 4, etc.). In health care, **Roman numerals** are used for some medications, solutions, and even for ordering systems. As a general guideline, use the following key points when using Roman numerals:

- All numbers can be expressed by using seven key numerals:
  I = 1
  V = 5
  X = 10
  L = 50
  C = 100
  D = 500
  M = 1000
- If a smaller numeral is placed after a larger numeral, the smaller numeral is *added* to the larger numeral. For example, VII = 7 (5 + 1 + 1 = 7).

- If a smaller numeral is placed in front of a larger numeral, the smaller numeral is *subtracted* from the larger number. For example, IX = 9 (10 − 1 = 9).
- When the same numeral is repeated in succession (no more than three numerals can be repeated in succession), the numbers are *added* together, for example, III = 3 (1 + 1 +1 = 3) and XX = 20 (10 +10 = 20).

Table 4-5 shows conversions between Arabic and Roman numerals. Of note in healthcare calculations and dosages is that the lowercase version of Roman numerals (ii = 2) is frequently used rather than the capital letters.

Military Time

Errors in recording times are unacceptable in health care because they may lead to patient harm. **Military time** is often used in health care to avoid the confusion created by the a.m. and p.m. designations used in the traditional system. Recording time on a patient chart, for example, can easily be misrepresented if a healthcare professional forgets to write down the a.m. or p.m. designation or if the incorrect designation is used. This can lead to serious errors in patient care.

The military clock is based on a 24-hour day, meaning that the 12th hour represents 12 noon and the 24th hour represents 12 midnight. Time is always expressed using four digits (i.e., 0300, 1200, 2100, etc.), and times are verbalized using a specific method, for example 1800 is pronounced eighteen hundred hours and 1630 is pronounced sixteen thirty hours (Fig. 4-3).

In military time, the morning (a.m.) hours are expressed in a way similar to how they are expressed using a traditional clock, for example, 9 a.m. = 0900. One easy way to convert afternoon (p.m.) hours is to add the time to 1200. For

TABLE 4-5

CONVERSION CHART FOR ARABIC AND ROMAN NUMERALS

Arabic	Roman	Arabic	Roman
1	I	21	XXI
2	II	22	XXII
3	III	23	XXIII
4	IV	24	XXIV
5	V	25	XXV
6	VI	30	XXX
7	VII	35	XXXV
8	VIII	40	XL
9	IX	50	L
10	X	100	C
15	XV	500	D
20	XX	1000	M

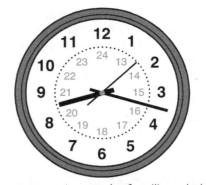

FIGURE 4-3 An example of a military clock.

example, 9 p.m. = 1200 + 0900 = 2100 hours, and 11 p.m. = 1200 + 1100 = 2300 hours. Table 4-6 will help you practice converting between traditional and military time.

Systems of Measurement

When learning and using the various systems of measurement found in health care, basic skills in calculation are used, with each system having its own terminology for designating mass (weight), capacity (volume), and distance (length). The three systems used in health care are the metric, household, and apothecary systems. Each system has its own method of naming, also known as **nomenclature.** The skills needed to convert between these systems are outlined here.

Metric System

The **metric system** is most familiar to those learners educated outside the United States. This system is a more accurate system than the household

TABLE 4-6			
CONVERSION CHART FOR MILITARY (24-HOUR CLOCK) VS. TRADITIONAL TIME			
Traditional	24-Hour Time	Traditional	24-Hour Time
12:05 a.m.	0005	12:05 p.m.	1205
12:45 a.m.	0045	12:45 p.m.	1245
1:00 a.m.	0100	1:00 p.m.	1300
2:30 a.m.	0230	2:30 p.m.	1430
3:00 a.m.	0300	3:00 p.m.	1500
6:25 a.m.	0625	6:25 p.m.	1825
9:30 a.m.	0930	9:30 p.m.	2130
12 noon	1200	12:00 midnight	2400

system, and it is easier to convert between numbers because everything is based on a unit of 10. Here is the nomenclature used for the metric system:

- Distance/length: meter (m)
- Capacity/volume: liter (l or L)
- Mass/weight: gram (g)

The meter, liter, and gram are modified by adding the appropriate prefix to express larger or smaller units (Table 4-7).

Using multiples of 10, conversions within the decimal system are calculated by multiplying by 10, 100, 1000 and so forth. For example:

- 4 kiloliters = 4000 × 1 liter = 4000 liters
- 2 hectoliters = 200 × 1 liter = 200 liters
- 5 decaliters = 50 × 1 liter = 50 liters
- 5 deciliters = 0.5 × 1 liter = 0.5 liter
- 4 centiliters = 0.04 × 1 liter = 0.04 liter

A shortcut for performing these operations is to move the decimal point the number of places indicated by the prefix. See Table 4-7 for common prefixes of the metric system. Consider the following examples:

- **Example 1:** When multiplying 1 × 10, move the decimal point one place to the right. This may require adding one or more zeroes.
- **Example 2:** Multiplying 6.3 × 10 = 63

Converting units within the metric system is accomplished by moving the decimal point. Here are two examples:

- **Example 1:** The physician orders 5000 milligrams of a medication, and this amount needs to be converted to grams. Make the conversion like this: Since milli- is the third place to the right of grams (1000 times), move the decimal point three spaces to the left toward gram: 5000 = 5.000, or 5. Change the unit name to "grams," for example, 5 grams. The proper dose would be 5 grams or five 1-gram tablets.
- **Example 2:** You want to convert 2000 centimeters to kilometers. Centi- is five decimal points to the right of kilo-, so move the decimal point five spaces to the left toward kilo-, and add zeroes as needed: 2000 = 0.02. Do not forget to change the unit name to "kilometers": 0.02 kilometers.

Flashpoint

Some students find it helpful to use a phrase to recall the name and order of prefixes for metric conversions, such as **K**ing **H**enry **D**ied **D**rinking **C**hocolate **M**ilk (**K**ilo, **H**ecto, **D**eca, **D**eci, **C**enti, **M**illi).

TABLE 4-7		
COMMON PREFIXES OF THE METRIC SYSTEM		
Prefix	Meaning	Examples
micro-	1/1,000,000	microgram (1,000,000 of a gram) = 0.000001
milli-	1/1000	milliliter (1/1000 of a liter = 0.001)
centi-	1/100	centimeter (1.100 of a meter = 0.01)
deci-	1/10	decigram (1/10 of a gram = 0.1)
deca-	10 times	deciliter (10 liters)
hecto-	100 times	hectogram (100 grams)
kilo-	1000 times	kilogram (1000 grams)

Flashpoint

In health care, medications are commonly measured using the metric system. Two units that are often seen and that represent the same amount are milliliters (mL) and cubic centimeters (cc). Both sets of units measure volume and they are often interchanged when dispensing liquids.

Just as important as moving the decimal point the correct number of places, is ensuring that it is moved in the correct direction. The easiest way to accomplish this is to first determine whether your answer should be a smaller or larger number, and then move the decimal point accordingly. For instance, if you are converting from hecto- to micro-, then you are converting from a larger to a smaller prefix. Thus, your answer will be larger. Using the same logic, your answer will be smaller when converting from a smaller to a larger prefix, for example when converting from micro- to kilo-.

Household System

Flashpoint

The various units of measurements in the household system relate to each other and can be converted among themselves.

Learners educated in the United States are generally most familiar with the **household system** of measurement. See Table 4-8 for types of measurements found in this system. Note that "ounce" is used as both a measurement of capacity/volume and mass/weight, with both being used by healthcare professionals. For instance, liquids such as a 6-ounce glass of water are measured in terms of capacity or volume. When assessing weight and mass, you would weigh a 6-pound, 10-ounce infant using a scale.

When basic equivalents are known, healthcare professionals can use proportions to determine unknown measurements. For example, suppose that 3 tablespoons of liquid are needed, but the only measuring device available is a cup marked in ounces (oz). How many ounces are in 6 tablespoons (6T)? You know that 2T = 1 oz, so you can set up your proportion as follows:

$$\frac{2T}{6T} = \frac{1\ oz}{x\ oz}$$

Then cross multiply:

$2x = 6$ oz

Divide each side by the number in front of the x to find the answer:

$2x \div 2 = 6\ oz \div 2$

$x = 3$ oz

TABLE 4-8

HOUSEHOLD MEASUREMENT SYSTEM

Type of Measurement	Nomenclature	Common Equivalents
Capacity/Volume	drop (gtt)	60 gtt = 1 t
	teaspoon (t or tsp)	3 t = 1 T
	tablespoon (T or tbsp)	2 T = 1 oz
	ounce (oz)	8 oz = 1 C
	cup (C)	2 C = 1 pt
	pint (pt)	2 pt = 1 qt
	quart (qt)	4 qt = 1 gal
	gallon (gal)	
Mass/Weight	ounce (oz)	
	pound (lb)	16 oz = 1 lb
Distance/Length	inch (in.)	
	foot (ft)	12 in. = 1 ft
	yard (yd)	3 ft = 1 yd
	mile (mi)	1760 yd = 1 mi

Apothecary System

The **apothecary system** is the least used and oldest of the three systems used for measurement. Because some physicians write prescriptions using the apothecary system, healthcare professionals must become familiar with these units of measurement (Table 4-9) and be able to convert within the system and to the metric system.

Roman numerals can be used in conjunction with the apothecary system, and they may be used in uppercase or lowercase. If lowercase is used, the Roman numeral I is written as a lowercase *i*.

Converting Systems of Measurement

Healthcare work sometimes requires that units from one system of measurement be converted to another. This requires knowledge of the equivalencies between the units of the different systems. There are frequently no exact equivalents, so when converting between systems, the answer is considered to be a close approximation.

Using the appropriate equivalencies, a proportion is then set up to identify and solve for the unknown quantity. The following steps are used to perform conversions:

1. Identify an equivalent between the two systems.
2. Set up a proportion so unit measurements on each side of the equation are the same.
3. Use *x* for the unknown value being calculated.
4. Cross-multiply.
5. Solve for *x*.
6. Verify if the answer is reasonable. When converting from a smaller unit to a larger unit, the answer will be smaller, for example, as when converting three quarters to dollars. When converting from a larger unit to a smaller unit, the answer will be larger, for example, as when converting $3 to quarters.

TABLE 4-9		
APOTHECARY MEASUREMENT SYSTEM		
Type of Measurement	**Nomenclature**	**Common Equivalents**
Capacity/volume	minim (♏︎) fluid dram (fl dr or f ʒ) fluid ounce (fl oz or f ℥) pint (pt) quart (qt)	1 minim = 1 drop 60 minims = 1 fl dr 8 fl dr = 1 fl oz 16 fl oz = 1 pt 2 pt = 1 qt
Mass/Weight	grain (gr.) dram (dr or ʒ) ounce (oz or ℥)	60 gr. = 1 dr 480 gr. = 1 oz

Consider the following examples when performing conversions:

- **Example 1:** Convert 21 inches to centimeters:
  1. Identify equivalency: 1 inch = 2.5 centimeters
  2. Set up a proportion with same units on each side of the equation. Use x for the unknown.
     $$\frac{1 \text{ in.}}{21 \text{ in.}} = \frac{2.5 \text{ cm}}{x \text{ cm}}$$
  3. Cross-multiply.
     $1x = 52.5$ cm
  4. Solve for x.
     $1x \div 1 = 52.5 \div 1$
     $x = 52.5$ cm
  5. Verify if the answer is reasonable. It takes a greater number of centimeters ($2\frac{1}{2}$ times) to measure the same distance as 1 inch; therefore, it makes sense that the answer is larger than 21.
- **Example 2:** Convert 6 teaspoons (tsp) to milliliters (mL):
  $$\frac{1 \text{ tsp}}{6 \text{ tsp}} = \frac{5 \text{ mL}}{x \text{ mL}}$$
  $x = 30$ mL
- **Example 3**: Convert 130 pounds (lb) to kilograms (kg):
  $$\frac{2.2 \text{ lb}}{130 \text{ lb}} = \frac{1 \text{ kg}}{x \text{ kg}}$$
  $2.2x = 130$ (When solving for x, each side is divided by 2.2.)
  $x = 62.9$ kg (Round to nearest 10th.)
- **Example 4**: Convert 20 grams (g) to milligrams (mg):
  $$\frac{1 \text{ g}}{20 \text{ g}} = \frac{60 \text{ mg}}{x \text{ mg}}$$
  $x = 1200$ mg

Temperature Conversion

Thermometers using **Fahrenheit** (F) as the measuring unit are more familiar to people living in the United States, although the Celsius or **centigrade** (C) system of measurement is frequently used in medical and healthcare practice. One way to understand the difference between the two systems is to compare how each expresses the boiling and freezing points of water (see Fig. 4-4).

Boiling points: 212°F = 100°C
Freezing points: 32°F = 0°C

Healthcare workers frequently need to convert between the two systems. Table 4-10 offers such a conversion chart. In addition, often the same results can be expressed using fractions or decimals, and deciding which to use depends on the healthcare professional's level of skill using either approach. Table 4-11 contains the formulas for conversion.

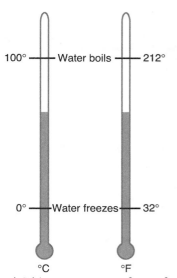

100° —— Water boils —— 212°

0° —— Water freezes —— 32°

°C   °F

FIGURE 4-4 Fahrenheit and Celsius temperatures of water freezing and boiling points.

TABLE 4-10
FAHRENHEIT TO CELSIUS CONVERSION CHART

Fahrenheit (degrees)	Celsius (degrees)
32 (freezing)	0 (freezing)
95	35
96	35.6
97	36.1
98	36.7
98.6	37
99	37.2
99.4	37.4
100	37.8
101	38.3
102	38.9
103	39.4
104	40
212 (boiling point)	100 (boiling point)

TABLE 4-11

TEMPERATURE SCALE CONVERSION FORMULAS

Convert From:	Fraction Formula	Decimal Formula
Fahrenheit to Centigrade	($°F - 32$) $\times$ $5/9$ = $°C$ Example: 101$°F$ ($101 - 32$) $\times$ $5/9$ = $°C$ $69 \times 5/9$ = $°C$ $345/9$ = 38.3$°C$ (rounded to nearest 10th)	($°F - 32$) $\div$ 1.8 = $°C$ Example: 101$°F$ ($101 - 32$) $\div$ 1.8 = $°C$ $69 \div 1.8$ = 38.3$°C$ (rounded to nearest 10th)
Centigrade to Fahrenheit	($°C \times 9/5$) + 32 = $°F$ Example: 25$°C$ ($25 \times 9/5$) + 32 = $°F$ $225/5$ + 32 = 77$°F$ $45 + 32$ = 77$°F$	($°C \times 1.8$) + 32 = $°F$ Example: 25$°C$ (25×1.8) + 32 = $°F$ $45 + 32$ = 77$°F$

Summary

The skills covered in this chapter will be invaluable to you in your healthcare career. Even though technology is available to calculate many of the formulas, it is important that you understand the basics of when and why we use these formulas. Medications and treatments are often based on the patient's body weight, and the physician may depend on you to provide correct information. Learning the formulas now will help you succeed in the future.

INTERNET RESOURCES

Organization/Service	Web Address	Description
Home School Math	http://homeschoolmath.net/online/algebra.php	Discover online resources for algebra, including tutorials, lessons, and calculators at this site.
Milken Family Foundation	http://mff.org	Check out this fascinating site by going to the website and then clicking on the Mike's Math Club link.
Internet French Property Company	http://french-property.co.uk	This site offers a metric conversion calculator that enables you to view conversion tables for the metric system.
S.O.S. Mathematics	http://sosmath.com	S.O.S. Mathematics is a free resource for math review material from algebra to differential equations.
Math.com	http://math.com	This site is an excellent resource to review basic math principles, examples, and exercises.
Purplemath	http://purplemath.com	Purplemath is a free resource for students focusing on algebra. Site includes tutoring, quizzes, and study tips.

Practice Exercises

Multiple Choice

1. Numbers used in counting that do not contain fractions or decimals are known as:

   a. Percentages

   b. Whole numbers

   c. Partial numbers

   d. Prime numbers

2. When rounding to the 10ths place, 24.384 becomes:

   a. 24

   b. 20

   c. 24.38

   d. 24.4

3. In the metric system, the prefix "deca-" refers to:

   a. 1/10

   b. 10 times

   c. 1/100

   d. 100 times

4. If 1 tablespoon equals 15 milliliters, then 4 tablespoons would equal:

   a. 10 mL

   b. 30 mL

   c. 45 mL

   d. 60 mL

5. The patient's weight is 165 lb. What is the weight in kilograms?

   a. 363

   b. 82.5

   c. 75

   d. 16.5

Fill in the Blank

1. The top number in a fraction that represents the actual number of parts of a whole is the _____.

2. _____ _____ have numerators that are larger than the denominators.

3. The _____ system of measurement is based on units of 10.

Short Answer

1. **Why is military time used in health care?**

2. **Which measuring system is most commonly used in health care and why?**

2 Human Body Basics

LEARNING THE LANGUAGE

5

Learning Outcomes

5.1 Define the terms "word root," "prefix," and "suffix"

5.2 Construct medical terms using the correct word parts

5.3 Follow rules for combining word parts and forming plural terms

5.4 Distinguish body planes and directional terms

5.5 Differentiate between acceptable and unacceptable abbreviations

Competencies

CAAHEP

- Describe structural organization of the human body. (CAAHEP I.C.1)
- Identify body systems. (CAAHEP I.C.2)
- Describe body planes, directional terms, quadrants, and cavities. (CAAHEP I.C.3)

ABHES

- Define and use entire basic structure of medical words and be able to accurately identify in the correct context, i.e., root, prefix, suffix, combinations, spelling, and definitions. (ABHES 3.a)
- Build and dissect medical terms from roots/suffixes to understand the word element combinations that create medical terminology. (ABHES 3.b)
- Understand the various medical terminologies for each specialty. (ABHES 3.c)
- Recognize and identify acceptable medical abbreviations. (ABHES 3.d)

Every successful healthcare practitioner must begin by learning a new language. Mastering the basics of medical terminology provides the foundation for communicating effectively. The history of medicine goes back to the Greeks and Romans, which is why medical terms have both Greek and Latin origins.

Medical terminology combines a series of prefixes, word roots, and suffixes to create the language of medicine. There are terms that describe body systems, diseases, and disorders of the body, as well as procedures and other treatments. As new diseases emerge and new procedures are developed, the language of medicine also changes. Some medical terms have become obsolete and

Key Terms

abduction Moving an arm or leg away from the body's midline

adduction Moving an arm or leg toward the midline of the body

adjective suffix A suffix that further describes a condition, a procedure, or even a disease

anatomical position A baseline for all healthcare professionals to use when referring to the body; this position is standing straight, facing forward with arms at the side, and palms and toes facing forward

combining form/combining vowel A vowel to make two or more word parts fit together; the vowel *o* is the most common combining form used between prefixes, word roots, and suffixes

eversion A directional term that means turning the foot outward

Continued

Key Terms—cont'd

extension A directional term that means pushing a joint out, such as straightening the knee

flexion A directional term that means curling a joint inward, such as pulling in the forearm

inversion A directional term that means curling the foot inward

Flashpoint

The forward slash (/) is used to indicate the division of word parts.

have been replaced by new terms. An example is "apoplexy," which is the term that was once used to describe the loss of neurological function as the result of a cerebral hemorrhage. This term has been replaced with the more current and descriptive term "stroke" or "cerebrovascular accident."

Word Roots

The foundation of medical terms is the ***word root.*** The word root designates the body part, organ system, or a process. Some medical terms require the use of more than one word root to indicate multiple related body organ systems. An example is the combination of two word roots to describe a condition of the stomach and the small intestine. The word "gastroenteritis" is dissected as follows:

Gastr/means stomach
Enter/means -intestine

Each body system has a unique set of word roots used to build medical terms. Prefixes and suffixes (defined below) remain the same for all body systems. It is also necessary at times to create words that involve more than one body system. For example, an orthopedist may treat a condition of both a muscle and a bone. This is a musculoskeletal condition. Table 5-1 lists each body system and the most common word roots associated with it.

TABLE 5-1

BODY SYSTEMS AND THE MOST COMMON WORD ROOTS ASSOCIATED WITH EACH

Organ System	Word Root	Meaning
Integumentary (skin)	derm/; dermat/; cutane/	skin
	adip/	fat
	cyt/	cell
	onych/	nail
	pil/; trich/	hair
	scler/	hardening
	xer/	dry
Nervous	cerebr/; encephal/	brain
	mening/	meninges
	myel/	spinal cord
	neur/	nerve
Cardiovascular (heart, blood, and blood vessels)	angi/; vas/	blood vessel
	arteri/	artery
	ven/; phleb/	vein
	cardi/	heart
	hem/; hemat/	blood

TABLE 5-1

BODY SYSTEMS AND THE MOST COMMON WORD ROOTS ASSOCIATED WITH EACH—cont'd

Organ System	Word Root	Meaning
Lymphatic system (lymph vessels and nodes)	aden/	gland
	lymph/	lymph
Respiratory (lungs, breathing)	bronch/; bronchi/	bronchus
	laryng/	larynx
	rhin/; na/	nose
	pharyng/	throat
	pneum/; pneumon/; pulmon/	lung, air
	thorac/	thorax
	aer/	air
	trache/	trachea
Digestive (stomach and intestines)	gastr/	stomach
	cholecyst/	gallbladder
	col/; colon/	colon
	dent/	teeth
	enter/	small intestines
	hepat/	liver
	lingu/; gloss/	tongue
	lapar/	abdomen
	or/	mouth
Urinary	cyst/	bladder
	nephr/; ren/	kidney
	ureter/	ureter
	urethr/	urethra
	ur/; urin/	urine
Reproductive (male)	balan/	penis
	orch/; orchi/; orchid/; test/	testes
	prostat/	prostate gland
	spermat/	sperm
Reproductive (female)	cervic/	cervix
	colp/; vagin/	vagina
	gynec/	woman, female
	hyster/; uter/	uterus
	mamm/; mast/	breast
	men/	menses
	oophor/; ovari/	ovary
	salping/	fallopian tube

Key Terms—cont'd

prefix A word part placed at the beginning of a word root that can change the meaning of the word by indicating a number, such as *bi-* (two), *tri-* (three); a direction, *epi-* (above), or *intra-* (within); or a time, *pre-* (before) or *post-* (after)

pronation A directional term that means turning the palm upward

suffix Found at the end of all words, it further describes a condition, a procedure, or a disease

supination A directional term that means turning the palm downward

word root Designates the body part, organ system, or a process

Prefixes

Some medical terms require the use of a **prefix** to describe a process, a number, or a location. A prefix is always at the beginning of the word ("pre-" means "before"). The prefix can change the meaning of the word by indicating a number, such as bi- (two), tri- (three); a direction, epi- (above) or intra- (within); or a time, pre- (before) or post- (after).

 STOP, THINK, AND LEARN.
Divide the following words into their separate parts, and label the parts.
tachycardia
hypertension
bilateral

Suffixes

At the end of all medical terms, you will find a **suffix** that further describes a condition, a procedure, or a disease. With a suffix, many word roots are changed into adjectives that describe a body part or condition. The word root *gastr/* means "stomach." By adding an **adjective suffix,** "-ic," meaning "pertaining to," the word becomes "gastric" and means "pertaining to the stomach." Surgical procedures are specified by a suffix. Using the root word *gastr/* and adding the suffix *–ectomy,* which means "removal of," produces the word "gastrectomy," meaning "removal of the stomach." Suffixes may also indicate a procedure, recording, or equipment. The suffix *–scope* refers to an instrument used to view. Adding this suffix to the word root *gastr/* and using the combining vowel, the word "gastroscope" is formed, which indicates an instrument that is used to view the stomach. Changing the suffix slightly to *–scopy,* the word becomes "gastroscopy" and refers to the procedure of looking into the stomach with the gastroscope. All medical terms have a suffix, which will change the meaning of the word.

 STOP, THINK, AND LEARN.
Divide the following words into separate parts, and label them.
gastroenteritis
cardiologist
gastropexy

Combining Forms

Once the individual word parts are mastered, the next step is to combine them to form medical terms. Not all word parts fit together easily, and many times they are difficult to pronounce. In these instances, a **combining form** or **combining vowel** is used to make two or more word parts fit together. The vowel *o* is the most common combining form used between prefixes, word roots, and suffixes. When learning to use the combining vowel, implement this helpful tip: Does the suffix begin with a vowel? If it does, the combining vowel is usually not necessary. An example is "gastrectomy." The word root is *gastr/* and the suffix is *-ectomy.* It does not require the use of a combining vowel. When combining multiple word roots, the combining vowel is usually necessary.

STOP, THINK, AND LEARN.

For each pair of word parts, decide if the combining form is necessary.

phleb/ + -otomy

gastr/ + enter/ + -itis

The combining vowel is an important part of medical terminology and will make many terms easy to pronounce and therefore easier to spell. A "gastroenterologist" is a physician who specializes in the treatment of disorders of the stomach and intestines. The word has two word roots, *gastr/* and *enter/*, and a suffix, *-logist.* Without the use of the combining vowel, the word would appear as "gastrenterlogist" and would not be easy to pronounce. By adding the combining vowel, the word becomes "gastroenterologist," which is much easier to sound out.

Directional Terms

When describing a body part or motion, directional terms help define an area or an action. ***Anatomical position*** is a baseline for all healthcare professionals to use when referring to the body. This position is standing straight, facing forward, with arms at the side and palms and toes facing forward. From this position, a specific area of the body can be described.

The body is divided into planes, or sections, to denote front and back, top and bottom, and side to side. Each of these body planes is given a directional term (Fig. 5-1).

Within each body plane are cavities containing organs or organ systems. The frontal cavity contains the abdominal and pelvic organs, and the dorsal, or back, cavity contains the brain and spinal cord. A good understanding of the directional terms and body cavities helps when learning the location of the body structures. You will continue to build your medical knowledge as you learn to combine the terms with the body structures.

Directional terms are used to determine where a structure lies in reference to the center of the body. Terms such as **proximal** and **distal** indicate if a structure is close to the center of the body or if it is distant from the center (see Fig. 5-1).

Medical terms can also give direction of movement. Moving an arm or leg toward the body or away from the body is described as ***adduction*** and ***abduction,*** respectively. A quick way to distinguish these terms is to remember that when moving an extremity toward the body, the extremity is being "added" back. Likewise, when turning a palm upward, ***supination*** is performed. The opposite term, ***pronation,*** indicates turning the palm downward. ***Flexion*** and ***extension*** are terms that indicate pulling an extremity

Flashpoint

An easy way to remember the term "dorsal," which means "back," is to remember that a shark is known for the dorsal fin on its back.

Flashpoint

It is easy to remember the term "distal," which means that a body part is a greater "distance" from the center of the body.

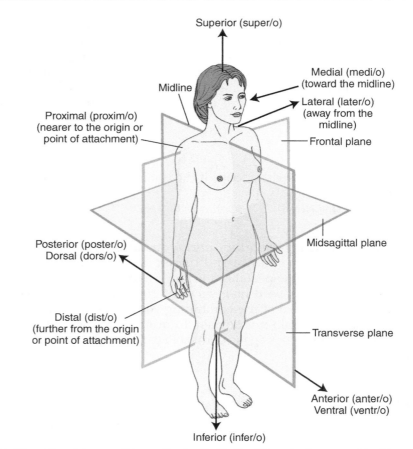

FIGURE 5-1 **Directional terms.** (From: Eagle, S. *Medical Terminology in a Flash! An Interactive, Flash-Card Approach,* Ed. 2. Philadelphia: FA Davis, 2011. Used with permission.)

forward and pushing it back out, such as flexing arm muscles or bending and straightening the knee. Curling a foot inward is ***inversion,*** and turning it out is ***eversion.*** Learning terms as opposites increases your vocabulary in half the time. Table 5-2 lists the most common directional terms and their opposites.

TABLE 5-2	
DIRECTIONAL TERMS, PAIRED IN OPPOSITES	
Anterior (front) (ventral)	Posterior (back) (dorsal)
Superior (top)	Inferior (bottom)
Lateral (side)	Medial (middle)
Adduction (toward the body)	Abduction (away from the body)
Supine (lying on back facing up)	Prone (lying on stomach facing down)
Supination (turning palm upward)	Pronation (turning palm downward)
Inversion (turning foot inward)	Eversion (turning foot outward)
Proximal (close to body center)	Distal (distant from body center)

Pronunciation

Some words have more than one correct pronunciation. Some regional dialects determine the pronunciation of medical terms, and some practitioners pronounce words as they learned them. An example of a word that may be pronounced differently is "angina." Some people put the accent on the first syllable (an' gi na), and others accent the middle syllable (an gi' na). Either pronunciation is correct.

Other medical terms may be confusing to pronounce because of their spelling. Look at the word "pneumonia." Although the word looks like it would start with a *p* sound, it is pronounced with the *n* sound. Words that begin with *p* may carry the silent *p* and are pronounced with the *s* sound, such as for *psoas muscle.* It is acceptable to ask for a word to be spelled if unsure about how to spell it based on another person's pronunciation. Many online or CD-based medical dictionaries offer alternate pronunciations for words that have multiple ways to say them.

Plural Terms

There are guidelines that determine how a medical term changes from singular to plural. Because many of these words are of Greek and Latin origins, Greek and Latin grammar rules are used to change a word from singular to plural. However, some words use English language rules to pluralize, so it is important to evaluate each term separately to determine the plural ending. If you are unsure, you may find the alternate ending in a medical dictionary to determine which ending is correct. For example, the rule for a word that ends in *-ix* or *-ex* is to change the ending to *-ices.* The preferred plural for "appendix" is not "appendixes," but rather "appendices." Changing from singular to plural may also change the pronunciation of the term. The word "phalanx" (fay' -lanks), which means the tip of the finger or toe, changes to "phalanges" (fa-lan' -geez) to indicate multiple fingers or toes.

In addition to understanding medical terminology, the ability to spell the terms correctly is essential. Medical records are legal documents and must contain accurate documentation, including the correct spelling of medical terminology. It is next to impossible to learn all of the medical terms used in health care today; however, by systematically learning the word roots, prefixes, and suffixes, you will be able to create thousands of medical terms for your career in health care.

STOP, THINK, AND LEARN.
The word "musculoskeletal" contains two word roots, a combining vowel, and a suffix. Can you identify each part?

What does the word "orthopedist" mean? Can you identify the individual parts of this word and what each part means?

Abbreviations

Abbreviating medical terms is becoming less acceptable in health care. When a healthcare professional begins to abbreviate words, it leaves others to wonder what the abbreviations mean. For example, MS can mean "multiple sclerosis" or "morphine sulfate." Medical records are legal documents, and it is best to write out all words for clarity. Healthcare accreditation agencies suggest that few, if any, abbreviations be used in patient records. "Do not use" abbreviation lists are provided by the Joint Commission, a healthcare accreditation agency, to ensure that medical errors are not made in the interest of patient safety. These suggestions should be followed in all healthcare facilities (Tables 5-3 and 5-4). It is important that healthcare personnel use only an approved list of abbreviations from their facility, and they must always make sure that patient notes are factual and legible.

Summary

Having a basic knowledge of word roots, prefixes, and suffixes and the ability to combine them correctly will give you the power to build your medical vocabulary and become comfortable using this new language.

TABLE 5-3

"DO NOT USE" ABBREVIATIONS AND SYMBOLS*

Do Not Use	Reason	Use Instead
U, u (unit)	Mistaken for the numbers 4 (four) and 0 (zero), and for cc (cubic centimeters).	Write out "unit."
IU (international unit)	Mistaken for IV (intravenous) or the number 10.	Write the words "international unit."
Q.D., QD, q.d., qd (daily) Q.O.D., QOD, q.o.d., qod (every other day)	These are often mistaken for each other. The period after the Q and the O are mistaken for an I.	Write out "daily," "every day," or "every other day," as appropriate.
Trailing zero: X.0 mg**	Decimal point is missed.	Write "X mg."
Lack of leading zero: .X mg	Decimal point is missed.	Write "0.X mg."
MS MSO_4 and $MgSO_4$	Can mean morphine sulfate or magnesium sulfate.	Write "morphine sulfate" or "magnesium sulfate."

*These guidelines are presented by the Joint Commission and are intended to apply to all medication orders and medication-related documentation that is handwritten, free text computer entry, or on preprinted forms.

**Exception: A trailing zero may be used only when required to demonstrate the level of precision of the value being reported, such as for laboratory results, imaging studies that report the size of lesions, or catheter/tube sizes. It may not be used in medication orders or medication-related documentation.

TABLE 5-4

ADDITIONAL ABBREVIATIONS, ACRONYMS, AND SYMBOLS UNDER CONSIDERATION FOR THE "DO NOT USE" LIST

Do Not Use	Reason	Use Instead
> (greater than) < (less than)	Misinterpreted as the number 7 or the letter L; often confused with each other	Write "greater than." Write "less than."
Abbreviations for drug names	Misinterpreted due to the similarity of many drug names	Write out drug names in full.
Apothecary units	Unfamiliar to most healthcare professionals; often confused with metric unit	Use metric units.
@	Mistaken for the number 2	Write "at."
cc	Mistaken for U (units) when poorly written	Write "mL," "ml," or "milliliters." The preferred abbreviation is "mL."
μ	Mistaken for mg (milligram), which would result in a 1000-fold overdose	Write "mcg" or "micrograms."

Practice Exercises

Multiple Choice

1. Which of the following terms indicates a physician who specializes in diseases of the skin?

   a. Pulmonologist

   b. Skinologist

   c. Integumentologist

   d. Dermatologist

2. The term "colectomy" means:

   a. Removal of the colon

   b. Removal of the gallbladder

   c. Removal of the stomach

   d. Removal of the kidney

3. Creating an opening in the stomach is called:

   a. Gastrectomy

   b. Ileostomy

   c. Gastrostomy

   d. Cholecystotomy

4. Turning the palm upward is:

   a. Pronation

   b. Suppination

   c. Flexion

   d. Extension

5. Which of the following organs is not found in the ventral cavity?

   a. Stomach

   b. Gallbladder

   c. Liver

   d. Spinal cord

Fill in the Blank

1. The hand is _____ to the elbow.

2. The plural form of "appendix" is _____.

3. Moving your leg away from your body is called _____.

4. Curling your forearm forward is an example of _____.

Short Answer

1. **Why is it a bad idea to use abbreviations in the medical record?**

2. **How is a combining vowel used, and what makes it important?**

3. **How is a medical term that ends in -*ix* or -*ex* changed into the plural form of the word, and what other change takes place?**

INTERNET RESOURCES

Organization/Service	Web Address
Free Medical Dictionary (also provides pronunciation)	www.medical-dictionary.thefreedictionary.com
Medical Dictionary Online	http://online-medical-dictionary.org
Medicine Net	http://medterms.com/script/main/hp.asp
Free Medical Dictionary (download from CNet)	http://download.cnet.com/Free-Medical-Dictionary/3000-2129_4-10329654.html
The Joint Commission	http://jointcommission.org

6
BASIC ANATOMY AND PHYSIOLOGY

Key Terms

adenosine triphosphate (ATP) The body's energy source

adipose Fatty tissue

afferents Neurons that bring information to the central nervous system from receptors throughout the body; also called sensory neurons

amphiarthroses Joints that exhibit only slight movement

anatomy Study of the body and its parts

arteries Vessels that carry oxygenated blood away from the heart

atom The smallest unit of matter

axon The portion of a nerve cell that transmits an impulse to the next cell

capillaries Blood vessels that connect arteries and veins

cell The basic unit of biological organization that is capable of all processes necessary to life

cerebellum A portion of the brain that is similar in structure to the cerebrum but is smaller than and posterior to the cerebrum; coordination of muscle movements, posture, and balance are its functions

Learning Outcomes

6.1 Describe the structural organization of the human body

6.2 Define homeostasis

6.3 Describe each body system and the organs included in the system

6.4 Explain the relationship of structure (anatomy) to function (physiology) of each body system

Competencies

CAAHEP

- Describe structural organization of the human body. (CAAHEP I.C.1)
- Identify body systems. (CAAHEP I.C.2)
- List major organs in each body system. (CAAHEP I.C.4)
- Describe the normal function of each body system. (CAAHEP I.C.5)

ABHES

- Identify and apply the knowledge of all body systems, their structure and functions, and their common diseases, symptoms, and etiologies. (ABHES 2.b)

The study of anatomy and physiology is essential to all health care–related fields. As you learn more about the **anatomy** (structure) and **physiology** (function) of the human body, you become more conscious of your own health. As you look at each body system, the process of **homeostasis** becomes apparent. Homeostasis is the ability of the body to maintain a stable internal environment, within limits, while the outside environment changes.

Some basic anatomical directional and regional terms are necessary to understand body structure locations. Knowing the benchmark of anatomical position is essential for understanding directional terms. **Anatomical position** is used as a reference diagram and indicates that the body is standing straight, facing forward with arms at the side and palms and toes facing forward. Directional terms are discussed in Chapter 5 (see Fig. 5-1).

Some key directional terms include superior/inferior, medial/lateral, proximal/distal, and anterior (ventral)/posterior (dorsal). See Table 5-2 in Chapter 5 for more information on directional terms.

Cells

Foundations in basic chemistry and biology are necessary to understand the changes in both the structure and function of the body. **Atoms,** the smallest units of matter, combine to form *molecules.* Molecules, particles containing at least two atoms, are arranged in an orderly fashion to build the basic unit of biological organization, the *cell.* The cell is capable of all processes necessary to life; in fact, some organisms, such as a **bacteria,** are composed of only one cell. Cells with similar structure and function are arranged in groups known as *tissues.*

Tissues

Structure

Tissues are classified into four groups: epithelial, connective, muscle, and nervous. **Epithelial** tissue forms coverings, linings, and glands. A good example of epithelial tissue is the *epidermis,* or outermost layer of the skin. The epidermis protects the body by providing a natural antibacterial and waterproof covering. *Glands* are a type of tissue formed by epithelial tissues that fold over themselves. There are two types of glands. *Exocrine glands,* such as sweat glands, secrete their product through a duct onto the surface. *Endocrine glands,* like the pancreas, have no ducts and secrete their product directly into the blood or the fluid between cells.

Connective tissue is the most diverse of the tissue groups as it binds structures together and offers support. Some examples of connective tissue are bone, cartilage, *adipose* (fat), and blood.

Muscle tissue is composed of cells that have the ability to shorten and contract, thus producing movement. **Nervous tissue** is the most highly organized tissue, and it is capable of transmitting quick electrochemical impulses. These four tissue types are arranged by structure and function into **organs.** Organs are structures made up of two or more types of tissue that perform specialized functions. For example, the heart comprises cardiac muscle tissue, various types of membranes, and special nervous tissue. Many organs and related structures function together as body systems to accomplish a specific purpose. For example, the heart acts as a pump and along with a complex network of arteries, veins, and capillaries composes the cardiovascular system. This system circulates blood throughout the body for an entire lifetime. There are 11 different **organ systems** in the human body.

Organ Systems

Integumentary System

The **integumentary system** provides a boundary, or interface, between the body and the outside world, which is essential to homeostasis. An average adult has 18 to 20 square feet of skin with an estimated weight of 6 pounds, making the integumentary system the largest of all body systems.

The integumentary system is an arrangement of skin and associated structures such as hair and nails. The skin is composed of epithelial and connective tissues. It is an excellent protective barrier to many substances and

Key Terms—cont'd

cerebrum The primary processing area of the brain; it has motor areas for control of movement and sensory areas for interpretation of stimuli; it is the intellectual and emotional center of the body

cornea The clear anterior portion of the sclera that is the first structure in the eye through which light rays pass

dendrites Short branching processes off the neuron's cell body that receive information and carry it to the cell body

dermis The inner, vascular layer of the skin

diarthroses Freely moving joints surrounded by a fibrous capsule containing synovial fluid for lubrication; also called synovial joint

efferent The neuron that carries a response back to the body (muscles or glands) from the central nervous system; also called motor neuron

endocrine glands Glands that have no ducts and that secrete their product directly into the blood or the fluid between cells

epidermis The uppermost layer of the skin

erythrocytes Red blood cells

exocrine glands Glands that secrete their product through a duct on to the surface, such as sweat glands

Continued

Flashpoint

The skin is the body's largest organ, and it is the first line of defense against bacteria.

Key Terms—cont'd

hematopoiesis The formation of red blood cells

homeostasis The ability of the body to maintain a stable internal environment, within limits, while the outside environment changes

hypothalamus The portion of the brain that is the major center for control of homeostasis, such as body temperature regulation

insertion The movable point of attachment of a muscle

iris The colored anterior portion of the choroid layer of the eye

leukocytes White blood cells

ligament Connective tissue that attaches bone to bone

meninges Three layers of protective connective tissue that surround the brain and spinal cord

molecules Particles containing at least two atoms

neurons Nerve cell

neurotransmitters A chemical stored in axon terminals of the neuron to transport the impulse across the synapse

origin The fixed point of attachment of a muscle

ovaries Glands that produce estrogen and progesterone and regulate secondary sex characteristics and the menstrual cycle in females

parasympathetic The division of the nervous system that slows down vital activities after emergencies

physiology The study of body functions

prevents dehydration of the body. The skin has an outer avascular (without blood vessels) epidermis and an inner vascular layer, the ***dermis*** (Fig. 6-1).

A main protein associated with the skin and this system is **keratin,** which aids in providing a tough, semi-waterproof outer layer. The skin prevents some physical and chemical agents from entering the body and protects it from ultraviolet (UV) rays. UV rays are absorbed by the pigment melanin, which is produced by the skin. **Melanin** provides the color in skin. Skin's secretion of oil and sweat offers some protection from bacteria and fungi. Specialized nerve receptors in the skin alert you to sensations such as pain, pressure, touch, and temperature. The blood vessels in the dermis allow for temperature regulation. As the body gets hot, dermal blood vessels dilate to radiate excess heat. In addition, the sweat glands of the skin will release their product, and cooling by evaporation will take place. When exposed to cold temperatures, the dermal blood vessels constrict to restrict blood to deeper portions of the body to maintain the core, or body, temperature. Another important function of the skin is that when it is exposed to sunlight, it begins the production of vitamin D, which is necessary for calcium and phosphorous absorption by the digestive tract.

Hair, a main characteristic of mammals, is the first of the skin's accessory structures. A small pouch-like structure of the epidermal layer forms the hair follicle, which surrounds the hair shaft and provides the site of hair growth. Hair has some evolutionary protective functions. The eyebrows and lashes prevent foreign objects from entering the eye. Similar hair is found in the nose and the ears to provide this same protection for the delicate organs within these

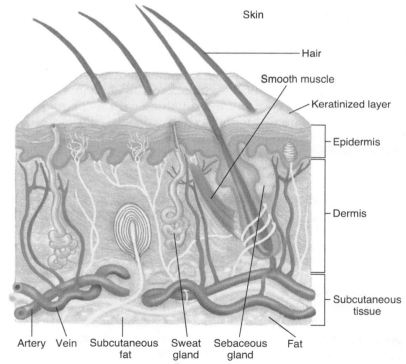

FIGURE 6-1 The skin. (From: Eagle, S. *Medical Terminology in a Flash! An Interactive, Flash-Card Approach,* Ed. 2. Philadelphia: FA Davis, 2011. Used with permission.)

structures. Body hair offers insulation from heat and cold by providing a cover between the skin and the outside temperature.

Nails are another of the accessory structures, and they are specialized keratin extensions of the epidermis that serve as protective structures on the tips of the fingers and toes. Nails are natural tools that help with everyday tasks, such as peeling labels and scratching an itch.

Sebaceous glands (oil glands) are associated with each hair follicle. The product of sebaceous glands is **sebum,** which serves as an oily substance for lubricating the surface of skin and keeping hair shafts supple. Sweat glands are exocrine glands that excrete their product onto the surface of the skin. Sweat serves as a minor form of waste excretion.

Skeletal System

How would any structure exist without its framework? The **skeletal system** is a classic example of how structure (anatomy) and function (physiology) are interrelated. One can look at the structure of the skeletal system and tell that it serves both support and protective functions. The body remains upright with the support of the skeleton. Skeletal structures provide protection for internal organs. The skull protects the brain, and the ribs protect the heart and lungs. Additionally, in conjunction with the muscular system, the skeletal system allows body movement. *Tendons* serve as attachments for muscle to bone. *Ligaments* are connective tissue that attach bone to bone. Other functions are for mineral storage, such as for calcium and phosphorus, as well as blood cell formation *(hematopoiesis)* in bone marrow. The two types of bone tissue are the hard compact bone and the spongy bone, which is located inside bone and provides space for marrow. There are three main types of bone cells. **Osteoblasts** are bone formation cells, **osteoclasts** are for bone reabsorption, and **osteocytes** are mature bone cells.

The skeletal system is composed of 206 bones. Bones range in size and shape from the largest long bone of the leg (femur) to the small, irregular bones inside the middle ear (malleus, incus, and stapes).

Articulations, or joints, occur where two or more bones come together. Joints are classified into three groups according to their function: synarthroses, amphiarthroses, and diarthroses. *Synarthroses* are immovable joints, such as sutures between cranial bones. *Amphiarthroses,* such as the pubic symphysis, exhibit slight degrees of movement. *Diarthroses,* or synovial joints, are the freely moving joints surrounded by a fibrous capsule containing synovial fluid for lubrication. Most joints in the body fall into the category of diarthroses or synovial joints. The bones of these joints usually have cartilage on the ends, which provides a smooth gliding surface. Movable joints are classified as hinge, ball and socket, sliding, and pivot, based on the amount of their movement (Table 6-1).

Muscular System

The **muscular system** is responsible for movement and production of body heat (Fig. 6-2). Muscle tissue is composed of special cells that have the ability to shorten and contract. This ability is possible because of the proteins myosin and actin, and the way they use *adenosine triphosphate (ATP),* the body's

Key Terms—cont'd

platelets Blood cells responsible for clotting; also called thrombocytes

sebaceous glands Oil glands associated with each hair follicle

sympathetic The division of the nervous system that speeds up vital activities during emergencies

synapse The gap between the axon terminals and the dendrites of the adjacent neuron

synarthroses Immovable joints such as sutures between cranial bones

Continued

Key Terms—cont'd

tendon Connective tissue that serves as an attachment for muscle to bone

testes Glands that produce testosterone, which produces muscle and bone mass as well as secondary sex characteristics in males

tissues Cells with similar structure and function

ureters Tubes that drain urine from the kidney to the bladder

urethra Tube that drains urine from the bladder to the outside

vein A blood vessel that carries unoxygenated blood

zygote One cell with a full genetic complement of the species that is formed when one egg and one sperm unite

TABLE 6-1
THE DIFFERENT KINDS OF JOINTS AND THEIR MOVEMENT

Category	Movement	Type	Description	Examples
Synarthrosis	Immovable	Suture	Fibrous connective tissue that joins bone surfaces	Skull
Amphiarthrosis	Slightly movable	Symphysis	A disk of fibrous cartilage located between bones	Pubic bones Vertebral bones
Diarthrosis	Freely movable	Ball and socket	Movement in all planes	Hip sockets, shoulder sockets
		Hinge	Movement in only one plane	Elbows, knees, fingers
		Condyloid	Movement in one plane with some lateral movement	Temporomandibular joint
		Pivot	Rotates	Neck (1st and 2nd vertebrae); radius and ulna
		Gliding	Moves side to side	Wrist bones
		Saddle	Moves in several planes	Thumb

energy source. Muscle contraction cannot occur without getting a signal from a nerve.

Muscle tissue is classified as **skeletal, smooth,** or **cardiac.** Skeletal muscle is under conscious, or voluntary, control and attaches to bones. These muscles are responsible for body movements. The fixed point of attachment is the ***origin*** and the movable point of attachment is the ***insertion.*** Smooth muscle is involuntary, or under unconscious control, and it is found in the walls of most body tubes such as the intestines, arteries, and the urinary bladder. As alternating layers of smooth muscle contract, it pushes substances through body tubes. **Cardiac muscle** is also involuntary, and it forms the muscle of the heart. Cardiac muscle cells have special connections that allow them to work in unison.

There are over 600 muscles in the human body. Naming of muscles is, in itself, a lesson in medical terminology. Muscles are named according to the following parameters:

- *Their origin and insertion:* The **sternocleidomastoid** connects from the sternum, clavicle, and mastoid bones.
- *Their location:* The **tibialis anterior** is located on the front of the tibia in the lower leg.
- *Their action:* The **flexor** muscle allows us to flex our hand or our foot.
- *The number of divisions:* The **biceps** have two origins but come together as a single muscle at the insertion.
- *The direction of muscle:* The **oblique** muscles cover the abdominal wall in a slanting position.

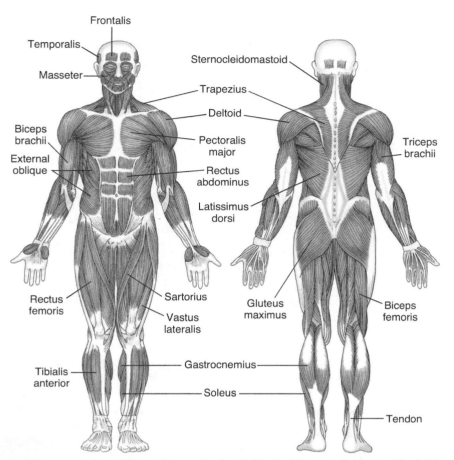

FIGURE 6-2 The muscular system. (From: Eagle, *S. Medical Terminology in a Flash! An Interactive, Flash-Card Approach*, Ed. 2. Philadelphia: FA Davis, 2011. Used with permission.)

Nervous System

The **nervous system** is one of the most highly organized body systems and is essential in the process of homeostasis. Through the use of quick electrochemical impulses it detects sensations, conducts mental and emotional functions, and stimulates muscles and glands. The two main divisions of this system are the central nervous system and the peripheral nervous system.

Central Nervous System

The **central nervous system (CNS)** is composed of the brain and spinal cord. Three layers of protective connective tissue known as the *meninges* surround both. The main function of the CNS is processing and interpreting information.

The brain is divided into four major portions: the brainstem, the diencephalon, the cerebrum, and the cerebellum (Fig. 6-3). The **brainstem,** beginning with the medulla oblongata and ending with the midbrain, is a connection between the brain and spinal cord. The brainstem is the center of important vital reflexes, such as breathing rhythm and rate of heartbeat. The **diencephalon** is composed of the **thalamus,** which relays incoming impulses to the proper area of the cerebrum, and the *hypothalamus,* which is a major center for control of homeostasis, such as body temperature regulation. The *cerebrum*

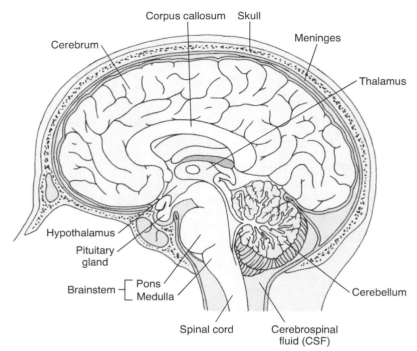

FIGURE 6-3 The brain. (From: Eagle, S. *Medical Terminology in a Flash! An Interactive, Flash-Card Approach,* Ed. 2. Philadelphia: FA Davis, 2011. Used with permission.)

is the primary processing area of the brain. It has motor areas for control of movement and sensory areas for interpretation of stimuli; it is the intellectual and emotional center of the body. The **cerebellum** is similar in structure to the cerebrum, yet it is smaller and posterior to the cerebrum. Coordination of muscle movements, posture, and balance are functions of the cerebellum.

Twelve cranial nerves arise from the base of the brain and service the head and neck area (Fig. 6-4). Thirty-one pairs of nerves arise from the spinal column and extend into the body as the bulk of the peripheral nervous system.

Peripheral Nervous System

The **peripheral nervous system (PNS)** consists of all the nerves that connect with the CNS. There are two main pathways for this system: afferent and efferent. The **afferent** or sensory pathway brings information to the CNS from receptors throughout the body. The **efferent** or motor pathway carries a response back to the body (muscles or glands) from the CNS.

Neurons, or nerve cells, contain four basic structures: dendrites, **axons,** cell body, and axon terminals. **Dendrites** are short branching processes off the neuron's cell body that receive information and carry it to the cell body. The cell body is where the nucleus and most of the organelles, the tiny organ-like structures, are located. As the impulse leaves the cell body, it travels along an axon until it reaches the axon terminals or endings. At the axon terminals, there is a gap **(synapse)** between those terminals and the dendrites of the adjacent neuron. It is the job of **neurotransmitters,** chemicals stored in axon terminals, to transport the impulse across the synapse.

The sector of the PNS that controls skeletal muscle is the **somatic system,** which is voluntary, or under conscious control. The **autonomic nervous system** is involuntary and connected to smooth and cardiac muscle, as well as many glands.

Flashpoint

The average male brain weighs 3 lb, and the average female brain weighs 2.8 lb. Albert Einstein's brain weighed 2.7 lb.

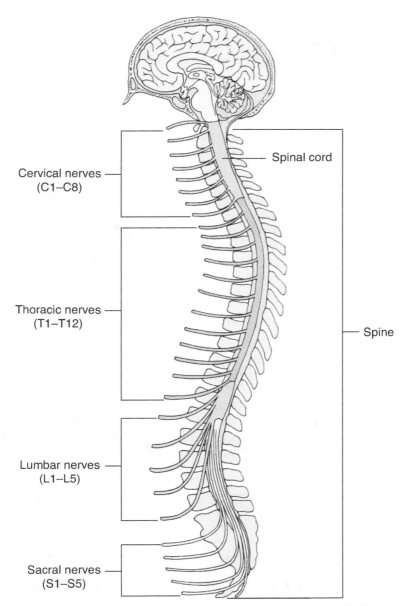

Cervical nerves
(C1–C8)

Thoracic nerves
(T1–T12)

Lumbar nerves
(L1–L5)

Sacral nerves
(S1–S5)

Spinal cord

Spine

FIGURE 6-4 The spinal cord. (From: Eagle, S. *Medical Terminology in a Flash! An Interactive, Flash-Card Approach,* Ed. 2. Philadelphia: FA Davis, 2011. Used with permission.)

The autonomic system consists of the **sympathetic division,** which speeds up vital activities during emergencies, and the **parasympathetic division,** which slows down vital activities after emergencies. The parasympathetic division also controls normal involuntary functions such as digestion, urination, and defecation.

Senses

Associated with the nervous system are the senses smell, taste, sight, and hearing. Receptors from these sense organs pick up stimuli and relay them to the CNS, which interprets the stimuli as sensations.

Flashpoint

Activation of the fight-or-flight response to emergencies is a function of the sympathetic division of the autonomic nervous system, after which you "rest and digest" through the parasympathetic division.

Smell

The sense of smell, or **olfaction,** arises from sensory receptors in the epithelial cells of the superior portion of the nasal cavity. These receptors are connected to the olfactory nerve, which transmits this information to the brain for interpretation. Odor molecules float into the nasal cavity, where they dissolve into the nasal mucosal lining and are detected by the dendrites of the olfactory neurons. The stimulus follows the sensory pathway to the brain for interpretation. Damage to nasal tissue or temporary swelling from an upper respiratory infection can greatly decrease the ability to smell.

Taste

Taste sensations come from receptors in the mouth commonly called **taste buds.** Most of these receptors are located along the sides of **papillae,** or small projections on the tongue shaped like small flasks. The five general types of taste receptors are sweet, salty, sour, bitter, and savory, or umami. Taste receptor cells are similar to olfactory receptors in that they have hairlike extensions that are bathed in saliva to dissolve the chemicals detected as taste. Taste sensations also follow the sensory nerve pathway to the brain for interpretation. Many foods contain combinations of flavors, which involve several receptors for interpretation. The aroma of food often stimulates the sense of taste.

Flashpoint

The human tongue has over 10,000 taste buds that are replaced about every 2 weeks. As people age, many of the taste buds are not replaced.

Sight

Vision is the predominant sense. Most of the sensory receptors are located in the eye, and the sense of sight involves more of the brain than do the other senses. The eye is composed of three layers. The white outer layer of the eye is the **sclera.** The clear anterior portion of the sclera is the *cornea,* which is the first structure that light rays pass through. The middle layer, or **choroid** layer, of the eye contains blood vessels and pigments. Attached to the anterior portion of the choroid layer is the ciliary body that attaches to the lens. The smooth muscle in the ciliary body allows the lens to adjust to incoming light rays. The colored anterior portion of the choroid layer is the *iris,* with an opening in the center known as the **pupil.** Smooth muscle in the iris controls the size of the pupil, depending on the amount of light available. Interior to the choroid layer is the **retina** (innermost layer), which contains the actual photoreceptors. There are two types of photoreceptors: **cones** for sharp color vision in bright light and **rods** for dim light conditions and peripheral vision. A properly functioning eye will adjust the light rays so they come to a focus point directly on the retina.

Flashpoint

Many forms of abnormal vision can be corrected with external lenses or surgical procedures.

Hearing and Balance

The fourth sense, arising from the ear, is hearing and balance. The ear is divided into the outer, middle, and inner portions. The outer ear includes the external portion of the ear, including the auricle or pinna, down to the tympanic membrane, or eardrum. The function of the outer ear is to capture sound waves and direct them to the tympanic membrane, causing it to vibrate. Sound vibrations are carried through the middle ear from the tympanic membrane to the oval window of the **cochlea.** Three small bones, known as the **malleus, incus,** and **stapes,** are the structures that transfer sound vibrations through the middle ear.

Also located in the middle ear is the auditory or **eustachian tube,** which runs to the **nasopharynx** and stabilizes atmospheric pressure on both sides of the tympanic membrane. The inner ear comprises the **cochlea, vestibule,** and **semicircular canals.** The cochlea is the organ of hearing. As the **ossicles** transfer sound waves to the oval window, this initiates vibrations in the fluid of the cochlea. As

Flashpoint

The bones in the ear are often called the hammer, anvil, and stirrup because they resemble these objects.

this fluid begins to vibrate, hairlike receptor cells pick it up and transfer the information to the vestibulocochlear nerve, which transfers it to the brain for interpretation. The vestibule and semicircular canals are in the inner ear, and they help you to hold your head up straight and maintain balance. Often called the human gyroscope, these structures relay the position of the head to the brain.

Endocrine System

The **endocrine system,** like the nervous system, is involved in control and communication of body functions and processes. Unlike the quick electrical impulses transmitted by the nervous system, this system transmits slower and more prolonged chemical signals: hormones. Most of the hormones work by a negative feedback mechanism, which means that the body has an automatic brake when the process is complete. An example of this is regulation of blood sugar levels. The body has a normal blood sugar level. As blood sugars rise above healthy levels, the pancreas releases the hormone insulin, which causes excess sugar to be removed from the blood to be stored in the liver, thus decreasing or reversing blood sugar levels. Likewise, if the blood sugar falls, glucagon is secreted to pull stored glucose back into the cells. Both processes stop when a healthy blood sugar level returns.

A major endocrine organ is the **pituitary gland,** which is located inferior to the hypothalamus of the brain (Fig. 6-5). The pituitary releases eight different hormones and is about the size of a pea. These hormones control such things as growth, milk production in females, development of eggs and sperm, and activity of the thyroid gland and the adrenal cortex. Other endocrine organs are the thyroid, parathyroid, adrenal, and pineal glands. The testes, ovaries, and sections of the pancreas also have endocrine functions.

The **thyroid gland** produces two hormones. Thyroxine, an iodine-based hormone, controls metabolic rates. Calcitonin regulates high calcium levels in the blood. The **parathyroid glands,** on the posterior surface of thyroid, release parathyroid hormone, which controls low blood calcium levels. Parathyroid hormone stimulates osteoclasts to remove calcium from the bone to be released to the bloodstream.

The **adrenal glands,** located superior to kidneys, produce and release several hormones. The **adrenal cortex,** or outer layer, produces three hormones. Aldosterone regulates mineral content of the blood, primarily sodium and potassium. This, in turn, regulates water balance in the body. The glucocorticoids, cortisol and cortisone, help the body deal with long-term stress by releasing and controlling blood glucose. They also affect inflammation by reducing edema or swelling. A third class of hormone produced by the cortex is the androgens, which are a type of male sex hormone. These androgens are produced in small amounts in both males and females. The **adrenal medulla,** or inner layer of the gland, is stimulated by the sympathetic nervous system and releases epinephrine and norepinephrine, which cause vital activities to speed up when dealing with emergencies. The fight-or-flight response to an emergency includes an increase in heart and respiratory rates, dilated pupils, and a general sense of fright. The parasympathetic nervous system calms this response by returning all hormones to normal levels and all body systems to the prestress function.

The **pineal gland** found on the posterior hypothalamus produces and secretes melatonin, a hormone that aids in regulation of the circadian rhythm, the body's 24-hour clock. The release of melatonin is stimulated by darkness, thus raising the levels at night to promote sleep. Some herbal products contain

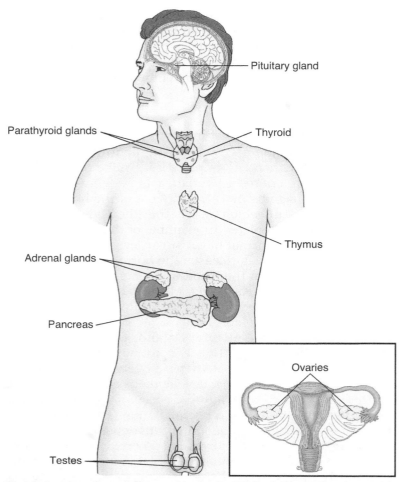

FIGURE 6-5 The endocrine system. (From: Eagle, S. *Medical Terminology in a Flash! An Interactive, Flash-Card Approach*, Ed. 2. Philadelphia: FA Davis, 2011. Used with permission.)

synthetic melatonin, which many people find helpful to support a good night's sleep. The pineal gland, which also helps with sexual development, is large in children and begins to shrink by puberty.

The **pancreas** serves an endocrine role in the regulation of blood glucose levels. Insulin is released from the pancreas when blood sugar is high, and glucagon is released when blood sugar is low. Insulin aids in the removal of excess glucose from the blood, to be stored in the liver. This stored glucose is released back into the blood, stimulated by glucagon when blood glucose levels are low.

The *testes* produce testosterone, which produces muscle and bone mass as well as secondary sex characteristics in males. The *ovaries* produce estrogen and progesterone, which regulate secondary sex characteristics and the menstrual cycle in females.

Cardiovascular System

The **cardiovascular,** or **circulatory system,** is a system that is capable of delivering life-sustaining fluids to every cell of the body. This system is composed of the heart, blood vessels, and blood, which is the major transport medium for substances traveling throughout the body (Fig. 6-6).

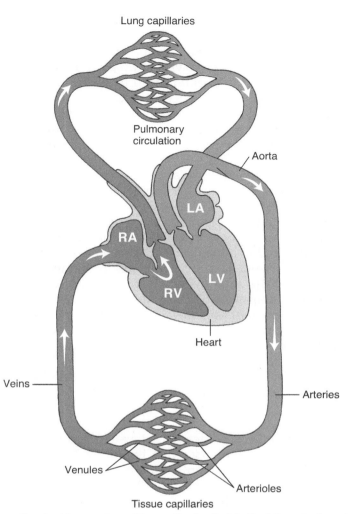

Lung capillaries

Pulmonary
circulation

Aorta

LA

RA

LV

RV

Heart

Veins

Arteries

Venules

Arterioles

Tissue capillaries

FIGURE 6-6 The cardiovascular system. (From: Eagle, S. *Medical Terminology in a Flash! An Interactive, Flash-Card Approach,* Ed. 2. Philadelphia: FA Davis, 2011. Used with permission.)

The **heart,** located in the thoracic cavity, is responsible for two cycles of circulation. Pumping deoxygenated blood to the lungs, where it loses carbon dioxide and picks up oxygen, is pulmonary circulation. The heart then pumps the oxygenated blood to the tissues and picks up carbon dioxide for removal; this is systemic circulation.

Four separate chambers compose the heart, including two upper chambers and two lower chambers, each with a different function. The **atria,** or upper chambers, are the receiving chambers. The right atrium receives blood returning from the tissues, and the left atrium receives blood returning from the lungs. The **ventricles,** or lower chambers, are the pumps of the heart. The right ventricle is the pump for pulmonary circulation, and the left ventricle is the systemic circulation pump. Systole refers to ventricular contraction, and diastole refers to ventricular relaxation. Blood pressure is highest during systole and lowest during diastole. When recording a blood pressure reading, the systolic measurement is the top number, and the diastolic measurement is the bottom number. Physicians monitor the diastolic measurement carefully as this is the pressure required for the heart to function during rest.

Flashpoint
During the body's lifetime, the heart will beat approximately 2.5 billion times.

The heart is equipped with valves that prevent backflow of blood to the chambers. The tricuspid valve is located between the right atrium and right ventricle. It prevents backflow into the atrium when the ventricle contracts. The pulmonary semilunar valve is located where the pulmonary artery arises from the right ventricle, and prevents backflow into it. The bicuspid or mitral valve is located between the left atrium and left ventricle, and it prevents backflow into the left atrium. The aortic semilunar valve is located where the aorta arises from the left ventricle, and it prevents backflow of blood into the left ventricle. Backflow of blood decreases the efficiency of the heart contraction and may lead to heart failure.

There are three types of blood vessels: arteries, veins, and capillaries. *Arteries* carry oxygenated blood away from the heart, and *veins* transport unoxygenated blood to the heart. There are two exceptions: the pulmonary artery transports unoxygenated blood from the right ventricle to the lungs, and the pulmonary vein transports oxygenated blood from the lungs to the left atrium. Arteries have a thicker middle muscle layer than do veins due to the fact they are under more pressure and must be more elastic to pump the blood. Veins have a larger channel so the same volume can be moved under lower pressure. Veins are equipped with flap-like valves to help return blood to the heart. The valves are necessary to prevent backflow due to the decreased pressure in the veins and the effects of gravity. Backflow of blood in the veins can lead to varicose veins. *Capillaries* are microscopic blood vessels, just one cell thick, and they serve as points of exchange for gases, nutrients, and waste. Arteries branch into smaller vessels known as arterioles, and veins branch into venules. The arterioles and venules branch into the capillaries.

Blood

The transport medium of the cardiovascular system is a specialized connective tissue called **blood.** Blood is composed of a liquid portion called **plasma,** which makes up 55%, and a cellular portion, which makes up the remaining 45%. Plasma is 90% water. The cellular portion of blood is composed of *erythrocytes* (red blood cells), *leukocytes* (white blood cells), and *platelets.* Red blood cells are the most numerous of all the blood cells, with an average person having five to six million of them. Red blood cells contain hemoglobin, which is an iron-containing pigmented protein; its main job is carrying oxygen. Hemoglobin gives oxygenated blood its bright red color. Anything that lowers the oxygen-carrying capacity of blood is a form of anemia. White blood cells are far less numerous than red blood cells. A person has 5000–10,000 white blood cells. There are five different types of white blood cells, all necessary for the function of the body's defense system. Platelets are fragments of cells used in the blood-clotting process. The average platelet count is 150,000–400,000. Hematopoiesis is the formation of blood cells and takes place in red bone marrow when stimulated by the lack of oxygen in the tissues, called **hypoxia.**

There are antigens on red blood cells that are used to classify the cells into certain groups. An antigen is a protein on the cell that recognizes an incompatible cell. The primary antigens are A, B, and Rh. If a person has the A antigen on his or her red blood cells, the blood is type A, and the A antigen will attempt to fight off any cell that contains a B antigen. When only the B antigen is present, the blood is type B. People who have both A and B antigens are type AB, and some have neither and are type O. When mismatched blood is transfused, agglutination, or clumping of cells, occurs. Blood cannot function properly when cells are clumped together, and the situation becomes a life-threatening condition. Type O is the universal donor and can be given to people with any blood type. Type AB is the universal recipient, because that type has both the A and B antigen and could receive O blood, which has no antigens. Red blood cells that have the Rh factor are considered positive, or when they lack the factor they are considered negative. For example, A-positive blood has the A antigen and Rh factor on the surface of the red blood cells. A person with O-negative blood type does not have the A antigen, the B antigen, or the Rh factor. Blood type is always described with both the antigen and Rh components.

Lymphatic System

The **lymphatic system** is probably the least understood of all the body systems. One of the main functions of the system is to return excess interstitial fluid, found between the tissues, to the bloodstream. Not all of the fluid that exists in capillaries in the tissues will return by way of capillaries. It is the job of lymphatic vessels to pick up this fluid as well as some larger particles and debris. As the fluid is returned to the bloodstream, it is processed and cleaned as it passes through lymph nodes.

Another main function of the lymphatic system is to provide the body with a system of **immunity,** or the ability to resist infection and certain diseases. There are two types of cells, called lymphocytes, that are produced to deal with foreign cells and proteins or antigens. One of these, the B lymphocytes, produce antibodies. T lymphocytes help with cellular immunity to virus-infected tissue and cancer cells. Both B and T lymphocytes produce memory cells, which allow quicker future responses to previously exposed antigens.

There are four types of immunity. The most effective type is **active natural immunity,** such as actual exposure to a foreign substance or disease. Most people are exposed to childhood diseases such as chickenpox and have therefore developed active natural immunity to them. Once someone has had the disease, the body remembers the virus and protects against recurrence. **Active artificial immunity** occurs when vaccines are received, such as the hepatitis vaccine. Healthcare workers are encouraged to keep immunizations up-to-date in order to protect themselves from communicable diseases to which they may be exposed during normal working conditions. **Passive natural immunity** occurs between a mother and a fetus or a nursing newborn. The mother's immunity is passed to the fetus through maternal-fetal circulation or through breast milk in the nursing infant. **Passive artificial immunity** is acquired by receiving an injection of immune serum or gamma globulin as soon as possible after exposure to a disease. Immune serum and gamma globulins are blood proteins obtained from blood donations to give a temporary boost to a person's immune system in an effort to prevent the development of the disease associated with the exposure. Healthcare workers exposed to conditions such as hepatitis would benefit from such an injection.

Respiratory System

The **respiratory system** is a gas exchange system. Through the main structures, the lungs, oxygen is added to the bloodstream, and toxic carbon dioxide is removed. The respiratory system consists of a series of air passageways known as bronchi and bronchioles, which warm and moisten air as it enters the body (Fig. 6-7). The actual points of gas exchange are in the **alveoli,** which

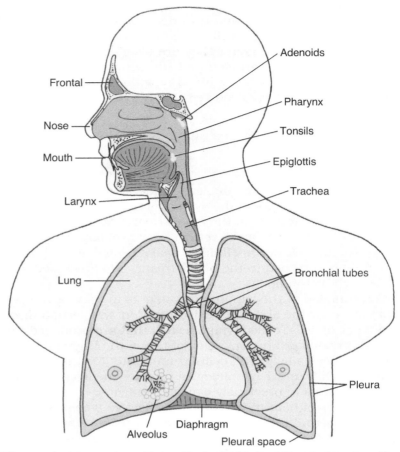

FIGURE 6-7 The respiratory system. (From: Eagle, S. *Medical Terminology in a Flash! An Interactive, Flash-Card Approach*, Ed. 2. Philadelphia: FA Davis, 2011. Used with permission.)

are small sacks one cell thick at the very ends of the terminal bronchioles in the lungs. Exchange of gases in the lungs is **external respiration,** and exchange in the tissue capillaries is **internal respiration.**

The diaphragm and the muscles between the ribs, called "intercostals," create expansion and compression of the thoracic cavity necessary for inhalation and exhalation. Air is about 21% oxygen. For most people, this concentration is sufficient to maintain life; in fact, research indicates that breathing 100% oxygen is harmful. To maintain the breathing process, healthy people exhale because of the buildup of carbon dioxide in the blood. People who develop long-term pulmonary disease inhale because of the low oxygen levels in their blood. Providing too much supplemental oxygen to these patients removes their stimulus to breathe.

Digestive System

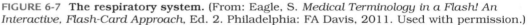

Processing of raw materials such as food for energy is a necessary life quality. Energy must be transformed from the raw source to the useable form, ATP. The body receives chemical nutrients through the **digestive system** (Fig. 6-8). This

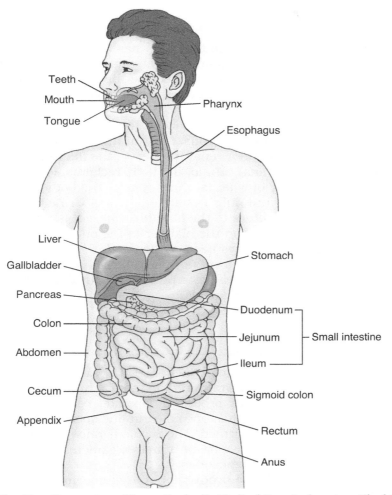

FIGURE 6-8 The digestive system. (From: Eagle, S. *Medical Terminology in a Flash! An Interactive, Flash-Card Approach*, Ed. 2. Philadelphia: FA Davis, 2011. Used with permission.)

system consists of a tube with specialized sections—the mouth, esophagus, stomach, small and large intestine—along its approximately 30-foot length. Food is broken down mechanically and chemically by the mouth and stomach into particles small enough to be absorbed by the blood. **Mechanical digestion** begins in the mouth with the mastication (chewing) of food.

Chemical digestion takes place as saliva and enzymes are mixed with the smaller food particles. **Carbohydrate digestion** begins in the mouth with salivary amylase, an enzyme that begins the breakdown. **Protein digestion** begins in the stomach, and **fat digestion** takes place in the first portion of the small intestine. The pancreas is an important accessory structure to the digestive system as it manufactures digestive enzymes. The liver produces bile, which is stored in the gallbladder for chemical digestion of fats. As food particles are broken down into molecules and absorbed, the energy in the food is transformed into ATP, which is the form of energy used by cells. Most nutrient absorption occurs in the small intestine, whereas the large intestine absorbs water.

Flashpoint

1 gram of carbohydrate contains 4 calories; 1 gram of protein contains 4 calories; and 1 gram of fat contains 9 calories.

Urinary System

The majority of the body is fluid, and that fluid has to be regulated in composition and volume. Eliminating nitrogenous waste and maintaining composition and volume of body fluids is the main function of the **urinary system.** The main structure of the system is the **kidney,** which filters about one-fourth of the body's blood every minute.

The process of urine formation takes place in the tiny nephrons of the kidney. Each kidney contains 1 million nephrons. Most of the fluid from the bloodstream leaves and is captured in a renal tubule. As the filtered material, or filtrate, travels through the renal tubule, the body reclaims what it decides is necessary and rids the body of what is unnecessary. The body produces about 150 liters of filtrate per day but only 1–2 liters of urine. Urine passes from the kidneys through a pair of **ureters** to the **bladder,** where it is temporarily stored. The **urethra** transports urine from the bladder to the outside in the process of urination. When a person's kidneys become diseased, the body can no longer maintain homeostasis. Toxins that are normally filtered out of the blood begin to increase in the body and may lead to a person's death if the person is not treated with dialysis or a kidney transplant.

Reproductive System

Elimination of this system results in extinction of the human race. Continuation of the species is the job of the **reproductive system.** Through a process called meiosis, **gametes,** or sex cells, are produced. Gametes contain half of the adult genetic material. When two gametes, one egg and one sperm, come together during fertilization, a **zygote** is formed. The zygote is one cell with a full genetic complement of the species. In the case of humans, gametes have 23 chromosomes, and a zygote has 46 chromosomes.

The testes of the male are the production site of sperm and the male hormone testosterone. Sperm are the carriers of the father's half of the genetic material. The ovaries of the female produce the ova, or eggs, which not only provide half of the species' genetic material but also provide the organism's first cell. As ova are released, they travel through fallopian tubes toward the uterus, where they may become fertilized by the sperm. Upon fertilization, chemical reactions occur that allow the uterus to receive the egg and provide it with a place and a system to develop over the next 9 months until birth. If the egg is not fertilized, chemical signals cause the inner layer of the uterus, the **endometrium,** to slough off and later be replaced for the next month's cycle. This process is **menstruation** and occurs on a 28-day cycle. Along with these metabolic changes of the uterus, there are hormones that cause the mammary glands to begin to prepare for milk production in anticipation of a pregnancy.

Summary

Structure and function together make up the human body. It is remarkable both in its anatomy and its physiology. The design of the body, with its interrelationships among the organs and organ systems, helps maintain a living, breathing organism. Although some of the organ systems may seem to be more important than others, it takes all of the systems to create and sustain life. Without the support of the skeletal and muscular systems, we would not be able to sit, stand, or move. The cardiovascular and respiratory systems provide life-saving oxygen. The ability to think and react is a product of the nervous system. We nourish our bodies and keep them clean with the digestive, urinary, and endocrine systems. The result is a finely tuned mechanism that can maintain a perfect balance within.

Practice Exercises

Multiple Choice

1. The study of the structure of the human body is:

   a. Physiology

   b. Anatomy

   c. Chemistry

   d. Psychology

2. The ability of the body to maintain a stable internal environment, within limits, while the outside environment changes is:

   a. Homeostasis

   b. Hematopoiesis

   c. Hematemesis

   d. Hemostasis

3. The basic unit of life is the:

   a. Cell

   b. Tissue

   c. Organ

   d. Organ system

4. Cells of a similar structure and function are:

   a. Mega-cells

   b. Tissues

   c. Organs

   d. Adipose tissue

5. Smooth muscle is also known as:

   a.   Voluntary

   b.   Involuntary

   c.   Peristaltic

   d.   Conscious

6. Which of the following bones provides protection?

   a.   Femur

   b.   Tibia

   c.   Ribs

   d.   Humerus

7. Your most predominant sense is:

   a.   Taste

   b.   Smell

   c.   Touch

   d.   Sight

Fill in the Blank

1. Our fight-or-flight reaction to emergencies is a function of the
   _____ nervous system.

2. The point where two bones come together is known as a
   _____.

3. We all have _____ pairs of cranial nerves.

4. _____ tissue forms coverings, linings, and glands.

Short Answer

1. **What is the main protein found in the skin, and what makes it important?**

2. **What parameters are used to name muscles?**

3. **Name the functions of the cerebellum.**

INTERNET RESOURCES

Organization/Service	Web Address
Inner Body/Your Guide to Human Anatomy	www.innerbody.com
Get Body Smart	http://getbodysmart.com
Instant Anatomy	http://instantanatomy.net/anatomy.html
Winking Skull Anatomy	http://winkingskull.com

7

HUMAN GROWTH AND DEVELOPMENT

Key Terms

birth order A child's ordinal position in the family, such as firstborn, middle child, baby

cephalocaudal Direction of growth in an infant; literally translated "head to tail," indicating growth occurs from head to toe

Denver Developmental Screening Test A standardized method of evaluating development in infants and children

development An increase in functionality of the child's physical, mental, and emotional abilities

DNA Deoxyribonucleic acid; a chemical substance that determines human characteristics at conception

failure to thrive An infant who is consistently below the predicted height and weight of the growth charts

fetal alcohol syndrome (FAS) A documented condition that occurs in infants whose mothers drink alcohol during pregnancy; the alcohol is passed directly to the fetus and causes growth delays, decreased muscle tone, poor coordination, and significant functional impairments after birth

Learning Outcomes

7.1 Distinguish between growth and development

7.2 Explain the importance of standardized growth charts

7.3 Identify factors that affect growth and development

7.4 Define birth order and the effects it has on development

7.5 Discuss the theories of development

Competencies

CAAHEP

- Compare body structure and function of the human body across the life span. (CAAHEP I.C.10)

ABHES

- Comprehend and explain to the patient the importance of diet and nutrition. Effectively convey and educate patients regarding the proper diet and nutrition guidelines. Identify categories of patients that require special diets or diet modifications. (ABHES 2.a)
- Identify and discuss developmental stages of life. (ABHES 5.f)
- Analyze the effect of hereditary, cultural, and environmental influences. (ABHES 5.g)

As humans, we all grow and develop in a systematic manner throughout life, with most changes occurring from conception to adolescence. In the early days of pregnancy, the embryo is less than $1/2$ inch in length and grows over the following 9 months to an average length of 20 inches and from less than 1 ounce to an average of 8 pounds.

Although the terms "growth" and "development" are often used interchangeably, they have different meanings. **Growth** is a measurable increase in physical size, and **development** describes an increase in functionality of the child's physical, mental, and emotional abilities. Growth and development occur in parallel, and changes in each attribute depend on changes in the other. People are different in many ways, but patterns of growth and development are much the same. Growth and development are predictable and occur on an expected timetable. In infancy, babies learn to roll over, crawl, pull up, and then walk. As their bodies grow and change, their abilities become more complex, and parents have a general idea of when to expect their child to reach certain milestones. These milestones are based on years of research and are well documented in medical publications.

Children are not little adults and should not be treated as such. Children have special growth and development needs that adults do not have. For example, a child's body is continually growing, which makes medication administration, often based on the child's weight, more exacting. Depending on the child's age, patient teaching must be directed to both the child and the parents to ensure cooperation with treatments. Physically, children must provide their body with sufficient nutrients for proper growth. All body systems in a child are constantly changing to keep up with the child's growth and developmental demands.

Growth

There are predictable patterns of growth in a continuous sequence of spurts and plateaus, but growth varies from child to child, even within the same family. Physical growth progresses in a cepahalocaudal direction. **Cephalocaudal** is a term that literally means "head to tail." At birth, an infant's head is disproportionately larger than the body, approximately one-fourth of the body length. By adulthood, that proportion becomes only one-eighth of the height. Adequate growth and development are measured through body length, head circumference, and chest circumference at birth and at regular intervals throughout the first years to determine whether the child is progressing in an acceptable pattern of growth. During the first year, the head, chest, and torso show significant growth, but the legs remain short. The legs begin to lengthen during a child's second year of life, leading to an increase in development when the child begins to walk (Fig 7-1).

Height

The **height** of children up to the age of 2 years is measured in a supine or flat position, allowing the healthcare provider to straighten the child's knees and fully extend the legs for a correct measurement. Once the child can stand independently, the height is measured using a standard scale. The average length of an infant at birth is 20 inches. Infants grow about 1 inch per month for the first 6 months of life, and by age 1 year the infant's length should increase by 50% from the length at birth, with most of this growth occurring in the torso. **Genetics** may become a factor in a child's height; however, a preteen who undergoes a rapid growth spurt and grows taller than average is still a child

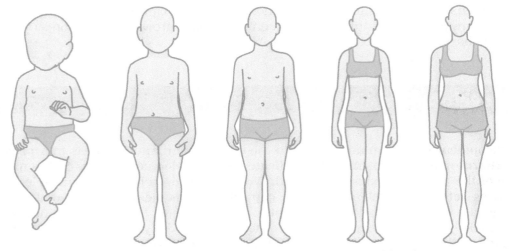

FIGURE 7-1 **Relative head sizes, from infancy to adulthood.**

Flashpoint
Rapid growth spurts are often followed by plateaus.

Key Terms—cont'd

genetics The branch of biology that deals with heredity and genetic variations, including eye color, hair color, and height

growth A measurable increase in the physical size of an infant or child

height The distance between the lowest and highest points of the body, measured in inches, feet, or centimeters

heredity The transfer of genetically controlled characteristics, such as hair or eye color, from one generation to the next

hierarchy of needs A list of human needs from the most basic needs of survival to the highest level of self-actualization necessary for development into a fully functioning adult

metabolism A series of processes by which food is converted into the energy and products needed to sustain life

nutrition The process of absorbing nutrients from food and processing them within the body in order to keep healthy or to grow

personality Your attitude, interests, behavioral patterns, emotional responses, social roles, and other individual traits that endure over long periods

Continued

and should be treated as such. In these preteen years, be cautious in using the term "average" when discussing height as this is the most variable period of growth in a child's life.

Weight

Weight is also an indicator of growth. Infants are weighed immediately after birth, and a full-term infant should fall within the average of 6 to 9 pounds. In the first few days of life, an infant will lose almost 10% of body weight, which is a normal transition to life outside the womb. This weight is regained within 2 weeks of birth, and by 6 months of age, the birth weight should double. By the infant's first birthday, the birth weight will have tripled. Proportionately, infants will gain more weight during the first year than any other time in their growing years. Children have a much higher metabolic rate than do adults, which means they need more fluid, calories, vitamins, and minerals in proportion to their body mass in the early years. Healthy eating habits and proper exercise routines must be developed early in a child's life to prevent childhood and adult obesity. Today's trend is to encourage all children to be more physically active in an effort to curb childhood obesity.

Measuring Growth

Growth is measured in two dimensions, weight in pounds or kilograms and height in inches or centimeters. For a person's measurements to have value, baselines must be established early in life. Pediatricians measure and document all areas of growth on standardized growth charts prepared by the National Center for Health Statistics of the Centers for Disease Control and Prevention (CDC). These charts were developed in 1977 after extensive research, and they allow healthcare practitioners to compare the child's growth with that of children of the same age and gender. Plotting the child's height and weight will show healthy children progressing at a more consistent rate than those with chronic illnesses or developmental delays. Growth charts have pre-established percentiles for height and weight, which allow physicians to gauge a child's growth against the 50th percentile, or the median level of height and weight for children. The growth charts are not intended to diagnose illness but can be used as one tool for healthcare practitioners to use when a child develops growth-related concerns. These charts are available in Appendix A.

Development

Development is human adaptation to the environment and proceeds in a **proximodistal** manner. Proximodistal indicates that development begins in the midline of the body and extends outward. We learn to control our large muscle masses before we develop fine motor control, such as picking up a cup off the table with our hands before we can pick up small items like coins with our fingers. Like growth, human development follows an orderly pattern. Development begins in the womb with the embryo and continues through the fetal period and the early years after birth. Many of the same factors that influence growth

---

Flashpoint

Most boys and girls have a very noticeable growth spurt when they reach puberty.

Key Terms—cont'd

prenatal care Routine care received by a pregnant woman from a healthcare professional to ensure a healthy pregnancy and outcome

proximodistal Development that begins in the midline of the body and extends outward, allowing the body to develop large muscle movements before fine motor control can be mastered

Punnett square A diagram used to see all the possible combinations of genotypes two parents can pass on to their offspring

weight The heaviness of a person measured in ounces, pounds, or kilograms

Flashpoint

A baby is considered an infant until he or she is 1 year old.

during these critical periods also affect development. Just as the growth charts gauge a baby's growth, there are tools that are used to measure development based on a standardized platform. The most common one is the **Denver Developmental Screening Test,** which was revised in 1990 to include new language skills. The newest revision of the test is known as Denver II, and it is intended to screen children from birth to 6 years old, but it is not used as a specific diagnostic study. Healthcare professionals use the results to chart a child's development in specific areas such as language, motor skills, social skills, and comprehension. Lack of progression or failure to perform in any area of the Denver II test indicates a need to further evaluate the child's development pattern.

Factors That Affect Growth and Development

Mother's Health

Even before birth, there are factors that affect growth and development. Early and continuous **prenatal care** is essential to a successful pregnancy. A mother's health and habits during pregnancy will influence the growth, development, and health of the newborn. Mothers who follow a proper diet and a healthy lifestyle increase the chance for a healthy newborn. Mothers who maintain this healthy lifestyle may also increase their chances of an uncomplicated delivery. Studies have proved that mothers who smoke during pregnancy risk having a baby with low birth weight, and mothers who drink alcohol or use recreational drugs deliver babies who are addicted at birth and suffer significant delays in growth and development. **Fetal alcohol syndrome (FAS)** is a documented condition that occurs in infants whose mothers drink alcohol during pregnancy. The alcohol is passed directly to the fetus and causes growth delays, decreased muscle tone, poor coordination, and significant functional impairments after birth. Facial structure defects are characteristic of FAS as are some heart defects. No "safe" levels of alcohol have been established for pregnant women, and heavy or binge drinking increases the risks of multiple defects. Certain diseases during pregnancy also affect the health of a newborn. Rubella, or German measles, during the mother's first trimester of pregnancy may result in birth defects such as physical deformities or mental insufficiencies. It is important for a woman to know her rubella immunity status prior to becoming pregnant, and if she is not immune, the rubella vaccine should be administered 3 months prior to conception.

Environment

The newborn's home environment influences growth and development. Problems arise when the family's financial resources are not sufficient to provide healthy food, a safe environment, or adequate educational opportunities. Parents who lack the understanding of the importance of well-baby care and routine immunizations may subject their newborn to otherwise preventable diseases. In a stable and secure environment where the infant is provided with love and attention, the infant is more likely to thrive. The term **failure to thrive** describes an infant who is consistently below the predicted

Flashpoint

Regular prenatal care helps to ensure a healthy outcome for mother and baby.

height and weight of the growth charts. It is important to determine the cause of the delay and develop a plan of care. Nutritional factors can be resolved by educating parents about proper feeding; however, if the issue is environmental, the family dynamics must be evaluated and improved. Research suggests that while intelligence is believed to be an inherited trait, the environment in which a child is raised also plays an important part. Reading to infants or providing music and color in their surroundings helps stimulate their minds.

Nutrition

The **nutrition** of an infant and toddler affects the rate of growth and development. Infants and children of families who cannot afford formula or healthy foods may suffer delays in both growth and development. Most physicians suggest breastfeeding the infant because it provides advantages such as a full range of necessary nutrients, easy digestion, natural immunity through the transfer of maternal antibodies, and development of a close mother-child relationship. Breastfeeding is convenient and economical and, even when done for only a few weeks after birth, provides benefits that bottle-fed babies do not get. Some infants have milk allergies or lactose intolerance and are unable to digest regular milk products such as formula. For these infants, soy-based products provide the necessary nutrition without the side effects of cow's milk. Feeding problems early in life may contribute to underfeeding or overfeeding and subsequent nutritional deficiencies. In extreme cases, such deficiencies can result in health problems such as rickets, goiter, or anemia. In most cases, however, problems caused by nutritional deficits can be corrected by a balanced diet, which, combined with exercise during the ensuing years, should result in proper growth and development into a healthy adult.

We live in a fast-food society that encourages people to grab a quick meal while running errands or during extracurricular activities. In moderation, these usually high-fat, processed meals are not dangerous, but when eaten frequently in the place of home-cooked meals, they can lead to serious health concerns. When children are less active and are fed these fast-food meals regularly, the combination can lead to obesity. Learning to plan meals around activities may be helpful in providing more healthy meals on a regular basis. The U.S. Department of Agriculture periodically provides updated food guides to healthy eating (http://choosemyplate.gov/). These dietary guidelines are established to help consumers follow a healthy diet that includes an emphasis on fruits, vegetables, whole grains, and fat-free or low-fat dairy products. Additionally, lean meats, poultry, fish, beans, eggs, and nuts are recommended. Items to be avoided include saturated fats, trans fats, cholesterol, salt, and added sugars. MyPlate is not a specific diet but rather is a guideline to make smart choices in the food groups to balance diet and physical activity and to make the most of the calories taken in. MyPlate also encourages you to examine your portion size and avoid the use of unnecessary empty calories. You should be able to enjoy your food while eating smaller portions. Table 7-1 provides more information on MyPlate basics.

Physical activity is just as important as nutrition for good health. Physical activity is movement of the body that uses energy. For health benefits, physical activity should be moderate or vigorous and add up to at least 30 minutes a day.

TABLE 7-1

MYPLATE GUIDELINES

Food Group	Examples
Grains At least half of the grains that you choose should be *whole* grains.	*Whole* grains: • whole-wheat flour • bulgur (cracked wheat) • oatmeal • whole cornmeal • brown rice *Refined* grains: • white flour • degermed cornmeal • white bread • white rice Serving size is based on age, sex, and activity level.
Vegetables Any vegetable or 100% vegetable juice is included in this group. The vegetables may be eaten raw or cooked. Fresh, frozen, canned, and dehydrated forms are acceptable. Vegetables are further divided into groups based on their nutrient content.	Dark green vegetables: • broccoli • kale • mustard greens • spinach Red and orange vegetables: • carrots • pumpkin • red peppers • sweet potatoes • tomatoes Beans and peas: • black beans • garbanzo beans (chickpeas) • kidney beans • lentils • soybeans Starch vegetables: • corn • green peas • green lima beans • potatoes • plantains Other vegetables: • artichokes • asparagus • avocado • beets • cabbage • celery • onions At least half of your plate should be fruits and vegetables.
Fruits Any fruit or 100% fruit juice may be eaten raw, cooked, canned, or frozen.	Fresh fruits: • apples • bananas

Continued

TABLE 7-1

MYPLATE GUIDELINES—cont'd

Food Group	Examples
	• oranges ✓ • berries ✓ • grapes ✓ • melon ✓ Dried fruits: • raisins • prunes • pineapple All fruits can be included in your diet. Make sure that canned or frozen fruits are in natural juice and not syrups or sweetened juice. At least half of your plate should be fruits and vegetables.
Dairy All fluid milk products and many foods made from milk are considered part of the dairy group. Most dairy group choices should be fat-free or low-fat. Foods made from milk that retain their calcium content are part of the group. Foods made from milk that have little to no calcium, such as cream cheese, cream, and butter, are not. Calcium-fortified soymilk (soy beverage) is also part of the dairy group. Other calcium fortified foods such as orange juice, cereals, rice, or almond-based beverages may supply calcium, but they do not provide other nutrients as do the true dairy products.	Milk products: • skim milk • low-fat (2% or less) milk • lactose-free milk • flavored milk Cheese • hard, natural cheese (cheddar) • soft cheese (ricotta) • processed cheese (American) ✓ Yogurt: • low-fat ✓ • fat-free Milk-based desserts: • pudding • ice cream • frozen yogurt Soy-based: • calcium-fortified soy milk If you do not already use low-fat dairy products, you should begin to switch to the lower fat options.
Protein All foods made from meat, poultry, seafood, beans and peas, eggs, processed soy products, nuts, and seeds are considered part of the protein food group. Beans and peas are also considered a part of the vegetable group and are used by vegetarians for their protein requirement.	Meats: • lean cuts of beef, pork, veal, lamb ✓ • poultry ✓ • eggs ✓ • seafood such as finfish and shellfish • beans and peas • nuts and seeds • processed soy products Using higher fat choices of meats will add to your limited empty calories. One ounce of meat is considered a serving. A large chicken breast may contain 2–2.5 servings. A serving of meat is about the size of a deck of cards.
Empty Calories Empty calories come from many of the beverages we drink and from solid fats used in cooking. These foods add no nutritional value to our diets.	Beverages: • soda • energy drinks

TABLE 7-1	
MYPLATE GUIDELINES—cont'd	
Food Group	**Examples**
	• sweetened fruit juices/drinks
	• sports drinks
	Solid fats:
	• cakes, cookies, pastries
	• pizza
	• chips
	• ice cream
	• sausages, hot dogs, bacon, ribs
	By limiting your intake of empty calories, you can increase your intake of healthier foods. Many of these products have a low-fat version which will help minimize your empty calorie intake.

Moderate physical activities include:

- Walking briskly (about 3.5 miles per hour)
- Hiking
- Gardening/yard work
- Dancing
- Golf (walking and carrying clubs)
- Bicycling (less than 10 miles per hour)
- Weight training (general light workout)

Vigorous physical activities include:

- Running/jogging (5 miles per hour)
- Bicycling (more than 10 miles per hour)
- Swimming (freestyle laps)
- Aerobics
- Walking very fast (4.5 miles per hour)
- Heavy yard work, such as chopping wood
- Weight lifting (vigorous effort)
- Basketball (competitive)

Children should be encouraged to spend time outdoors engaging in physical activity.

Gender

By nature, males often weigh more at birth and grow taller than females. This difference is thought to begin in the womb during the second trimester of pregnancy. The weight begins to level out in the final trimester; however, studies have suggested this early weight gain is due to the maternal secretion of androgens during pregnancy.

Male children are often steered into more physically challenging activities, which increase **metabolism** and muscle growth, although today's trend is to encourage all children to participate in physical activities. Lack of physical exercise and an unhealthy diet are two of the most dangerous contributors to childhood obesity. The federal government supports an increase in physical exercise with the Title IX laws that prevent discrimination in all educational opportunities, including all sporting activities, for both sexes. Primarily a high school and collegiate issue, Title IX ensures that monies are available for male and female athletic equipment and scholarships. Children in elementary and middle school once enjoyed a time of exercise and free play during the school day, but that has been slowly absorbed by academics. Today, schools are encouraged to provide physical exercise in the form of recess or physical education classes. Health classes have also become a part of the school curriculum.

Culture

The United States has a very diverse population of ethnic culture that has a definite influence on the growth and development of children. Customs within a culture help shape a child's growth and development through dietary requirements and beliefs related to pregnancy and child rearing. An example is that of a Chinese diet rich in vegetables with small portions of meat and rice as a part of every meal. A Mexican family may consume large quantities of pork, chicken, and ground beef with beans, chilies, and corn as dietary staples. Japanese women do not follow the "eating for two" philosophy and as a result do not have a significant weight gain during pregnancy.

Table 7-2 lists some customs that may influence the growth and development of children. It is important for healthcare professionals to respect cultural differences and provide nonjudgmental care for anyone whose beliefs are different from one's own.

Birth Order

A child's ordinal position in the family, referred to as **birth order,** actually may have some effect on its development. Alfred Adler, a psychologist who studied child development during the early 20th century, believed that children born first in the family ended up having to take on an abnormal level of responsibility, which could result in psychological problems. He also believed that the youngest children in the family would lack any need to take responsibility for themselves or others and thus would have issues related to this lack. The birth order theories that have developed over time expand upon and alter those ideas. The first child is likely to develop language and motor skills more rapidly because the child may be exposed to more adult conversations and interaction. The first child may also become more independent because this child must master many tasks alone as he or she grows. Many new parents often have higher expectations of the first child and provide more encouragement to accomplish tasks at a very young age. Younger siblings watch the older child and develop knowledge and skills from him or her. The youngest child may be thought of as the baby of the family and be treated in a way that might delay development in speech and independence.

Some studies indicate that birth order can affect intelligence in terms of IQ ratings. Some studies have found that first-born children have higher IQs than their siblings. One theory why this is so is because parents give the first-born more books and educational toys. When subsequent siblings come along, the family financial resources that may have been available to the first child's development are no longer available to the other siblings. Another theory is that first-borns receive more parental and adult attention and thus learn language and concepts earlier than do their siblings. Also, first-borns are often in the position of having

Flashpoint
Many preschools and day-care facilities promote gender-neutral activities in play and learning.

Flashpoint
The cultural background of a family will have a significant impact on the birthing process and adaptation to the new infant.

Flashpoint
Different does not mean wrong.

TABLE 7-2

CUSTOMS THAT MAY INFLUENCE THE GROWTH AND DEVELOPMENT OF CHILDREN

Culture	Pregnancy Customs	Labor and Delivery Customs
Germany	Well-respected nurse-midwives provide prenatal care.	Cesarean sections are seen as a "failure" to deliver naturally. Pregnant women cannot be fired from their jobs and are not allowed to work for 8 weeks following delivery. The baby's name must come from a government-approved list.
Japan	Mother must always think "happy thoughts" during pregnancy.	Women usually do not receive pain medicine as tolerating the pain is thought to prepare the woman for the rigorous task of raising a child. New mothers are hospitalized for about 5 days but remain in bed for 3 weeks after delivery. New mothers and babies go to her parents' home for a month after birth.
Guatemala	No one should eat in front of the pregnant woman without offering her some of the food. Failure to do so may cause the baby to suffer hunger in its life. The mother must show the baby her country and what her life is like by walking while talking to the baby in the uterus.	The mother and baby are secluded in a special place for 8 days after the birth to protect the purity of a newborn baby. No one is allowed to visit except for people who bring food to the mother. Other children in the family are not allowed in the mother's room during this time. After the 8 days, the house is thoroughly cleaned and the baby placed in a new bed prior to visits from family and friends bearing gifts.
Turkey	A physician rather than a midwife provides prenatal care and delivery. No baby showers are allowed prior to delivery.	The rate of cesarean section delivery is 75% as women choose this method over natural deliveries. This is partially because epidural anesthesia is not readily available.

to explain things to younger siblings, which fosters communication and critical thinking skills. But these findings may not matter much because several studies have demonstrated that specific personality traits, such as conscientiousness and openness to experience, are up to 10 times more important than IQ ratings.

STOP, THINK, AND LEARN.

Are you an only child? Are you the oldest? Youngest? Middle child? List three positive aspects and three negative aspects of growing up in your birth order.

Research one of the following people to determine the famous sibling: Billy Carter, Billy Ripkin, Elliott Roosevelt, Tisa Farrow, Neil Bush, Roger Clinton. What is each person's birth order in the family? Does it coincide with the current theories of birth order?

Heredity

Heredity plays a large part in the growth and development of children. Human characteristics are developed at conception through a chemical substance known as deoxyribonucleic acid **(DNA)**. Physical resemblances such as eye color, hair color, height, and skin color are passed on from generation to generation through the DNA of the parents. Within the DNA is a gene for a certain characteristic, and every child inherits genes from each parent. One of the genes will be the dominant trait, and one will be recessive. As it implies, the dominant gene will mask or hide the recessive trait. When a child receives a tall gene from the father and a short gene from the mother, the result will be a tall child because the tall gene is dominant. A **Punnett square** is a diagram used to see all the possible combinations of genotypes two parents can pass on to their offspring. In a Punnett square (Fig. 7-2A), there is a 100% chance that the children of these parents will be tall because the tall gene is dominant and appears in each of the combinations of genes. In the scenario depicted in Figure 7-2B, however, each parent carries a recessive short gene, so there is a 25% chance that the offspring will be short.

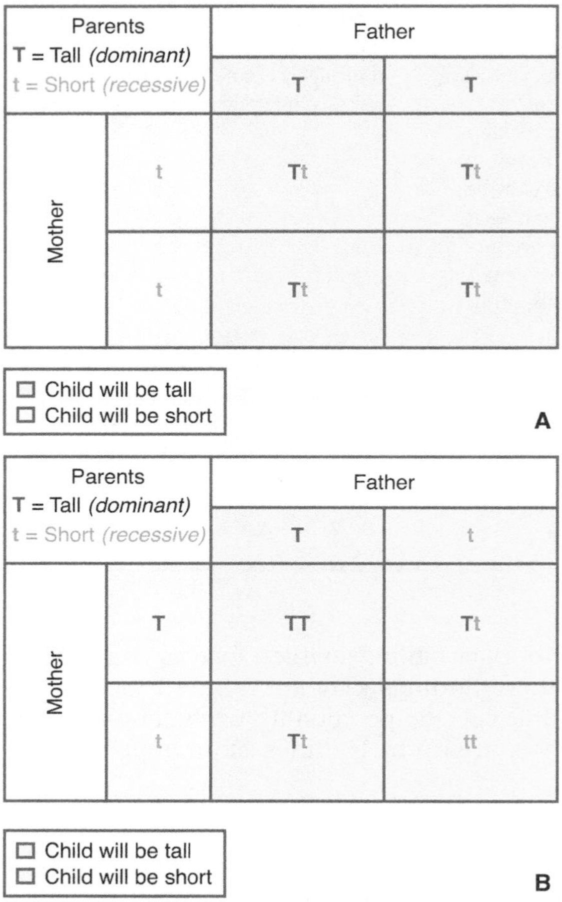

Parents **T** = Tall *(dominant)* t = Short *(recessive)*		Father	
		T	**T**
Mother	t	Tt	Tt
	t	Tt	Tt

☐ Child will be tall
☐ Child will be short

A

Parents **T** = Tall *(dominant)* t = Short *(recessive)*		Father	
		T	t
Mother	T	TT	Tt
	t	Tt	tt

☐ Child will be tall
☐ Child will be short

B

FIGURE 7-2 **Punnett squares depicting the likelihood of a child's being tall or short based on the parents' genotypes. In (A), a child has a 100% chance of being tall, but in (B) that chance is reduced to 75% because both parents have a "short" gene.**

Personality

In addition to physical growth and development, humans also develop social and moral characteristics based on many of the factors that have been discussed. There has been significant research conducted on how and why people develop their own individual **personality.** It is interesting to note that even within families, when exposed to the same conditions, children will develop their personalities at different times and in very different ways. Are you like your siblings? Are you energetic and adventurous while your brother or sister is content to sit reading a book for hours? What makes you unique in your family?

One link in physical and social development may lie in early skills. Some children may have vision or hearing problems and not be able to read and write correctly or even throw a ball straight. Without proper evaluation, this child may be seen as being "developmentally delayed," and teachers and other children often label the child as such. Being treated as "delayed" may cause the child to believe it, too, and the child will then perform to those expectations. In fact, the child may be developmentally and intellectually sound, and the potential for success may be stunted due to a simple lack of proper evaluation. Tests such as the Denver II are helpful in preventing such occurrences.

Occasionally, a child will be compared with an older sibling. Have you ever heard someone say to a child, "you sure aren't like your big sister"? This can be a damaging statement when the child thinks that he or she is either not as good as or better than the older sibling. Healthcare professionals need to remember that this is unfair to both the child and the sibling. Each child should be given the respect of being his or her own person. For example, when working with children, focus on the younger patient's unique character traits by asking questions about the individual and not his or her siblings. Questions such as, "Did you have a good day at school today?" or "What do you like to do in your free time?" are more appealing to the younger patient than questions such as "How many brothers and sisters do you have?" or "What sports does your brother play?" Focusing on the individual child establishes a connection that makes the experience more enjoyable for the patient.

Theories of Development

Abraham Maslow was an American humanistic psychologist, believing that humans strive to be their best. Maslow developed what he called a **hierarchy of human needs** that must be met in order to develop into a fully functional adult. These needs are portrayed on a pyramid, starting at the broad base with the most basic needs (Fig 7-3).

- *Physiological needs:* These are the most basic survival needs of food, water, and shelter. Consider the family that does not have adequate resources to provide these basic needs. What developmental delays would you expect a child to have?

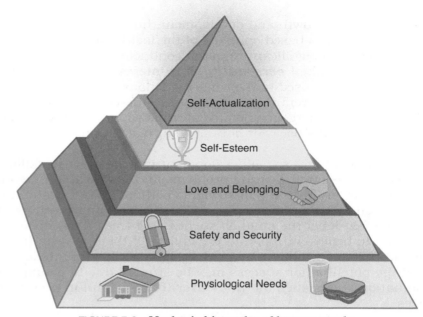

FIGURE 7-3   **Maslow's hierarchy of human needs.**

- *Safety and security:* Most adults never question their physical safety, whereas infants and children need constant assurance that they are safe in their environment. Can you think of a time when a child may experience separation anxiety?
- *Love and sense of belonging:* Everyone wants to feel loved and that they belong in a family unit. Children who receive little or no attention and no change in scenery may become despondent and develop a failure-to-thrive syndrome or be unable to develop trust. The inability to trust others may prevent a child from developing healthy relationships with family or friends. What ways can a family involve a newborn or a young child to make him or her feel loved?
- *Self-esteem:* Children can cultivate a positive self-esteem only when the first three levels of the hierarchy are met and they begin to respect themselves and others. Self-respect is important in molding a child's moral character.
- *Self-actualization:* At the pinnacle of the pyramid is the stage of a young adult's life when that person becomes comfortable with himself or herself. Realizing one's full potential and setting sights on a career path is the final step in Maslow's hierarchy. Do you remember when you felt self-sufficient and began to realize your full potential?

Many other researchers developed theories of development that are used today to evaluate a child's development. Table 7-3 briefly describes the most important aspects of developmental research. Identifying areas that a child has missed in his or her early years may help the healthcare professional understand and explain a behavior that the child may be exhibiting. Using these theories, a plan of care can be developed that may help the child and family resolve developmental issues.

TABLE 7-3
THEORIES OF HUMAN DEVELOPMENT

Researcher	Theory of Development	Stages
Jean Piaget 1896–1980	Cognitive Behaviors	*Sensorimotor:* From birth to two years, children use their five senses to discover their world. *Preoperational:* Ages 2 through 7, children do not have logical thinking skills. *Concrete operational:* Children from ages 7 to 11 can now think logically, but they are very concrete in their thoughts. *Formal operational:* After age 11, children begin to think logically but with reason.
Lawrence Kohlberg 1927–1987	Moral Development	*Pre-conventional:* The child learns discipline through consequences. *Conventional:* The child strives to live up to the "good girl/ good boy" image. During this stage, children also learn about rules. *Post-conventional:* Older children learn that everyone is an individual within a social network and that universal fundamental values rarely exist.
Erik Erickson 1902–1994	Social Development	*Trust vs mistrust:* An infant must learn to trust its caregivers. This is the stage of hope. *Autonomy vs shame and doubt:* Young children have the need to explore their world. This is the stage of will. *Initiative vs guilt:* Children are learning to do things for themselves. This stage is referred to as purpose. *Industry vs inferiority:* This is the stage of children comparing themselves to others. The stage is of competence. *Identity vs role confusion:* As children become teenagers, they begin to question themselves. Questions such as "am I popular?" and "do you think he/she likes me?" are paramount in their lives. This is the stage of fidelity. *Intimacy vs isolation:* In the later teen years and young adulthood they begin to experience first loves. The stage is love. *Generativity vs stagnation:* Commonly referred to as a midlife crisis, this stage is referred to as caring. *Integrity vs despair:* The final stage of social development, and it is the time in people's lives that they wonder if they accomplished what they set out to do and if they made a difference in the world. This final stage is that of wisdom.

Summary

Growth and development occur simultaneously in an orderly fashion and are measured using established charts and tools. Although the patterns are predictable, there will always be variations in children, in families, and in cultures regarding a child's growth and development. Healthcare professionals must always be observant and nonjudgmental in their evaluation and care of children and families.

Practice Exercises

Multiple Choice

1. In what manner does physical growth proceed?

   a. Proximodistal

   b. Parallel

   c. Cephalocaudal

   d. Proximocaudal

2. Adaptation to our environment is known as:

   a. Growth

   b. Development

   c. Heredity

   d. Genetics

3. By the age of 6 months, a baby's birth weight should be:

   a. Doubled

   b. Tripled

   c. Halved

   d. 20 pounds

4. At birth, an infant's head is approximately _____ of its total body length.

   a. $^1/_4$

   b. $^1/_2$

   c. $^1/_3$

   d. $^2/_3$

5. One of the primary factors of childhood obesity today is:

   a. Standardized school lunches

   b. Lack of physical exercise

   c. Vegetarian diets

   d. High fructose corn syrup

6. Beans and peas fall into what category in the USDA's MyPlate?

   a. Protein

   b. Dairy

   c. Vegetable

   d. Both a and c

Fill in the Blank

1. _____ is a measurable increase in physical size.

2. _____ describes an increase in functionality of the child's physical, mental, and emotional abilities.

3. The psychologist who developed the hierarchy of human needs was _____.

Short Answer

1. **What does the term "failure to thrive" mean?**

2. **What are "growth charts" and why are they significant?**

3. **What are the physiological needs of an infant?**

INTERNET RESOURCES	
Resource	Web Address
Choose MyPlate	http://choosemyplate.gov
Denver Developmental Screening	http://denverii.com
Title IX laws	http://usdoj.gov/crt/cor/coord/titleixstat.php
U.S. Department of Agriculture	http://usda.gov
National Center for Health Statistics of the Centers for Disease Control and Prevention	http://cdc.gov/nchs

8 WORKING SAFELY

Key Terms

body mechanics The way in which the body moves and maintains balance while making the most efficient use of all its parts

ergonomics The correct placement of furniture and equipment, training in required muscle movements, efforts to avoid repetitive motions, and an awareness of the environment to prevent injuries

infectious waste Any item or product that has the potential to transmit disease, such as linens, sharps, and trash

material safety data sheet (MSDS) Printed information that must be made available to employees outlining precautions to take when handling chemical agents and first-aid measures to take if exposure occurs

National Fire Protection Agency (NFPA) An international nonprofit organization that develops and publishes consensus codes that minimize the effects of fire and other risks

PASS (pull, aim, squeeze, sweep) Acronym that describes proper steps in the use of a fire extinguisher

Learning Outcomes

8.1 Demonstrate the use of proper body mechanics

8.2 Describe the importance of ergonomics in the workplace

8.3 Recognize potential occupational hazards

8.4 Demonstrate the importance of fundamental safety practices

8.5 Understand emergency plans for fire and other disasters

Competencies

CAAHEP
- Identify personal safety precautions as established by the Occupational Safety and Health Administration. (OSHA) (CAAHEP III.C.4)
- Identify safety techniques that can be used to prevent accidents and maintain a safe work environment. (CAAHEP XI.C.2)
- Describe the importance of Materials Safety Data Sheets (MSDS) in a healthcare setting. (CAAHEP XI.C.3)
- Identify safety signs, symbols, and labels. (CAAHEP XI.C.4)
- Describe fundamental principles for evacuation of a healthcare setting. (CAAHEP XI.C.7)
- Discuss fire safety issues in a healthcare environment. (CAAHEP XI.C.8)
- Discuss requirements for responding to hazardous material disposal. (CAAHEP XI.C.9)
- Identify principles of body mechanics and ergonomics. (CAAHEP XI.C.10)
- Discuss critical elements of an emergency plan for response to a natural disaster or other emergency. (CAAHEP XI.C.11)
- Identify emergency preparedness plans in your community. (CAAHEP XI.C.12)
- Discuss potential role(s) of the medical assistant in emergency preparedness. (CAAHEP XI.C.13)

ABHES
- Perform risk management procedures. (ABHES 4.e)
- Dispose of biohazardous materials. (ABHES 10.c)

Importance of Safety in Health Care

Healthcare professionals must constantly observe safety rules in healthcare settings to prevent injuries to themselves and others. Never underestimate the importance of demonstrating good, fundamental safety practices, which include the following:

- Using proper body mechanics to prevent injuries and the basic rules of good body mechanics

- Having a solid foundation of knowledge regarding occupational hazards, such as chemical hazards, radiation hazards, infectious waste, and administration of oxygen
- Understanding the regulatory requirements imposed by the Occupational Safety and Health Administration (OSHA), a federal agency that regulates workplace safety; in the healthcare setting, OSHA's Occupational Exposure to Chemical Hazards and Bloodborne Pathogens standards help protect healthcare workers
- Knowing the principles of ergonomics and environmental safety, general safety guidelines, and safety guidelines regarding computer use in healthcare settings
- Understanding fire safety principles, how to operate fire extinguishers, and how to implement your institution's fire emergency plan
- Ensuring you are aware of how to participate in your institution's emergency disaster plan, how a triage system works, and what to do in case of a bioterrorism attack

Preventing Accidents and Injuries

Because healthcare workers perform many mechanical movements with their bodies that can lead to injuries, following safety guidelines is of utmost importance to reduce the chance of injuries and prevent unnecessary pain and suffering. Injuries are usually the result of poor practices over time involving repetition of improper movements.

Risk Factors and Preventive Practices

Healthcare workers face certain risk factors just as do employees in any other profession, and these risk factors increase the possibility of work-related injuries. Some of these risk factors include the following:

- Poor posture and poor body mechanics
- Low level of fitness
- Obesity
- Stress, both mechanical and psychological

By following simple and commonsense preventive practices regarding sitting and standing (Box 8-1 and Box 8-2), many injuries can be avoided. These measures include the following:

- Using good posture during all activities
- Staying fit by exercising regularly
- Maintaining flexibility with stretching exercises
- Staying trim by eating properly
- Reducing mental stress through good lifestyle habits

Most injuries are a result of habitual activities repeated over years, so it is important that healthcare workers build good habits and safe practices into their everyday lives.

Key Terms—cont'd

RACE (rescue, activate, contain, extinguish) Acronym used to remember steps in a fire emergency

repetitive motion injuries (RMIs) Injury that is generally based on the overuse of one part of the body and that generates undue stress on tendons, nerves, or joints while causing inflammation; also called cumulative trauma injury

triage systems Guidelines used to assess patients' conditions and determine where they should be sent and what treatments should be administered

Flashpoint

The chance of sustaining injuries increases with age as flexibility decreases and recovery time increases.

Box 8-1 Proper Sitting Techniques

1. Keep head and shoulders aligned over hips and avoid bending the neck forward for long periods.
2. Avoid pressing the back of the knees against the edge of the chair seat.
3. When possible, minimize twisting and bending motions. Position equipment and work so that the body is directly in front or close to them.
4. When turning is necessary, pivot the entire body in unison. Use a swivel chair if one is available.
5. Change positions frequently.
6. Use a chair that supports the normal curves of the back (use a lumbar support if needed). Avoid sitting on stools, and avoid slouching in chairs or on couches.
7. Position your chair so work is at eye level and feet are flat on the floor.
8. When using the telephone for extended periods, use a speakerphone or a headset.

Box 8-2 Proper Standing and Walking

1. Keep your neck in a neutral position. Avoid slouching.
2. Wear cushioned shoes with good support if work requires standing or walking frequently.
3. When standing, shift your weight often. If standing in place for long periods, use a footstool. Alternate placing one foot up on the stool to take the strain off of the back.
4. Be aware of your posture. Maintain the three normal curves of the back.

Workplace Activities and Injuries

Healthcare professionals engage in numerous activities daily in work settings that can lead to injuries; for example, nurses lifting patients, staff sitting and working long hours at computer stations, and surgical technicians standing during long surgical procedures. As a result, healthcare workers commonly suffer musculoskeletal or nervous system injuries such as strained back muscles or pinched nerves.

Repetitive motion injuries (RMIs), or cumulative trauma disorders, encompass many different injuries that are generally based on the overuse of one part of the body, generating undue stress on tendons, nerves, or joints, while causing inflammation. Common RMIs include tendonitis, carpal tunnel syndrome, and thoracic outlet syndrome (see Table 8-1).

Healthcare professionals should follow these general guidelines to help prevent injuries to the musculoskeletal and nervous systems:

- Warm up and stretch before and after activities that are repetitive, lack movement, or are prolonged.
- Use the largest joints and muscles to do the work, such as squatting down and using the legs, as opposed to the back, to lift a box.
- Avoid static positions for prolonged periods. Make sure to take a break every 20–30 minutes to move around and stretch stiff muscles.
- Practice proper posture by maintaining the three normal curves of the back.
- Change positions or stop whenever activities cause pain.

TABLE 8-1

COMMON REPETITIVE MOTION INJURIES (RMIS)

Condition	Signs and Symptoms	Etiology (Cause)
Tendonitis	Swelling, tenderness, or weakness in the tendons of the shoulder, elbows, wrists, or hands	Repeated motion in a joint inflames tendons
Thoracic outlet syndrome	Poor blood circulation in the hands and fingers Weakness in arms and hands Tingling, numbness, and pain in the neck, shoulder, arms, or hands	Repeated motion causes bones or disks to compress nerves in the neck
Carpal tunnel syndrome	Inability to make a fist Loss of strength in the hand Tingling, numbness, and pain in the hand	Repeated hand motions cause inflammation and swelling, which pinch nerves that pass through a tunnel of bones and ligaments in the wrist

- Use splints and wrist supports only upon recommendation of a physician or therapist.

Preventing the types of injuries outlined above and practicing solid safety standards are paramount in healthcare settings.

Body Mechanics

To prevent injury to yourself and others while working in the health field, it is important that you observe good body mechanics. **Body mechanics** refers to the way in which the body moves and maintains balance while making the most efficient use of all its parts.

Basic rules for body mechanics are provided as guidelines to prevent strain and help maintain muscle strength. There are four main reasons for using good body mechanics:

1. Muscles work best when used correctly.
2. Correct use of muscles makes lifting, pulling, and pushing easier.
3. Correct application of body mechanics prevents unnecessary fatigue and strain and saves energy.
4. Correct application of body mechanics prevents injury to self and others.

Healthcare professionals are advised to follow eight basic rules of good body mechanics, especially when lifting (Box 8-3 and Fig. 8-1):

1. Maintain a broad base of support by keeping the feet 6–8 inches apart, placing one foot slightly forward, balancing weight on both feet, and pointing the toes in the direction of movement.
2. Bend from the hips and knees to get close to an object, and keep the back straight. Do not bend at the waist.
3. Use the strongest muscles to do the job. The larger and stronger muscles are located in the shoulders, upper arms, hips, and thighs. Back muscles are weak.
4. Use the weight of the body to help push or pull an object. Whenever possible, push, slide, or pull rather than lift.

Box 8-3 Tips on Lifting

1. Move in close to the object to be lifted.
2. Increase the base of support by positioning your feet 6–8 inches apart.
3. Squat down by bending your hips and knees, maintaining normal curves of the back.
4. Position your hand underneath the object to be lifted, take a deep breath and tighten your abdomen muscles prior to lifting, and lift the load with your legs (**not** with the back). Use two hands to lift the object. Tilt containers or objects to avoid bending the wrist when picking up objects.
5. Carry objects close to body at waist level.
6. When turning, avoid twisting and turn your body in unison, using the feet rather than the back.
7. Avoid reaching overhead with heavy loads. Be sure to use step stools, ladders, etc.
8. Do **not** attempt to pick up or carry loads that are too heavy. Use carts and dollies instead to carry these heavy loads.

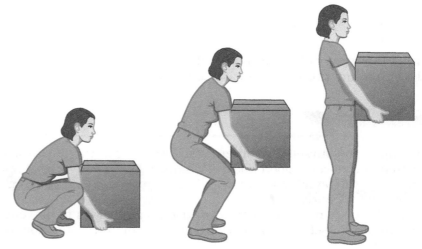

FIGURE 8-1 **Proper lifting technique.**

5. Carry heavy objects close to the body. Also, stand close to any object or person being moved.
6. Avoid twisting your body as you work. Turn with your feet and entire body when changing direction of movement.
7. Avoid bending for long periods.
8. If a patient or object is too heavy to lift alone, always get help. Mechanical lifts, transfer (gait) belts, wheelchairs, and other similar types of equipment are also available to help lift and move patients.

Back Belts

Some healthcare facilities now require healthcare workers to wear back belts while lifting or moving patients (Fig. 8-2). The supports are intended to help prevent back injuries, but their use is controversial and they are not recognized by OSHA as effective in preventing back injuries.

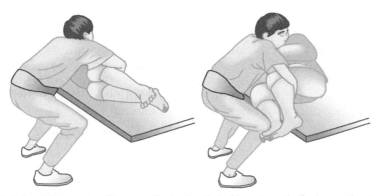

FIGURE 8-2 **A healthcare worker wearing a back belt and assisting a patient out of bed.**

Those who support their use feel that back belts increase intraabdominal pressure and create support for the spine and back muscles when lifting heavy objects, increase flexibility of the stomach and back muscles, and serve as a reminder for workers to follow proper safety techniques. Those who oppose back belts point out that the belts increase the worker's blood and pelvic pressure, which can lead to cardiac problems. It is also believed that back belts cause heat rashes and provide a false sense of security when workers attempt to lift heavier objects.

Occupational Exposures

In healthcare settings, professionals face exposure to potential occupational exposures on a routine basis. These include chemical hazards, radiation hazards, infectious waste, and administration of oxygen. These are described below.

Chemical Hazards

Chemical agents are found throughout healthcare settings, and these agents can cause harm to workers and patients if swallowed, inhaled, or absorbed into the skin. Great care must be taken when working with or near these agents. OSHA requires that *material safety data sheets (MSDSs),* which is printed information that includes precautions to take when handling chemical agents and first-aid measures to take if exposure occurs, be available to all employees. In addition, it is best to follow other general guidelines such as the following:

- Do not use any chemicals in containers that are not properly labeled, and recheck labels at least three times.
- Never mix any two chemicals together without first verifying their compatibility.
- Avoid eye and skin contact with chemicals, and do not inhale these agents. Ensure precautions are taken not to splash or spill solutions.
- Wear personal protective equipment (PPE) as indicated.
- Do not pour toxic or irritating chemicals that may be poisonous or flammable down a drain. Instead, place them in the proper container per policy and procedure.

Flashpoint

If you wear a back belt at work, don't try to lift heavier objects than normal as the back belt does not ensure freedom from injury.

Radiation Hazards

Healthcare workers employed in areas where x-rays or radiation therapy are administered must practice safety precautions to avoid exposure to radiation waves and particles. Excessive exposure can cause tissue damage and put employees at risk for contracting cancer or becoming sterile. Some strict safety guidelines must be followed, including the following:

- Wearing safety-monitoring film badges that record and measure amount of exposure.
- Placing radioactive waste in a special container, labeling it as "radioactive," and never placing the container in the regular trash or down a drain.
- Ensuring that only employees from a licensed facility remove these wastes from the healthcare facility.

Infectious Waste

Similar to other hazardous waste, strict guidelines must be followed when handling infectious waste in healthcare facilities. ***Infectious waste*** is any item or product that has the potential to transmit disease, such as linens, sharps, or trash. Infectious waste must be handled using standard and transmission-based precautions, be placed in bags or containers labeled appropriately, and be decontaminated on site. Alternatively, the waste must be removed by a licensed removal facility for decontamination.

Healthcare workers have the responsibility of following their facility's policies and procedures in the proper handling, containment, and cleanup of spills, as well as disposal of infectious waste. Any contact with infectious waste must be reported according to facility policy.

Oxygen Precautions

Patients sometime require the administration of oxygen when unable to breathe properly on their own. A physician will order how much oxygen to give, what device to use to deliver the oxygen, and how long to administer the oxygen. Special precautions must be in effect when administering oxygen, including posting signs that oxygen is in use in a given area. The following precautions must also be observed:

- Never use any electrical appliances, equipment, or toys without first checking with the supervisor, as sparks might emerge from their use.
- Never use flammable liquids such as alcohol or oils when oxygen is in use.
- Smoking is forbidden when oxygen is in use, and all smoking materials must be removed from the area where oxygen is being administered.
- Ensure that the oxygen tank is secured tightly in place so it does not fall over.
- Avoid use of materials that might cause static electricity, such as wool or synthetics; instead, use cotton blankets, gowns, or clothing.

National Fire Protection Agency Exposure Warnings

The ***National Fire Protection Agency (NFPA)*** is an international nonprofit organization that develops and publishes consensus codes to minimize the effects of fire and other risks. They have developed a warning label that identifies the hazards and the degree of severity of the health risks, the flammability, and the stability of a substance. The four-part diamond-shaped label (Fig. 8-3) indicates the hazard by color and the severity by a numerical scale, ranging from 0 for minimal risk to 4 for higher risk. The lower portion of the label is white and may indicate what protective equipment is necessary when handling the substance or other special hazards.

OSHA Safety Standards

OSHA, a division of the U.S. Department of Labor, establishes and enforces safety standards for the workplace. Two main standards affect healthcare workers:

1. The Occupational Exposure to Hazardous Chemicals Standard
2. The Bloodborne Pathogen Standard

   Following is a description of both standards.

Occupational Exposure to Hazardous Chemicals Standard

The Occupational Exposure to Hazardous Chemicals Standard requires that employers inform employees of all chemicals and hazards in the workplace. In addition, all manufacturers must provide material safety data sheets (MSDSs) with any hazardous products they sell. The MSDSs must provide the following information:

• Instructions for safe use of the chemical
• Product identification information about the chemical

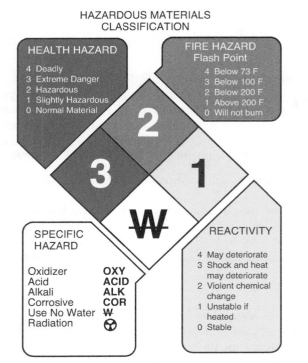

FIGURE 8-3 **NFPA hazardous materials symbol.** (From: Strasinger, S.K., and Di Lorenzo, M.S. *Urinalysis and Body Fluids*, Ed. 5. Philadelphia: FA Davis, 2008., Used with permission.)

- Protection or precautions that should be used while handling the chemical (for example, wearing protective equipment or using only in a well-ventilated area)
- Procedures for handling spills, cleanup, and disposal of the product
- Emergency first-aid procedures to use if injury occurs

The Occupational Exposure to Hazardous Chemicals Standard also mandates that all employers train employees on the proper procedures or policies to follow with regard to the following:

- Using personal protective equipment (PPE) such as masks, gowns, gloves, and goggles
- Identifying the types and locations of all chemicals or hazards
- Locating and using the MSDS manual containing all of the safety data sheets
- Reading and interpreting chemical labels and hazard signs
- Reporting accidents or exposures and documenting any incidents that occur
- Locating cleaning equipment and following correct methods for managing spills and/or disposal of chemicals

Bloodborne Pathogen Standard

The Bloodborne Pathogen Standard provides mandates intended to protect healthcare providers from diseases caused by exposure to body fluids. Body fluids include blood and blood components, urine, stool, and semen. Two diseases that can be contracted by exposure to body fluids include hepatitis B, caused by the hepatitis B virus, and AIDS, caused by the human immunodeficiency virus.

Ergonomics and Environmental Safety

The science of **ergonomics** looks at what kind of work you do, what tools you use, and what your whole job environment comprises. The application of ergonomics includes the correct placement of furniture and equipment, training in required muscle movements, efforts to avoid repetitive motions, and an awareness of the environment to prevent injuries. Examples of ergonomic changes to your work might include the following:

- Adjusting the position of the computer keyboard to prevent carpal tunnel syndrome
- Being sure that the height of a desk chair allows the feet to rest flat on floor
- Learning the right way to lift heavy objects to prevent back injuries
- Using handle coatings or special gloves to suppress vibrations from power tools

 STOP, THINK, AND LEARN.
While sitting at your desk, take a few minutes to practice the following "deskercises" that may be helpful in preventing RMIs.

- *Shoulder rolls:* Raise your shoulders and rotate them in a circle.
- *Arm stretch:* Interlace your fingers and stretch your arms straight out in front of you as far as you can reach. Hold for 10 seconds. Repeat.
- *Tilt:* Relax your shoulders and tilt your head to the right for 10 seconds, then repeat on the left.
- *Shake your fingers out:* Stretch your fingers out as far as possible and hold for 10 seconds, clinch your fists as tight as you can for 10 seconds, then shake your hands vigorously for 10 seconds. Repeat.

General Safety Guidelines

There are many ways in which healthcare workers can address environmental safety issues, but the best way is always prevention. There are several general guidelines to follow:

- *Moving safely to prevent accidents:* For example, do not run in an emergency, stay to the right in hallways, remove any loose rugs from the floor to prevent tripping, and use handrails when climbing or descending stairs.
- *Dressing for safety:* For example, wear long hair tied back to prevent contact with contaminated material, do not wear earrings that extend beyond the earlobe, keep fingernails short, and limit jewelry to a wedding band.
- *Working safely with patients*: For example, do not perform any patient procedures until you have received proper training, note conditions in patients that might increase their risk for an accident, ensure you are working with the correct patient, verify that the patient has given consent for treatment, and keep the work area clean and organized.
- *Protecting yourself and others:* For example, follow OSHA standard precautions as outlined in this chapter, do not leave cabinet doors open to prevent someone from bumping into them, and keep floors clean by immediately picking up dropped objects and wiping up spills.
- *Reporting for safety:* For example, report any unsafe conditions to your supervisor immediately, including equipment that needs to be repaired, and report any accidents or injuries immediately by completing an incident report.
- *Being prepared for potential workplace violence:* For example, violence ranging from verbal abuse by patients to physical attacks by agitated, psychotic patients or even family members.

Computers

The advent of computers in the workplace also has created an increased awareness of ergonomics because of the large number of injuries being reported and the increase in RMIs, which may occur with the extensive use of a computer keyboard and mouse. Visual problems and discomfort also arise with the use of computer screens. All healthcare workers using computers should follow the measures found in Box 8-4 to protect themselves from potential RMIs.

One major contributor to RMIs is the extensive use of a mouse as a pointing device. The mouse should be within easy reach of the user, and the mouse should be positioned at the same level as the keyboard. Additionally, using keyboard shortcuts can reduce the use of the mouse. A list of common shortcuts is presented in Table 8-2.

Flashpoint

Workers can cut down on the possibility of injuries by using the keyboard for common commands, such as saving a document using the Ctrl + S function on your keyboard.

Box 8-4 Tips While Using the Computer

1. During your entire work session, place both feet on the floor to reduce back strain. Keep your back in total contact with the back of the chair. Position your abdomen close to the edge of the desk to prevent poor posture.
2. Position the screen at arm's length to reduce eyestrain and head-forward posture. Position the top of the monitor just below eye level directly in front of the body.
3. Place a document holder next to the screen rather than working from a document placed flat on the desk.
4. Maintain your wrists in a neutral (straight) position when keying or using a pointing device. Avoid resting wrists against hard surfaces and sharp edges. Use wrist rests during pauses to help maintain neutral position.
5. Position the keyboard so your elbow is at the same height as the keyboard. Slant the keyboard as necessary to maintain your elbows at an angle of 90–100 degrees and a neutral wrist position. Try using an ergonomically designed keyboard.
6. Stretch frequently; for example, arch your back and shrug your shoulders.

TABLE 8-2
COMMON KEYBOARD SHORTCUTS

PC	Mac	Action
Ctrl+C (or Ctrl+Insert)	Command-C	Copy the selected item
Ctrl+X	Command-X	Cut the selected item
Ctrl+V (or Shift+Insert)	Command-V	Paste the selected item
Ctrl+Z	Command-Z	Undo an action
Ctrl+Y	Command-Z	Redo an action
Ctrl+Shift with an arrow key	Shift-Command with any arrow key	Select a block of text
Shift with any arrow key	Shift with any arrow key	Select text within a document
Ctrl+F4	Command-W	Close the active document (in programs that allow you to have multiple documents open simultaneously)
Alt+Tab	Command-Tab (switch application forward) Shift-Command-Tab (switch application backward)	Switch between open items
Ctrl+P	Command-P	Open the print screen

In addition, visual discomfort is frequently associated with computer use, with eyestrain and headaches reported as common problems. The eyes tire quickly when looking at a computer screen as opposed to reading printed materials, and computer glare contributes to eye discomfort. See Box 8-5 for suggestions on preventing eyestrain.

Box 8-5 Preventing Eyestrain

1. Adjust the contrast on the computer screen to a comfortable level.
2. Keep the computer screen clean.
3. Position the screen to avoid glare from surrounding lights and windows. Consider using a glare screen on the monitor.
4. Use a paper holder so you can view the text directly in front of you.
5. Look away from the computer screen and focus on other objects in the environment at frequent intervals.
6. Rest the eyes every 20 minutes by blinking your eyes rapidly, closing them, or focusing on another object farther away from the computer screen for 20 seconds.

Equipment and Solutions Safety

Basic rules must be followed when working with equipment and solutions in the workplace. Two key rules are (1) to ensure that you have been trained in the use of equipment and (2) to follow all operating instructions for the equipment as outlined by the manufacturer. See Table 8-3 for suggested safety measures to follow when operating healthcare equipment and working with solutions.

TABLE 8-3

SAFETY SUGGESTIONS FOR WORKING WITH EQUIPMENT AND SOLUTIONS

Equipment	Solutions
• Do **not** operate any equipment until you have been instructed on how to use it. When handling any equipment, observe all safety precautions that have been taught. • Read and follow the operating instructions for all major pieces of equipment. Ask for assistance if you do not understand the instructions. • Do **not** operate any equipment unless your instructor/immediate supervisor is in the room. • Report any damaged or malfunctioning equipment immediately and make no attempt to use it. • Do not use frayed or damaged electrical cords. Do not use a plug if the third prong for grounding has been broken off. Never use excessive force to insert a plug into an outlet. • Never handle any electrical equipment with wet hands or around water. • Store all equipment in its proper place. • Unused equipment should not be left in a patient's room, a hallway, or a doorway.	• Read MSDS before using any hazardous chemical solutions. • Never use solutions from bottles that are not labeled. • Read the labels of solution bottles at least three times during use to be sure you have the correct solution. • Do **not** mix any solutions together unless instructed to do so by your instructor/immediate supervisor or until you can verify that they are compatible. • Some solutions can be injurious or poisonous. Avoid contact with your eyes and skin. Avoid inhaling any fumes displaced by a solution. Use only as directed. • Store all chemical solutions in a locked cabinet or closet following the manufacturer's recommendations. For example, some solutions must be kept at room temperature, whereas others must be stored in a cool area. • Dispose of chemical solutions according to the instructions provided on the MSDS for the solution. • If you break any equipment or spill any solutions, immediately report the incident to your instructor/immediate supervisor. You will be told how to dispose of the equipment or how to remove the spilled solution.

Patient and Personal Safety

Basic rules must be followed to enhance both patient safety as well as personal safety in the workplace. Just as in operating equipment, healthcare professionals must adhere to simple but important guidelines in both these areas, such as ensuring proper authorization to perform a procedure and observing a patient closely during a procedure.

See Table 8-4 for suggested measures to enhance patient and personal safety in healthcare settings.

Fire Safety

This section provides you with basic facts about fires, how they start, and how to prevent them. This information is important for fire safety in the laboratory and the work environment.

Fires need three sources in order to start: oxygen, fuel, and heat. Oxygen is present in the air; fuel sources are found in any material that burns; and heat sources include sparks, matches, and flames.

TABLE 8-4
MEASURES TO ENHANCE PATIENT AND PERSONAL SAFETY

Patient/Resident Safety	Personal Safety
• Provide privacy for all patients such as knocking on the door before entering any room and asking for permission to enter before going behind closed privacy curtains.	• Use correct body mechanics while performing any procedure.
• Always identify your patient. Be absolutely positive that you have the correct patient. Check the name on the patient's bed and on the patient's record. Check the identification wristband, if present. Ask the patient's name at least twice.	• Wear the required uniform. • If you see an unsafe situation or a violation of a safety practice, report it to your instructor/immediate supervisor promptly. • Keep all areas clean and neat with all equipment and supplies in their proper location at all times.
• Always explain the procedure so the patient knows what you are going to do. Make sure you have the patient's consent before performing any procedure.	• Walk—do **not** run—in the laboratory or clinical areas, in hallways, and especially on stairs. • Promptly report any personal injury or accident, no matter how minor, to your instructor/immediate supervisor.
• Do **not** perform any procedure on patients unless you have been instructed to do so. Make sure you have the proper authorization. Follow instructions carefully.	• Wash your hands frequently. Hands should always be washed before and after any procedure and any time they become contaminated during a procedure. Dry your hands thoroughly before handling any electrical equipment.
• Observe the patient closely during any procedure. Be alert to the patient's condition at all times.	• Keep your hands away from your face, eyes, mouth, and hair.
• Frequently check the patient area, waiting room, office rooms, bed areas, or home environment for safety hazards. Report all unsafe situations immediately to the proper person or correct the safety hazard.	• Wear safety glasses when instructed to do so and in situations that might result in possible eye injury. • While working with your partner in patient simulations, observe all safety precautions taught in caring for a patient.
• Before leaving a patient/resident in a bed, observe all safety checkpoints, for example, check the bed to be sure that the side rails are elevated, if indicated; the bed is at the lowest level to the floor; and the wheels on the bed are locked to prevent movement of the bed.	• If any solutions come in contact with your skin or eyes, immediately flush the area with cool water. Inform your instructor/immediate supervisor. • If a particle gets in your eye, inform your instructor/immediate supervisor. Do **not** try to remove the particle or rub your eye.

The major cause of fires is carelessness with smoking and with matches. Other causes include defects in heating systems, spontaneous ignition, misuse of electricity (overloaded circuits, frayed electrical wire, and/or improperly grounded plugs), improper rubbish disposal, and arson.

Fire Emergency Plan

By following the fire emergency plan, knowing the location of fire extinguishers and exit doors, and remaining calm, the healthcare worker can help prevent loss of life or serious injury during a fire.

Know and follow the fire emergency plan established by your facility. The plan usually states that all patients and personnel in immediate danger should be moved from the area. The alarm should be activated as quickly as possible. All doors and windows should be closed, if possible, to prevent drafts, which cause fire to spread more rapidly. Electrical equipment and oxygen should be shut off. Elevators should never be used during a fire. The acronym **RACE** is frequently used to remember these important steps.

- **R = Rescue** anyone in immediate danger, such as moving patients to a safe area.
- **A = Activate** the alarm, such as sounding the alarm and giving the location and type of fire.
- **C = Contain** the fire, such as closing windows and doors to prevent drafts.
- **E = Extinguish** the fire or evacuate the area.

Preventing fires is everyone's job. Constantly be alert to causes of fires, and correct all situations that can lead to fires. Some rules for preventing fires are in Table 8-5.

Electrical Hazards

Electrical hazards pose an ongoing risk of fire in healthcare facilities due to the use of medical equipment. Most electrical hazards can be avoided by following basic safety precautions.

- Be familiar with the operation of any equipment before attempting to use it, including reviewing manufacturer operating instructions.

TABLE 8-5

RULES FOR PREVENTING FIRES

- Dispose of all waste materials in proper containers.
- Do not allow clutter to accumulate in rooms, closets, doorways, or traffic areas. Make sure no equipment or supplies block any fire exits.
- Before using electrical equipment, check for damaged cords or improper grounding. Avoid overloading electrical outlets.
- Obey all "No Smoking" signs. Most healthcare facilities are now smoke-free environments and do not permit smoking anywhere on the premises.
- Extinguish matches, cigarettes, and any other flammable items completely. Do not empty ashtrays into trashcans or plastic bags that can burn. Always empty ashtrays into separate metal cans or containers partially filled with sand or water.
- Store flammable material such as kerosene or gasoline in proper containers and in a safe area. If you spill a flammable liquid, wipe it up immediately.
- When oxygen is in use, observe special precautions. Avoid the use of electrically operated equipment whenever possible. Do not use flammable liquids such as alcohol, nail polish, and oils. Avoid static electricity by using cotton blankets, sheets, and gowns.

- Ensure that damaged equipment is reported and not used until the equipment has been repaired.
- Do not use electrical cords that are not completely intact or force plugs into outlets.
- Do not handle electrical equipment around water or use wet hands to handle electrical equipment due to the potential of electrocution.

Fire Extinguishers

Healthcare workers must become familiar with the types and locations of fire extinguishers in their place of employment before a fire occurs so they are prepared to act when faced with this type of situation.

In case of fire, the main rule is to remain calm. If your personal safety is endangered, evacuate the area according to facility procedure and sound the alarm. If the fire is small, confined to one area, and your safety is not endangered, determine what type of fire it is and use the proper extinguisher, detailed below.

Fire extinguishers are classified and labeled according to the kind of fire they extinguish, and many different types of fire extinguishers are available and used in healthcare settings. The main classes of fire extinguishers are:

- *Class A:* Used on fires involving combustibles such as paper, cloth, plastic, and wood
- *Class B:* Used on flammable or combustible liquids such as gasoline, oil, paint, grease, and cooking fat fires
- *Class C:* Used on electrical fires such as fuse boxes, appliances, wiring, and electrical outlets
- *Class D:* Used on burning or combustible metals; often specific for the type of metal being used and are not used on any other types of fires

Most fire extinguishers are labeled with a diagram and/or a letter showing the type of fire for which they are effective. Many extinguishers are used on different types of fires and are labeled with more than one diagram and/or letter.

When using a fire extinguisher, use the acronym **PASS** to help you remember its proper operating sequence:

1. **P**ull the pin.
2. **A**im the nozzle at the base of the fire.
3. **S**queeze the handle.
4. **S**weep back and forth along the base of the fire.

Emergency Disaster Plans

As required by OSHA, healthcare professionals are legally responsible for being familiar with an institution's emergency disaster plan policies in the event of disasters such as tornadoes, hurricanes, or earthquakes. In any type of disaster, stay calm, follow the policy of the healthcare facility, and provide for the safety of yourself and the patients.

Some of the required knowledge found in emergency disaster plans may include the following:

- Whether you should report to work
- Your specific duties

- Measures to protect yourself and your patients
- How to obtain communications and updates

During implementation of any emergency disaster plan, it is imperative that healthcare workers stay calm, report to the person in charge at regular intervals, communicate, and be cooperative.

Triage System

Triage systems, which are used in the emergency room, are also used to effectively manage a disaster response. Specially trained personnel follow established triage guidelines to assess patients' conditions and to determine where they should be sent and what treatments are to be administered.

In the emergency room, triage systems are frequently used in situations in which multiple patients need medical care, for example, a bus accident with multiple passengers being treated. Triage personnel must determine who to treat first, what laboratory or diagnostic tests receive priority, and whom to send to surgery. They are also responsible for continually reassessing patients waiting for services and implementing care as appropriate.

Bioterrorism

Since the September 11, 2001, terrorist attacks on the United States, healthcare facilities around the country have prepared for the possibility of bioterrorism attacks. One key area of preparation has focused on potential attacks surrounding biological weapons such as anthrax, smallpox, and botulism.

Well-devised emergency disaster plans incorporate a biological exposure readiness plan. The first step in this plan is to become aware of an outbreak and report a suspected attack to your local law enforcement agency, who will in turn notify the appropriate agencies. The plan also calls for the appropriate type of transmission precautions to be in place in the event of a bioterrorism attack.

Summary

Safety is the responsibility of every healthcare worker. It is essential that established safety standards be observed by everyone. This protects the worker, the employer, and the patient.

Key safety aspects reviewed in this chapter include use of proper body mechanics, knowing and following basic safety standards, understanding ergonomics and environmental safety principles, and being familiar with fire safety causes and prevention along with your facility's fire emergency plan.

Practice Exercises

Multiple Choice

1. The federal agency charged with regulating workplace safety is:
   a. CLIA
   b. EPA
   c. OSHA
   d. FDA

2. Which of the following is a risk factor for work-related injuries?
   a. Poor posture and body mechanics
   b. Low level of fitness
   c. Obesity
   d. Stress
   e. a, b, and d only
   f. All of the above

3. Which of the following is an example of a repetitive motion injury?
   a. Back strain
   b. Poor posture
   c. Compartment syndrome
   d. Carpal tunnel syndrome

4. Triage systems are used to:
   a. Identify patients with insurance
   b. Prioritize the patients by age
   c. Prioritize treatment based on the patients' injuries
   d. Number the patients for treatment as they arrive

5. Ergonomics includes all of the following, except:
   a. Having your chair height adjusted so that your feet rest flat on the floor
   b. Learning the correct way to lift and carry heavy objects
   c. Using special gloves to suppress vibrations from power tools
   d. Using repetitive motions to get your job done more efficiently

6. The Bloodborne Pathogen Standard addresses exposure to:

   a. Blood and blood components

   b. Body fluids

   c. Used gloves

   d. A and B only

   e. All of the above

Fill in the Blank

1. Following _____ _____ is of utmost importance to reduce the chance of injuries and prevent unnecessary pain and suffering.

2. Never mix chemicals without verifying their _____.

3. Your back has _____ normal curves that you should maintain to ensure good posture.

Short Answer

1. **What are most injuries the result of?**

2. **The way in which the body moves and maintains balance while making the most efficient use of all its parts is known as what?**

3. **What can excessive exposure to radiation cause?**

INTERNET RESOURCES

Organization/Service	Web Address	Description
University of Virginia Office of Environmental Health and Safety	http://keats.admin.virginia.edu	This site presents an ergonomics quiz and reviews both correct and incorrect answers with the viewer.
U.S. Department of Labor Occupational Safety and Health Administration (OSHA)	http://osha.gov	Click on the ergonomics link and then FAQs for information when evaluating if an injury is work-related.
Ergoweb	http://ergoweb.com	This site presents news articles that can be used for writing reports.
Centers for Disease Control and Prevention	http://cdc.gov	Visit this government site's Workplace Safety & Health section.

ROLE OF GOVERNMENT AGENCIES IN HEALTH CARE

9

Learning Outcomes

9.1 Identify the governmental agencies that have a direct impact on health care

9.2 Discuss personal and governmental insurance plans

9.3 Differentiate forms of managed care

9.4 Compare utilization management and utilization review

Competencies

CAAHEP

- Identify types of insurance plans. (CAAHEP VII.C.1)
- Identify models of managed care. (CAAHEP VII.C.2)
- Describe procedures for implementing both managed care and insurance plans. (CAAHEP VII.C.4)
- Discuss utilization review principles. (CAAHEP VII.C.5)

ABHES

- Locate resources and information for patients and employers. (ABHES 8.e)

Key Terms

biohazard Infectious agents or hazardous biological materials that present a risk or potential risk to the health of humans, animals, or the environment

bloodborne pathogens Blood or body fluids that are potentially infectious

CDC Centers for Disease Control and Prevention

CHIP Children's Health Information Program

CLIA Clinical Laboratory Improvement Amendments

controlled substance A medication that is subject to statutory control, especially a drug that can be obtained legally only with a doctor's prescription

copay A preset amount that a patient must pay out of pocket for an office visit, prescription, or other healthcare service

Continued

Many countries around the world have government-sponsored health programs. The intention of this arrangement is to allow all citizens ready access to health care. The United States spends more on health care than any other country in the world, but health care in our country is not universal and leaves millions of citizens with little or no access to health coverage. High unemployment rates increase the number of families without insurance, and technological advances in medicine continue to escalate the costs of health care. Taken together, these factors create a disconnect between available benefits and the people who need them.

Before reviewing the healthcare system in the United States, it is important to understand the concept of government-sponsored health care in other nations. In 1948, Great Britain established the ***National Health Service (NHS)*** to provide medical care for its residents at little or no cost. Approximately 80% of this program was funded through taxation. Like other government projects, the

155

Key Terms—cont'd

DEA Drug Enforcement Agency

deductible A preset amount that an insured must pay before the insurance company provides any compensation

DHHS Department of Health and Human Services

EPA Environmental Protection Agency

FDA Food and Drug Administration

group policy An insurance policy that employees may subscribe to as a benefit of an organization

individual policy An insurance policy that an individual purchases

insurance An agreement in which a company provides healthcare benefits in return for a payment premium

managed care A program that focuses on quality care for a reduced rate

Medicare A program funded by the federal government that provides health insurance for citizens age 65 and over, those under 65 with certain disabilities, and all citizens with end-stage renal disease (ESRD) requiring dialysis or a kidney transplant

National Health Service (NHS) A service established in Great Britain in 1948 to provide medical care for residents at little or no cost

NIH National Institutes of Health

OSHA Occupational Health and Safety Administration

start-up and early costs exceeded the estimated program costs by $100 million, and over the ensuing years, the healthcare program suffered shortfalls in patient care, supplies, and equipment. In the late 1980s, the program was reviewed, and British citizens were offered some relief through market-based competition in health care through advertising by physicians and healthcare facilities, which allowed patients to choose where they would receive care. The NHS is the largest health service and the third largest employer in the world today. Other European countries followed suit with a national plan for health care, and they too fell victim to the financial pitfalls when some healthcare consumers began taking advantage of free care. In many of these countries, the limited number of practitioners, inadequate hospital beds, and older technology still prevent some citizens from accessing quality health care.

Modern medicine in the United States began in the 1920s when doctors and hospitals started charging more than most Americans could afford, and the effect of the costs was compounded by the Great Depression during the 1930s. Blue Cross, the health insurance company, started in Dallas, Texas, at Baylor Hospital during the Great Depression to help bridge the gap between rising healthcare costs and Americans' decreasing ability to pay for medical services. In the 1940s, private insurers entered the market seeking ways to get around wartime wage controls by competing for labor by offering health insurance. During this time, employers were offered a tax break from the government for supplying healthcare benefits to employees, allowing insurance companies to grow. In order to make a profit, the insurance companies became particular about which patients they would insure and which medical services and treatments they would cover. This, coupled with advances in technology, medical practice specialization, and an aging population, caused health insurance premiums to rise.

In a response to rising healthcare costs, health maintenance organizations (HMOs) became popular in the 1970s and 1980s. These HMOs started out as nonprofits in an attempt to control healthcare costs, but they eventually evolved into for-profit organizations. To increase profits, the HMOs became aggressive about denying patient treatments.

Private insurance companies continued to grow in the United States in the 1990s and 21st century, and they are still profitable businesses today. Many private **insurance** companies provide healthcare coverage for those citizens in the United States who can afford the premiums. Health insurance may be an **individual policy,** purchased by the **subscriber,** or **group policy,** which may be partially funded by an employer. Each person who purchases coverage from a private insurance company pays a monthly **premium** for specified coverage. When combined with the premiums from all subscribers, the money is used to pay claims submitted on behalf of the subscribers. The monthly premium does not cover healthcare costs completely. Each policy requires that the patient pay an annual **deductible,** or preset amount, before the insurance company pays its portion. Also included in the policy may be a per-visit copay. The monthly premium will vary based on the amount of these out-of-pocket expenses. In addition to private insurance companies, the U.S. government has many organizations or branches that are involved with financial and regulatory aspects of health care.

Today, employers are reducing healthcare benefits to employees due to cost, while hospitals are consolidating and becoming less accommodating to low-income patients because these patients typically have limited or no health insurance. Hospitals are also faced with the challenge of whether to maintain, cut, or add services in response to patient demand. The challenge is heightened when the same services are also offered by other hospitals in the local community. Duplication of inpatient services, services that occur within the hospital, are associated with higher healthcare costs but also with more profit for the hospital. These deficits have spurred the demand for a national healthcare plan in the United States. To date, many different types of national health care plans have been proposed, including a system like NHS, with none being signed into law.

The Centers for Medicare and Medicaid

The Centers for Medicare and Medicaid (CMS), formerly known as the Health Care Financing Administration (HCFA), is the federal agency that administers Medicare, Medicaid, and CHIP (Children's Health Insurance Program). Approximately one in three Americans receives benefits through CMS.

Medicare

Medicare is a program funded by the federal government that provides health insurance for citizens aged 65 and over, those under 65 with certain disabilities, and all citizens with end-stage renal disease (ESRD) requiring dialysis or a kidney transplant. Medicare offers three separate services. **Medicare Part A** coverage is paid through payroll taxes and thus is available only to those who have worked and paid into Social Security. When a person reaches the age of eligibility, this benefit covers inpatient hospitalization, some home health care, and hospice care. **Medicare Part B** requires the beneficiary to pay outright a small monthly premium and covers physician care and other medically necessary outpatient services such as physical therapy. Medicare has a component that covers prescription drugs. New to Medicare in 2006, beneficiaries now choose a **Medicare Prescription Drug Plan** and pay a monthly premium to ensure lower prescription prices. This benefit allows Medicare consumers to purchase their medications at a reduced rate based on their income and the chosen plan. Also helpful are new pharmacy drug plans that offer generic medications at a fraction of the normal cost for a 3-month supply.

Medicaid

Medicaid is a program managed independently by each state to provide health care and medications for low-income families that meet certain criteria. Criteria used to determine Medicaid eligibility includes income and resources; age; certain conditions such as pregnancy, disability, and blindness; and U.S. citizenship. Medicaid recipients in some states are responsible for a small monetary payment when receiving benefits, known as the **copay.** Like many other healthcare programs, Medicaid has developed a **managed care** format to help control rising healthcare costs by restricting unnecessary or wasteful services. Managed care in the United States is a result of the Health Maintenance Organization Act of 1973; but today, managed care is used by a variety of private health-benefit programs. Managed care organizations (MCOs) comprise physicians, and others comprise a combination of physicians, hospitals, and other providers. These MCOs provide an array of health services to the enrollees (patients) in the MCO,

Flashpoint

The *Federal Register* is the official daily publication of rules, proposed rules, and notices of federal agencies and organizations, as well as executive orders and other presidential documents (see www. gpoaccess.gov).

Flashpoint

Many elderly live on a fixed income, and before prescription drug plans were available, some often had to choose between food and medications.

Key Terms—cont'd

premium A monthly payment made to an insurance company in return for coverage

subscriber The individual who purchases an insurance policy and agrees to pay the premium

utilization management The process used to determine if the future services used by the patient in terms of medical services and procedures, facilities, and practitioners are necessary, appropriate, and the most cost-effective

utilization review A process used to review medical treatment already received by the patient to evaluate if the medical services were appropriate and cost-effective

whistle-blower A person who identifies safety or other concerns in his or her place of employment and reports them to the appropriate personnel

with an emphasis on financial incentives to encourage the enrollees to use care services efficiently.

Managed care focuses on quality care at reduced costs, often by using a primary care physician to direct the patient's overall care. This results in decreased unnecessary physician visits by the patient and limits the patient's access to specialists. Managed care programs also offer financial incentives to physicians and patients to select less costly forms of care as well as programs that review the medical necessity of specific services. Inpatient admissions and lengths of stay are also decreased to help contain costs.

Managed care organizations use the process of **utilization management** to determine if the services to be used by the patient in the future, in terms of medical services and procedures, facilities, and practitioners, are necessary, appropriate, and the most cost-effective. For example, if you are going to have your appendix removed, the insurance company reviews your request for this procedure prior to the surgery to determine if it is necessary, how much it will cost, and if your insurance plan covers the cost of the procedure. The insurance company can deny coverage of the procedure if it feels you do not meet its criteria for the surgery. Utilization management is the process of preauthorization for medical service. It also may be used for approval for additional treatments while a patient is undergoing medical care (a concurrent review). Reviews of appeals also fall under utilization management. *Utilization review* is a process used to review past medical treatment received by the patient to evaluate if the medical services were appropriate and cost-effective. Utilization review also assesses medical files and compares them with treatment guidelines. Information retrieved during a utilization review can be used as part of a system that creates the insurance company's guidelines for a given condition. When creating these documents, insurance companies not only use patient experiences but also review how physicians, laboratories, and hospitals handle the care of their patients.

The opposite of managed care is a fee-for-service plan, which is a health insurance plan that allows the patient to make almost all healthcare decisions independently. The plan holder, or patient, pays for a service, submits a claim to the insurance company, and if the service is covered in the policy, receives reimbursement. Fee-for-service plans often have higher deductibles or copays than do managed care plans.

Capitation is a healthcare reimbursement model that is also used to help control medical costs. Capitation, which is used primarily by HMOs, occurs when the provider (typically the physician or nurse practitioner) is paid a fixed amount per person regardless of the number or type of services the person requires. It has been argued that an unintended consequence of capitation contracts is that healthcare providers working under them actually have an incentive to limit patient access to treatment and testing.

Children's Health Insurance Program

Under Title XXI of the Social Security Act and jointly funded by federal and state governments, the Children's Health Insurance Program, or **CHIP,** provides health insurance to children and pregnant women whose income does not qualify them for Medicaid coverage but is not sufficient to afford private insurance coverage. As with Medicaid, each state is responsible for determining eligibility criteria. In most states, the CHIP covers doctor visits, immunizations, emergency room visits, and hospitalizations. This program is essential for those families who fall through the cracks of available healthcare coverage. Statistics show that more than 7 million children and over 300,000 adults received assistance through CHIP in 2008.

Clinical Laboratory Improvement Amendments (CLIA)

CMS, along with the Food and Drug Administration (FDA) and the Centers for Disease Control and Prevention (CDC), regulates all laboratory testing done on humans through the Clinical Laboratory Improvement Amendments (CLIA). The goal is to provide quality testing for all specimens except those done for research. **CLIA** is responsible for governing over 180,000 laboratories on issues such as quality-control testing, proficiency testing, and classification of tests. Laboratory tests are classified as waived, moderate complexity, including provider-performed microscopy procedures, and high complexity. The more complex the test is to perform or interpret, the higher the complexity level it is assigned. Waived tests are those that require minimal interpretation and skill to perform and are often performed in the physician's office. Errors in waived tests would not pose any risk to the patient if performed or reported incorrectly. The majority of laboratory tests fall into the high-complexity category. Laboratories may be located within a physician's office, in a hospital, or function as a free-standing facility. More complex testing is done at regional reference laboratories. These larger laboratories have specialized equipment for performing highly complex tests that are not cost-effective for smaller laboratories to maintain. Laboratories must apply for and receive certification in order to perform testing. To acquire and maintain this certification, laboratories must test themselves on a regular basis to ensure quality results. In addition to internal quality control testing, all CLIA-certified laboratories must participate in proficiency testing. When a laboratory enrolls with a proficiency testing company, they are provided with testing samples on a regular basis. The testing company has pretested the samples and records the results. The laboratory performs the test and returns their results to the company, who compares those results to the known results.

CLIA helps our government improve the quality of testing on all specimens used in diagnosis and treatment of patients.

Flashpoint

Children need routine healthcare services to ensure their body's growth demands are being met.

Occupational Health and Safety Administration

The agency that protects healthcare workers from injury is the Occupational Health and Safety Administration, or **OSHA.** This agency is a division of the U.S. Department of Labor (DOL), and it protects all U.S. workers by setting standards for safety, providing education for employers and employees, and encouraging all industries in continuous work practice improvements. OSHA employs inspectors, investigators, engineers, and physicians, along with many technical and support personnel, to educate, inspect, and evaluate working conditions in all industries. With OSHA's guidance, healthcare institutions have decreased needlesticks and improved safety with the adoption of safety needles and acceptable sharps and **biohazard** waste disposal. Biohazards are infectious agents or hazardous biological materials that present a risk or potential risk to the health of humans, animals, or the environment. The risk can be direct through infection or indirect through the environment. Sharps waste disposal uses approved methods and containers to dispose of sharps or any device or object used to puncture the skin (such as a needle). Other biohazard waste safety products include signs alerting others to the existence of biohazard waste in the area, red plastic biohazard garbage bags, and biohazard garbage cans. One of the most important U.S. statutes for healthcare workers is 29 CFR 1910.1030. This standard addresses **bloodborne pathogens,** bloodborne diseases spread by contamination of blood and blood products, and the risk of exposure for healthcare workers. From this standard, we have adopted procedures to protect healthcare workers and patients alike.

Because of these standards, all healthcare workers may feel safe and protected in the work environment. To ensure that workers are free to participate in all matters related to safety, OSHA offers protection for **whistle-blowers** who identify safety concerns in their places of employment and report them to the appropriate personnel. OSHA protects employees who report employer violations from losing their jobs, losing benefits, disciplinary action, intimidation, threats, refusal to promote or offer pay increases, and decreased hours or pay. OSHA is an organization designed to protect us in our chosen field and should not be seen as punitive or insignificant.

Flashpoint

Safety in the workplace is essential to prevent accidents and exposure to communicable diseases.

STOP, THINK, AND LEARN.

Look around your classroom, laboratory, and school to identify any obvious safety hazards to you and your classmates.

Department of Health and Human Services

The Department of Health and Human Services **(DHHS)** is the government agency that is primarily responsible for protecting the health of Americans and providing health services for those who are not fully able to take care of themselves. There are approximately 11 agencies within this government agency, and their services account for about one-quarter of all federal expenditures and provide more grant dollars than any other federal agency. The following agencies are a sample of those that fall under the direction of the DHHS.

National Institutes of Health

Another essential agency under the auspices of the DHHS is the National Institutes of Health, or **NIH.** This agency is a world-renowned research organization that provides the medical community with documented studies on many of today's most devastating diagnoses. The agency conducts nationwide research to provide the most up-to-date findings and treatments to benefit patients who suffer from many diseases including debilitating diseases such as Alzheimer's, cancer, diabetes, and AIDS.

The Food and Drug Administration

The **FDA** is one of the more widely recognized agencies of the DHHS because of the wide array of services it provides. Many people associate this agency with the safety of their food, medications, and cosmetics; however, the agency regulates much more. The FDA is responsible for the safety of all medical devices such as pacemakers, joint replacements, hearing aids, and contact lenses. Vaccines used for immunization are also regulated by the FDA. The FDA regulates cellular telephones and other radiation-emitting devices. FDA also has responsibility for regulating the manufacturing, marketing, and distribution of tobacco products to protect the public health and to reduce tobacco use by minors. Other areas of expertise within the FDA are animal and veterinary supplies and devices. They also deal with cloning and animal-borne diseases such as "mad cow disease."

The FDA is also responsible for advancing the public health by helping to speed innovations that make medicines more effective, safer, and more affordable and by helping the public get the accurate, science-based information they need to use medicines to maintain and improve their health. The FDA regulates almost every facet of prescription drugs, including testing, manufacturing, labeling, advertising, marketing, efficacy, and safety. The FDA oversees three main types of drug products: new drugs, generic drugs, and over-the-counter drugs. New drugs undergo intensive research studies by the FDA and the drug companies that developed the drug; these drugs are available by prescription only. The FDA regulates the approval of new drugs before they become available to patients. Generic drugs are the chemical equivalent of name brand drugs whose patents have expired. For approval of a generic drug, the FDA requires scientific evidence that the generic drug is interchangeable with or therapeutically equivalent to the originally approved drug. Over-the-counter (OTC) drugs are drugs and medicine combinations that do not require a doctor's prescription. Many OTC drugs are previous prescription drugs that the FDA now deems safe for sale over the counter. Recalls are actions taken by a pharmaceutical company to remove from the market any product, including a medication, that is in violation of laws administered by the FDA. Recalls of a drug may be conducted on a pharmaceutical company's own initiative or by FDA request, but the FDA is not responsible for mandating drug recalls. However, the FDA can take more authoritative legal actions against pharmaceutical companies or manufacturers that persist in marketing a defective medication, such as that of seizure and injunction.

Centers for Disease Control and Prevention

A very important agency for all healthcare providers is the Centers for Disease Control and Prevention, or **CDC.** Established originally as an agency to prevent malaria during World War II, this agency now closely monitors and prevents the outbreak of disease, implements prevention strategies for disease, and maintains national health statistics through its mission "to promote health and quality of life by preventing and controlling disease, injury, and disability." As their mission, the CDC hopes to accomplish its vision of healthy people in a healthy world through disease prevention. In addition to being very active in the United States, the CDC maintains offices and personnel around the world in an effort to prevent international transmission of diseases. Citizens of the United States who wish to travel internationally can find information regarding necessary vaccinations and disease alerts at the CDC Web site when planning a journey or trip. For healthcare students and professionals, the CDC Web site offers a wealth of information on diseases, treatment, and prevention.

The DHHS offers other services to the people of the United States through various agencies specific to the needs of these people. These agencies include:

- The Indian Health Service, serving the over 560 recognized tribes
- The Health Resources and Services Administration, which provides medical care for low-income people around the United States and oversees the nation's transplant services

Flashpoint

In addition to the U.S. Department of Agriculture, the FDA and CDC are excellent references for food and product recall information.

- The Substance Abuse and Mental Health Services Administration, which works to improve the quality and availability of substance abuse prevention and treatment of addictions along with resources for those with mental health needs
- The Agency for Healthcare Research and Quality, whose job is to study healthcare cost and quality issues along with access to healthcare and the effectiveness of treatment

Each of these agencies operates on a multi-billion dollar budget within the direction of the Department of Health and Human Services to provide healthcare services to many Americans. There are still, however, many who do not have adequate coverage for their healthcare needs. The topic of health care continues to be a passionate debate in most political arenas.

Drug Enforcement Agency

The federal government delegates the responsibility of regulation of **controlled substances** (those substances with the potential for abuse) used in health care to the office of the Drug Enforcement Agency **(DEA)** under the Department of Justice. The DEA also works to prevent controlled substances from being distributed in an illegal manner. Physicians must register with the DEA in order to prescribe controlled substances for their patients. This registration is closely monitored by the DEA and must be renewed on a regular basis. In medical offices, the physician's blank prescription pads must be protected from fraudulent use by keeping extra pads locked away and the pads being used by the physician secure. It is an alarming fact that these pads are stolen by patients and employees and used in an illegal manner. A physician who engages in illegal controlled substance activity is subject to losing his or her license to practice medicine when indicted. Healthcare workers who choose to become involved in these schemes can also be indicted and lose not only licensure or certification but most likely the ability to ever work in health care again. There have been reports of healthcare workers who were brought into an illegal drug scheme against their will or knowledge. In most situations such as this, the employee's innocence was proven.

Environmental Protection Agency

Although not as obviously related to healthcare as the other agencies listed here, the Environmental Protection Agency **(EPA)** is a federal agency that strives to protect human health through research of our world. Studying the environment and its effects on diseases provides information to help protect us from pollutants in the air, water, and soil around us. The EPA monitors the quality of our air, water, and soil in hopes of reducing exposure to any contaminants. Air quality is especially important for people who suffer from pulmonary disorders such as asthma. The EPA works with local groups to notify swimmers and beachgoers who may be exposed to contaminated bodies of water as well as with farmers when planting food crops. After environmental disasters such as tornadoes, hurricanes, and earthquakes, the EPA evaluates the situation to alert people to possible hazards in the environment.

Summary

Our government is involved in health care for many reasons. Federal agencies conduct research and provide information that affects our health. Some agencies provide regulatory guidance for the development and use of new medications and equipment, and others provide healthcare benefits for certain populations. The idea of universal health care may sound enticing, but without proper funding and administration, it is not likely to happen. It will remain a hotly debated topic in current and future political races. The government strives to protect patients and healthcare workers with the research and regulations provided by the organizations discussed in this chapter. Your job is to follow the standards set forth by these agencies and stay current with any changes in order to provide the best health care possible.

Practice Exercises

Multiple Choice

1. Which of the following governmental agencies is responsible for safety in the workplace?

    a. OSHA

    b. CDC

    c. EPA

    d. FDA

2. The first known insurance plan in the United States was:

    a. Geico

    b. AFLAC

    c. Blue Cross

    d. Blue Shield

3. An insurance policy offered to employees as a part of a benefits package is known as:

    a. Individual policy

    b. Group policy

    c. Subscriber's policy

    d. Industrial policy

4. A federal program that is managed by each state to provide healthcare coverage for certain low-income families is:

   a. Medicare

   b. Medicaid

   c. Tri-Care

   d. CHIP

5. Before your insurance company pays benefits, you must meet an annual:

   a. Copay

   b. Coinsurance fee

   c. Deductible

   d. Premium

6. A reimbursement model that was put in place to control the costs of health care is:

   a. Capitation

   b. Major medical

   c. Coinsurance

   d. Deductible

Fill in the Blank

1. _____ helps our government improve the quality of testing on all specimens used in diagnosis and treatment of patients.

2. Approximately _____ Americans receive benefits through CMS.

3. The official daily publication of rules, proposed rules, and notices of federal agencies and organizations, as well as executive orders and other presidential documents, is the _____.

Short Answer

1. **How does utilization review help control the costs of health care?**

2. **In addition to regulating foods and drugs, what is another responsibility of the FDA?**

3. **What are two reasons why everyone in the United States does not have access to health care?**

INTERNET RESOURCES

Agency/Organization	Web Address	Resources/Functions
Agency for Healthcare Research and Quality	www.ahrq.gov	Researches quality and costs of health care.
Centers for Disease Control and Prevention (CDC)	www.cdc.gov	Monitors the outbreak and spread of diseases worldwide and provides research for prevention.
Centers for Medicare and Medicaid (CMS)	www.cms.gov www.medicare.gov (beneficiary site)	Oversees the Medicare, Medicaid, and Children's Health Insurance Programs.
Clinical Laboratory Improvement Amendments (CLIA)	http://cms.hhs.gov/CLIA	Responsible for the quality of all laboratory testing in the United States.
Department of Health and Human Services (DHHS)	www.dhhs.gov	Protects the health of Americans and provides assistance for those who are not fully able to care for themselves.
Department of Labor (DOL)	www.dol.gov	Provides information on all aspects of employer and employee rights and laws.
Drug Enforcement Agency (DEA)	www.doj.gov/dea	Responsible for enforcing controlled substance use.
Food and Drug Administration (FDA)	www.fda.gov	Oversees the safety of medicines, medical equipment, and cosmetics.
Health Resources and Services Administration	www.hrsa.gov	Oversees the organ transplantation program and provides health services.
Indian Health Services (IHS)	www.ihs.gov	Provides assistance to the established Indian tribes in the United States.
National Institutes of Health (NIH)	www.nih.gov	Governmental research agency for diseases.
Occupational Safety and Health Administration (OSHA)	www.osha.gov	Provides education, training, and enforcement of safety in the workplace.
Substance Abuse and Mental Health Services Administration	www.samhsa.gov	Works to improve the services available to those suffering with substance abuse or mental health issues.

10 INFECTION CONTROL POLICIES AND PROCEDURES

Key terms

airborne The passage of germs through the air by a cough or sneeze

aseptic Clean, without infection

autogenous Self-generation of a disease, such as scratching an infected lesion and transferring the infection to another part of the body

bacteria Single-celled organisms capable of causing disease

clean An object or surface that is free of all infectious organisms

direct contact Touching a contaminated person, object, or surface

disinfectant A chemical solution that kills pathogenic organisms but does not sterilize

droplet A particle produced by a cough or sneeze

engineering control Equipment that, when used properly, minimizes exposure to potentially infectious materials; engineering controls in the healthcare environment include equipment such as hand-washing sinks, sharps containers, autoclaves, and personal protective equipment (PPE)

Learning Outcomes

10.1 Describe common microorganisms and the distinct characteristics of each

10.2 Identify all components in the chain of infection

10.3 Summarize the methods of disease transmission

10.4 Discuss all components of effective infection control

10.5 Demonstrate proper hand washing technique

10.6 Distinguish between disinfection and sterilization

10.7 Demonstrate the correct application and removal of personal protective equipment

Competencies

CAAHEP

- Describe the infection cycle, including the infectious agent, reservoir, susceptible host, means of transmission, portals of entry, and portals of exit. (CAAHEP III.C.1)
- Define asepsis. (CAAHEP III.C.2)
- Discuss infection control practices. (CAAHEP III.C.3)
- Identify personal safety precautions as established by the Occupational Safety and Health Administration (OSHA). (CAAHEP III.C.4)
- List major types of infectious agents. (CAAHEP III.C.5)
- Compare different methods of controlling the growth of microorganisms. (CAAHEP III.C.6)
- Match types and uses of personal protective equipment (PPE). (CAAHEP III.C.7)
- Differentiate between medical and surgical asepsis used in ambulatory care settings, identifying when each is appropriate. (CAAHEP III.C.8)
- Discuss quality control issues related to handling microbiological specimens. (CAAHEP III.C.9)
- Describe standard precautions, including:
  - Transmission-based precautions
  - Purpose
  - Activities regulated (CAAHEP III.C.11)
- Discuss the application of standard precautions with regard to:
  - All body fluids, secretions and excretions
  - Blood
  - Nonintact skin
  - Mucous membranes (CAAHEP III.C.12)
- Identify the role of the Centers for Disease Control and Prevention (CDC) regulations in the healthcare setting. (CAAHEP III.C.13)
- Participate in training on standard precautions. (CAAHEP III.P.1)
- Practice standard precautions. (CAAHEP III.P.2)
- Select appropriate barrier/personal protective equipment (PPE) for potentially infectious situations. (CAAHEP III.P.3)
- Perform hand washing. (CAAHEP III.P.4)

ABHES
- Apply principles of aseptic techniques and infection control. (ABHES 9.b)
- Use standard precautions. (ABHES 9.i)
- Dispose of biohazardous materials. (ABHES 10.c)

Microorganisms, such as bacteria and viruses, are all around. They can lead to disease and, in some cases, death. **Germ** is a generic term that describes different microorganisms that may cause disease. **Microorganism** is a microscopic living organism too small to be seen with the unaided eye. Many microorganisms exist in the environment, and not all are associated with disease. One fact that will remain constant throughout your education and healthcare career is that you must do all that you can to control microorganisms and the diseases they cause. Cell phones, shopping carts, doorknobs, and most other common objects always harbor microorganisms. There are more microorganisms on a single individual's body than there are people in the United States, so it will be impossible to avoid them all. Most organisms are harmless when they remain outside, but once they enter the body, they may cause illness. Nevertheless, your responsibility is to take care of yourself and practice essential infection control procedures, such as hand washing. These procedures will not be effective if you use them only at home or just at work. You must be diligent in protecting yourself, your patients, and your family from disease-producing microorganisms.

Common Microorganisms

Bacteria

A bacterium (singular) is a single-celled microorganism responsible for many diseases. It contains a cell wall, cell membrane, and a nucleus; takes in nutrients from the environment; and reproduces by cell division. Thousands of different types of **bacteria** (plural form of bacterium), each classified by their shape, arrangement, and staining properties, exist (Table 10-1). "Staining properties" refers to **Gram staining,** in which bacteria are divided into two large groups, the gram-positive or gram-negative group, based on the bacteria's cell wall. The classification relies on the positive or negative results from the Gram-staining method, which uses complex purple dye and iodine to determine the complexity of the bacteria's cell wall. By classifying the bacteria's cell wall, a determination can be made as to which antibiotic is most effective in treating the bacteria. Each square inch of your body may contain as many as 100,000 bacteria that may cause disease in one of several ways.

Some bacteria have small hair-like projections called flagella, which allow the bacteria to move independently and to attach themselves to tissues. This attachment prevents attack by the body's white blood cells. Other types of bacteria secrete a slime material that provides a means of attachment to healthy tissues. The slime envelopes the bacteria and gives them a nourishing environment in which they can reproduce. A film-like coating that also provides the method of attachment protects this environment. For example, *Streptococcus pneumoniae,* the bacteria that causes pneumonia, seals itself off deep in the lung tissues. The bacteria multiply and resist attack by the person's white

Key Terms—cont'd

fungus A classification of organism that typically causes diseases of the skin, hair, and nails; examples include yeasts and molds

germ A generic term that describes different microorganisms that may cause disease

Gram staining The division of bacteria into two large groups—gram-positive or gram-negative—based on the bacteria's cell wall

Continued

Flashpoint

Sneezing or coughing into your elbow rather than your hands may help decrease the spread of disease.

Flashpoint

Bacteria are further classified by their shape and configuration.

TABLE 10-1
TYPES OF BACTERIA

Bacteria	Shape	Arrangement	Causes disease
Cocci	Round, spherical	Pairs = diplococci Chains = streptococci Clusters/groups = staphylococci	Gonorrhea Meningitis Pneumonia Strep throat Rheumatic fever Boils Urinary tract infection Wound infection Toxic shock syndrome
Bacilli	Rod	Single, pairs, chains	Tuberculosis, tetanus, pertussis (whooping cough), botulism, diphtheria, typhoid
Spirilla	Spiral, corkscrew, comma	Single	Syphilis, cholera

Flashpoint

Going to school or work when you have a fever is never a good idea.

Key Terms—cont'd

hand washing Using soap, water, and friction for a minimum of 20 seconds to remove all potentially harmful microorganisms from the hands

incubation period The period of time during which an infective pathogen can produce a disease once it is transmitted to another host

indirect contact Occurs when a piece of equipment is not cleaned properly between uses or someone picks up a contaminated object

microorganism A microscopic living organism too small to be seen with the unaided eye

blood cells, thus resulting in pneumonia symptoms of fever, cough, fatigue, and chills.

Still other bacteria cause disease by the production and release of toxins into the body. Tetanus, or lockjaw, is the result of the bacteria *Clostridium tetani*, which releases a very strong toxin that interferes with the transmission of nerve impulses, causing paralysis. The disease was coined "lockjaw" as it first affected the muscles of the face preventing the patient from opening the jaw. The bacteria *Mycobacterium tuberculosis*, which is transmitted by breathing in air droplets from a cough or sneeze of an infected person, can cause the disease tuberculosis (TB). Symptoms of TB include cough, excessive night sweats, fatigue, fever, and weight loss.

Most bacteria do cause disease, but there are also bacteria known as "normal flora" or "helper bacteria." This type of bacteria can help in processes such as digestion and absorption of food.

Virus

A *virus* is an ultramicroscopic infectious agent that cannot live without a host. It must reside in a plant, animal, or bacteria, where it uses the host cells' equipment to stay alive and reproduce. Sometimes during reproduction, the virus will change or mutate and make treatment more difficult. The virus is able to reproduce at a rapid rate; eventually, the cell ruptures and releases the virus to invade other cells within the body. This process continues and causes disease in the host. During this process, there may be as many as 100,000 virus particles within a single cell.

A virus causes common childhood diseases such as chickenpox, measles, and mumps. There have been over 300 viruses identified by researchers. All strains of influenza are viral in nature. Coughing, sneezing, and direct contact with an infected person are the most common ways of spreading a virus. There are vaccinations available to help prevent most childhood diseases and some strains of the flu. A common cold may be the result of any one of over 200 viruses, thus making a vaccination for this condition unlikely. Herpes, hepatitis, and AIDS are also viral diseases. There are very few antiviral drugs to treat these conditions, and treatment is aimed at relieving the symptoms of the disease. Antibiotics are ineffective against a virus.

Parasite

A **parasite** is a microorganism that lives on or in another living thing and receives all nutrition from the host. While living inside a human body's cells, a parasite deprives normal cells of the proper nutrients, invades and destroys tissues, and causes allergic or inflammatory reactions. Parasites vary greatly in size. Those causing diseases, such as malaria and amebic dysentery, an infection of the intestines, are microscopic, whereas larger parasites such as flukes or worms are visible to the unaided eye. Parasites may enter the body through food or water consumed. Transmission of malaria, a disease that involves a high fever, chills, and flu-like symptoms, is **vector-borne,** which means it is delivered by the bite of an insect, in this case, a mosquito, just as Lyme disease is transmitted through tick bites. The insect may not be infected, but rather it transfers the disease from one host to another. Tropical climates typically have the largest number of parasitic diseases, but there are also those diseases common to all areas of the world. Pediatricians in the United States see many cases of pinworms caused by a parasite in school-age and preschool children.

Fungi

Although not as dangerous as other microorganisms, a **fungus** can present a problem for some people. The more common fungal diseases affect the skin, mucous membranes, nails, and hair, and a few can lead to systemic disease. Athlete's foot and thrush are two of the more common fungal infections. The lungs and the central nervous system are susceptible to life-threatening fungal diseases such as histoplasmosis or cryptococcal meningitis. Persons with AIDS are more vulnerable to fungal diseases because of their decreased resistance to infection. Yeast, a common fungus, reproduces by a process known as budding from the original cell. Mold, another common fungus, copies itself into new cells known as spores.

Normal Flora

Microorganisms living in or on your body that are not dangerous are identified as **normal flora** (Table 10-2). They are both healthy and helpful to the vital functions of the body and help us to maintain homeostasis. Normal flora reside on the skin, in the upper respiratory system, and in the gastrointestinal and urogenital systems. Normal flora provide many benefits, such as making vitamins, aiding digestion, and feeding on cellular waste and dead cells of the body. A specific normal flora that maintains homeostasis of the gastrointestinal system is *Escherichia coli*, or *E. coli*. *E. coli* that live in the gastrointestinal tract is typically harmless to the body except when it comes into contact with the urinary tract due to diarrhea or improper wiping after toileting. When the *E. coli* migrate to the urinary tract, they can cause a urinary tract infection that includes symptoms of fever, frequent urge to urinate, burning upon urination,

Key Terms—cont'd

normal flora Bacteria that reside on and in the human body and perform useful and essential tasks to help the body function; under normal conditions, these bacteria do not cause disease

OPIM Other potentially infectious materials

parasite A type of microorganism that lives its entire life cycle in or on a host's body and receives all nutrition from that host

pathogen A bacteria, virus, or organism that is capable of causing disease

portal of entry The orifice of the body through which a pathogen may enter

portal of exit The orifice of the body through which a pathogen will exit

PPE Personal protective equipment, including gowns, gloves, masks/face shields, and head/shoe covers provided to employees for protection against blood and body fluid contamination

reservoir A place in which microorganisms reside, including plants, soil, and the human body

sharps Pieces of equipment that can penetrate the skin and cause a puncture or cut; examples are needles and scalpels

sterile Free of all microorganisms

Continued

Key Terms—cont'd

universal precautions The healthcare guidelines developed by the Centers for Disease Control and Protection (CDC) in 1987 that say that all blood and body fluids (except sweat) could contain transmissible infectious agents, meaning all patients are potentially infectious

vector-borne The transmission of a disease from one host to another, usually through the bite of an insect

virus An ultramicroscopic organism that cannot live without a host; it invades a cell and uses the cell's equipment to survive

work practice control The physical acts of hand washing, wearing PPE, and proper disposal of sharps and biohazard materials are work practice controls

TABLE 10-2

NORMAL BODY FLORA: EXAMPLES OF THE PREDOMINANT ORGANISMS FOUND ON AND IN THE HUMAN BODY

Body Site	Organisms
Skin	Alpha-hemolytic streptococci Nonhemolytic streptococci *Corynebacterium* species Diphtheroids
Throat, mouth, and nose (and subsequently sputum)	Alpha-hemolytic streptococci Lactobacillus Micrococcus Few *Haemophilus* species Few *Streptococcus pneumoniae* Few gram-negative rods
Colon	Alpha-hemolytic streptococci Nonhemolytic streptococci Enterobacteriaceae *Clostridium* species *Escherichia coli* *Proteus* species Yeasts
Vagina	Alpha-hemolytic streptococci Peptostreptococcus Gram-negative rods Yeast *Gardnerella vaginalis* Lactobacillus

and blood in the urine. As you study disease processes in your career, you will discover how these microorganisms play a role in our daily lives.

Chain of Infection

Certain conditions must be in place for an infection to occur. The **chain of infection** describes how organisms cause disease (Fig 10-1).

Pathogenic Agent

Bacteria, viruses, or other organisms capable of causing disease, called **pathogens,** can be a pathogenic agent. Bacteria can survive outside of a host; viruses can survive only within a living cell. Antibiotics can destroy bacteria, but viruses are more difficult to treat because they reside within the cell and there are fewer antiviral medications available. A pathogen's ability to cause disease depends on its capability to invade and reproduce within a host, the speed of reproduction, the ability to produce toxins that damage tissue, and the

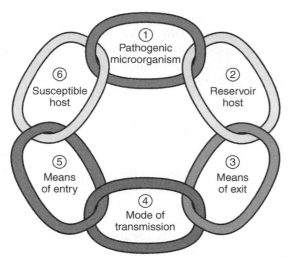

FIGURE 10-1 Chain of infection. (From: Eagle, S., et al. *The Professional Medical Assistant: An Integrative, Teamwork-Based Approach.* Philadelphia: FA Davis, 2009. Used with permission.)

ability to induce an immune response in the host. The stronger these characteristics are, the more likely the microorganism is to produce disease.

Reservoir

The organisms live and reproduce in a ***reservoir.*** Plants, soil, the human body, or other organic substances can act as the reservoir. When the organism infects the host, the host may exhibit signs of a clinical illness or may be asymptomatic. A patient who is asymptomatic may serve as a carrier of the organism and transmit it to others without ever having developed the disease.

Portal of Exit

The pathogenic organism must have a specific method of leaving the reservoir or host. The ***portal of exit*** in humans depends on the organism and may be by a single method or multiple methods. The gastrointestinal tract, the respiratory tract, open lesions or wounds, or any orifice through which blood, body fluids, or other potentially infectious materials ***(OPIMs)*** may escape, are examples of portals of exit.

Transmission

Direct contact, indirect contact, droplets, or autogenous contact (self-inoculation) may transmit the infectious organism. The hands of healthcare workers may transmit organisms directly from one patient to another or to another healthcare worker. ***Direct contact*** often occurs as a result of improper or lack of hand washing. ***Indirect contact*** may occur when a piece of equipment is not cleaned properly between uses or someone picks up a contaminated object. ***Droplet*** transmission occurs when a person coughs or sneezes without covering the mouth or nose. An example of ***autogenous*** contact is impetigo, an infection that spreads throughout the body when the patient scratches an infected lesion and rubs or scratches another area of the body. Insects such as ticks and mosquitoes can also be methods of disease transmission, known as vector-borne transmission. The time during which an infective pathogen can produce a disease once it is transmitted to another host, the **incubation period,** varies with each disease.

Portal of Entry

Just as a way for the organism to leave the host must exist, a method by which it enters the newly susceptible host, a **portal of entry,** must also exist. An organism can enter the new host by ingestion, inhalation, crossing the mucous membranes, or through a percutaneous injection. Medical procedures, such as intravenous therapy and urinary catheter insertion, may also provide methods of entry. However, exposure does not always mean that an infection will ensue. The exposed person's immune response and physical resistance determine a subsequent infection. Consequently, persons with a compromised immune system are more susceptible to the infection. Any break in the chain of infection prevents the transmission of the disease. As healthcare workers, we seek to break the cycle of infection.

Infection Control

Now that you know how organisms spread, you can take simple steps to make the healthcare environment cleaner and safer. It is much easier to develop good habits now than to break bad habits later. Protecting the environment and ourselves is not totally up to us; the government plays a large role in infection control. Standards are in place to aid infection control.

In 1970, President Richard Nixon established the Occupational Safety and Health Act, which created a governmental agency given the authority to develop baseline standards of safety and protection for all U.S. workers. This agency is the Occupational Safety and Health Administration (OSHA). OSHA has specific guidelines for the safety and protection of all workers, not just those in healthcare-related occupations.

In 1987, the Centers for Disease Control (CDC) developed guidelines specific to healthcare known as **universal precautions.** The general principle of universal precautions was that blood and all body fluids—except sweat— could contain transmissible infectious agents; therefore, all patients are considered potentially infectious. In 1996, the universal precautions were expanded and became known as **standard precautions.** The new statutes include a group of infection prevention practices that apply to all patients and healthcare workers. Healthcare workers are exposed to many infectious diseases on a daily basis, and a joint effort of OSHA, the CDC, employers, and employees to make the work environment as safe as possible must be present.

Methods of infection control have been developed to prevent the spread of infection in the healthcare arena. They include engineering controls and work practice controls.

Engineering Controls

Engineering controls include equipment that, when used properly, minimize exposure to potentially infectious materials. Engineering controls in the health-care environment include equipment such as hand-washing sinks, sharps containers, autoclaves, and personal protective equipment *(PPE).* Biohazard containers, fume hoods, and spill kits are more examples of engineering controls. To be compliant with OSHA guidelines, employers must provide all of the necessary engineering controls for the facility. New employees must be trained in the infection control policies and procedures of the facility, and all employees should be updated annually.

Most facilities maintain a spill kit to clean up spills or leaks. The kit is all-inclusive of the items you would need to clean up a spill without having direct contact with the material. Kits are designed for use with chemicals or for infectious waste. The infectious waste kits include latex gloves, absorbent material, bleach, boundary tape, biohazard bags for disposal, and a first-aid kit. These spill kits help prevent an accidental exposure to infectious materials and should be easily accessible in every area of schools and healthcare facilities.

A fume hood is a specialized piece of equipment that may help prevent exposure to *airborne* pathogens. Fume hoods are used primarily in the laboratory area when working with cultures that may become aerosolized. The hood offers a strong vacuum to pull airborne particles up and out, similar to a range hood in the kitchen. Another use for a hood is to protect workers when they are mixing chemicals or chemotherapeutic agents.

Work Practice Controls

The physical acts of hand washing, wearing PPE, and proper disposal of *sharps* and biohazard materials are *work practice controls.* These concepts are explained in detail later in this chapter. Disinfection and sterilization of equipment and instruments are other examples of using work practice controls. An employer must provide the engineering controls, and employees must participate by understanding the importance of these controls and using them in their daily work (see Appendix B for competency form and training checklist examples).

Employers must maintain a current safety manual for employees. This manual should include an infection control plan, categorization of all job titles according to OSHA, policies and procedures for safety issues, and postexposure information. These categories are discussed later in this chapter. The manual should also address employees' hepatitis B status. Each employee in categories I and II are offered the series of hepatitis B vaccines at no cost upon employment. The vaccine series is not mandatory, but it is strongly suggested. Not everyone converts to immune status after the series, so it is a good idea to have a hepatitis B titer drawn 1 to 2 months after the last injection. Revaccination is evaluated on an individual basis. Should an employee choose not to take the series, they sign a declination statement, which becomes a part of the employee's personnel file (see Appendix C). The safety manual should be readily available to all employees in the office and updated at least annually by the infection control coordinator. Healthcare facilities use a variety of chemicals and other potentially dangerous substances in infection control procedures. Examples may include chemical reagents for laboratory testing, bleach, detergents for cleaning, and even copy machine toner. A material safety data sheet (MSDS) is a compilation of material from the manufacturer describing in detail the make-up of these substances and the proper care, handling, storage, first aid, and any adverse health effects. An MSDS should be accessible if a leak or spill occurs or if an employee is exposed to the substance. MSDSs are also helpful to emergency personnel if there is a fire or other situation that requires evacuation of the facility. MSDSs may be requested from the manufacturer of the substance; however, some of the more common ones, such as sodium hypochlorite (bleach), are available on the Internet.

Destroying the Microorganisms

The most effective way to destroy microorganisms is thorough ***hand washing.*** Hand washing is an easy procedure, and it is the single most effective method of preventing cross-contamination in a healthcare setting. It requires these three components: soap, water, and friction. The American Medical Association (AMA) and the CDC currently do not suggest antibacterial soaps for routine hand washing because microorganisms can adapt to that environment, which may increase their resistance. In addition, antibacterial compounds in the soap must remain in contact with your skin for a minimum of 2 minutes to be effective. Hands must be washed properly and frequently to be an effective work practice control. Doing so will eliminate most microorganisms from the hands. When possible, use warm water. Add enough soap to provide a significant lather. Wash all surfaces of the hand, wrist, and fingers vigorously for a minimum of 20 seconds. Rinse thoroughly, and dry the hands with a clean towel. In most instances, paper towels are preferable. Keep the hands pointed downward so that the microorganisms are washed down the sink drain instead of up the forearms. Pay close attention to the fingernails. Extremely large numbers of microorganisms grow and multiply under long fingernails. Keeping the nails short allows for easier cleaning, is safer, and looks more professional. Artificial nails are strongly discouraged and even prohibited in some healthcare institutions due to the increased risk of hidden contamination. Be careful not to recontaminate the hands once they are clean. Jewelry also harbors microorganisms and is therefore discouraged in healthcare settings. Hands must be thoroughly washed before and after wearing gloves, as gloves never replace hand washing.

     ## STOP, THINK, AND LEARN.
Name at least three times you should wash your hands at work and three times you should wash your hands at home.

The newest product on the market is alcohol-based hand sanitizer. Research has determined that these products are effective against microorganisms when the alcohol content is 60%–90% and the hands are not visibly dirty. The advantage of using these cleansers is that they destroy almost all surface microorganisms in a matter of seconds. They are effective against many different organisms, provide rapid and broad-spectrum activity, and have excellent microbicidal characteristics. Unlike antibacterial soaps, these sanitizers lack the potential of becoming resistant to organisms. Hand sanitizer is readily available and requires no special equipment.

Alcohol-based products are recommended for use among persons who need immediate protection after touching contaminated surfaces or before and after contact with someone at high risk for infection when soap and water are not available. People should still wash their hands with soap and water as soon as possible after exposure. Because alcohol dries the skin, it is important to use a sanitizer that contains moisturizers or hand lotion afterward. Dry, cracked skin can break the protective skin barrier.

Disinfection and Sterilization

When an object is *clean,* it is free of all **infectious** organisms, whereas a *sterile* object is free of **all microorganisms.** Providing sterile one-time-use and reusable medical supplies decreases the risk of infection. Sterilizing instruments for reuse is a multistep process. As soon as possible after use, disinfect the instruments using physical and chemical methods. A *disinfectant* solution is a chemical that kills pathogenic organisms but does not sterilize. A bristle brush and an adequately prepared disinfectant solution can start the process. Utility gloves protect hands, as they are thicker than latex gloves and not as likely to allow a puncture. A face shield protects the eyes and mucous membranes from possible splatters and splashes of contaminated material or disinfectant solutions.

Once the instruments are disinfected, sterilization eliminates any transmissible organisms from all surfaces. Steam sterilization uses a combination of steam, pressure, and time to sterilize the instruments. A temperature of 250°F (or 121°C) at 15 lb of pressure per square inch for 15 minutes should be sufficient to kill or inactivate all bacteria, viruses, and fungi and their spores. Timing does not begin until the correct temperature and pressure are met. Biological indicators confirm autoclave proficiency where an indicator tape shows that the instrument was exposed to the conditions necessary for sterilization. Sterile instruments provide an additional level of protection against infection. Large equipment items or those with heat-sensitive parts that cannot be placed into a steam sterilizer or exposed to such high heat can be sterilized using a chemical or gas technique. Instruments that need to maintain sterility until used are packaged and sterilized by the chemical sterilization method, using either ethylene oxide gas or hydrogen peroxide plasma. These instruments are placed into packaging material that is compatible with the specific chemical sterilization method; the packaging must allow adequate chemical sterilant penetration to be effective.

Radiation is also a technique used to sterilize sensitive medical equipment. Equipment sterilization is imperative to prevent the spread of infection.

Personal Protective Equipment

PPE is a very important part of both engineering and work practice controls. Employers must provide it and train employees in its use, and employees must use it as an effective part of infection control. PPE is designed to protect healthcare workers from potential contamination when exposed to blood and body fluids, chemicals, radiation, physical, electrical, mechanical, or other hazards in the workplace. Healthcare workers should be most concerned with exposure to diseases through blood and body fluids. Types of PPE used in healthcare include, but are not limited to, gloves, gowns, safety shields/goggles, head/shoe covers, and masks/respirators (Fig. 10-2). The type of healthcare facility determines the use of PPE. Workers in the operating room use PPE on a daily basis, whereas workers in an ophthalmology office may find their use very limited.

Gloves

Never use gloves to replace hand washing. Always wear gloves when there is a potential for exposure to blood and body fluids. After use, remove gloves inside out, and discard them in a biohazard container if grossly contaminated. Never save and reuse gloves. Wash hands before and after using gloves. The gloves act as a physical barrier for both the patient and the healthcare worker.

Research has indicated that latex gloves are the most effective in eliminating the risk of exposure to blood and body fluids. In recent years, however, an increase in the number of latex allergies with repeated exposure among healthcare workers has surfaced. New technology has produced synthetic materials that provide adequate protection for those healthcare workers with known or suspected latex allergies. Two common substitutions are nitrile and vinyl. The

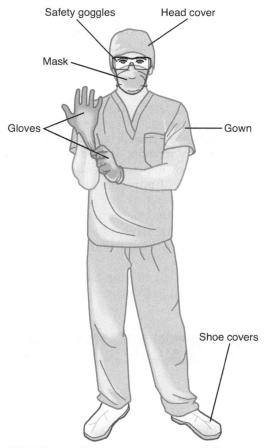

FIGURE 10-2 **Personal protective equipment.**

synthetic rubber, nitrile, is more puncture resistant; however, the fit and comfort is not comparable to that of latex. Vinyl gloves have not yet been proven to offer the same protection as latex and do not compare in fit and durability to the latex or nitrile gloves. Vinyl gloves cost about the same or even slightly less than latex gloves, and nitrile gloves are more expensive. Cost should not be a factor in providing employees with appropriate PPE.

Gown

When the potential for spraying or splashing of blood or body fluids is present, it is advisable to cover clothing with a nonpermeable gown. This prevents contamination of clothes. When removing the gown, it is important to remove it inside out. This prevents contamination from the outside of the gown. Soiled gowns should be disposed of in the biohazard container.

Goggles, Mask, or Face Shield

The face, eyes, and respiratory tract also need to be protected from potential splashes and airborne exposure. A surgical mask and safety goggles or a one-piece face shield offers protection. The operating room or dental offices are examples of facilities that require this type protection on a daily basis. Safety goggles not only protect the eyes from splashes or sprays but also against any flying objects. When sanitizing instruments in a chemical bath, the shield protects against splashes of both contaminated matter and chemicals.

Healthcare workers exposed on a regular basis to airborne diseases require the special protection of an N95 respirator mask as recommended by the CDC. Individually fitted masks provide the best possible protection from airborne diseases. The term "N95" indicates that these masks have a filter efficiency of 95% or greater. In an emergency situation when an N95 mask is not available, a surgical mask can be substituted.

Head and Shoe Covers

Shoe covers are designed to do just that, cover shoes in case of splashes or spills. Operating room personnel are some of the few healthcare workers that use these PPEs daily. All healthcare workers should pay close attention to their footwear. There is always the potential for an unexpected spill or splash. For this reason, nonpermeable shoes are a good idea. Be careful in selecting shoes as many of the newer styles are designed for style and not comfort and protection.

Protecting the head and hair is commonplace in an operating room, but situations may arise in other areas that require the use of a head cover. The lightweight head covers not only prevent hair from contaminating a sterile or clean surface but also protect you from splashes and aerosolized contaminants.

OSHA Guidelines for PPEs

OSHA has specific guidelines for the use of PPE. In Title 29 of the *Code of Federal Regulations* (CFR), parts 1910.1030(d)(3)(i-iii), we learn that employers have the responsibility for providing PPE for their employees based on each

Flashpoint
Laboratory coats serve different purposes for different healthcare professionals.

employee's potential for exposure. Each job description in the facility should address the PPE needs as follows:

- *Category I.* A task or activity in which direct contact or exposure to blood or other body fluids, to which universal precautions/standard precautions apply, is normal. Examples of category I tasks include specimen collection, applying or removing bandages, performing CPR, and disinfecting instruments.
- *Category II.* A task or activity performed without exposure to blood or other body fluids to which universal precautions/standard precautions apply, but from which exposure may occur as an abnormal event or an emergency. Examples of category II tasks are taking a medical history, assisting with exams, and transferring patients from bed to stretcher or wheelchair.
- *Category III.* A task or activity that does not entail normal or abnormal exposure to blood or other body fluids to which universal precautions/ standards precautions apply. Category III tasks may include filing insurance, scheduling appointments, or data input.

 STOP, THINK, AND LEARN.
What OSHA category will you be in once you graduate? Why?
Name two healthcare occupations that fall into each of these three OSHA categories.

When a healthcare facility hires someone new, the employer must provide training in infection control for this employee during normal working hours at no cost. This training must be completed within 30 days of employment or prior to any potential exposure. The training must be provided to all employees annually. Additional training is required for new and established employees when there are changes to the standards or the employee's job category changes. Many facilities choose to have an annual in-service day for updating and training all employees to comply with OSHA and CDC standards. Documentation of this training becomes a part of the employees' personnel folders.

Regardless of the OSHA requirements and employer mandates, there are individuals who either have become complacent in their attitude or have made a personal decision not to protect themselves or their patients by using PPE. One's attitude and decision about using PPE should reflect a true desire to succeed in the healthcare environment.

Biohazard Waste

OSHA defines regulated waste as "liquid or semi-liquid blood or other potentially infectious material (OPIM); contaminated items that would release blood or OPIM in a liquid or semi-liquid state if compressed; items that may be caked with dried blood or OPIM and are capable of releasing these materials during handling; contaminated sharps; and pathological and microbiological wastes containing blood or OPIM."

Healthcare facilities and training facilities must arrange for the safe and proper disposal of regulated waste. Large facilities may have their own disposal system, such as an incinerator, but smaller facilities will contract with a company specializing in the disposal of this material. These companies will develop a pickup schedule with each facility they serve based on the amount of biohazard waste the facility produces. Charges are based on weight, so it is important to pay close attention to what is placed in the biohazard containers.

It is important to develop good habits for disposal of biohazard waste. You must place all biohazard waste in specially marked red containers that are clearly marked with the universal biohazard symbol (Fig. 10-3).

All non-sharp objects are placed in a marked red plastic bag that is placed inside a sturdy container to prevent overflow or spillage. Once the bag is filled, it is tied securely and sealed in the sturdy container.

Sharps Disposal

Needles, scalpels, and other sharp objects are disposed of in a slightly different manner. To prevent injuries, you should place any sharp object in a closable, puncture-proof, leak-proof red container marked with the biohazard symbol (see Fig. 10-3). These canisters are placed everywhere a healthcare professional uses sharps. This includes the medication room, the patient's bedside, the operating room, the treatment room, and laboratory and triage areas. Sharps are disposed of at the site of use, and they are never transported to another area for disposal. Needles and other sharps are never to be recapped prior to placing in the container. Make it a habit to place the sharp in the container without attempting to recap. It is too easy to get distracted and end up with a needlestick. Sharps containers contain a "full" marking, and objects should never be forced into a full container. When full, the sharps container is sealed and prepared for disposal in a manner similar to the non-sharp waste.

All sharps are now equipped with a safety device to prevent needlesticks. These easily employed devices allow you to protect both yourself and the patient immediately after the sharp is used. Once you activate a safety device, never

Flashpoint

All needlesticks or exposures should be reported immediately to your supervisor or physician.

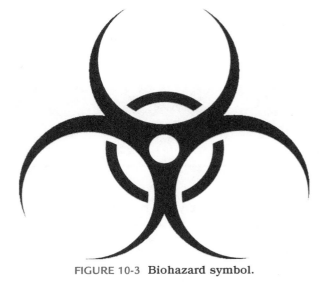

FIGURE 10-3 **Biohazard symbol.**

attempt to release it. If you find yourself with an exposed needle that does not have a safety device, do not attempt to recap the needle using two hands. Even a brief interruption increases the chance of a needlestick. Slowly scoop the cap back onto the needle using one hand and dispose of it immediately in the sharps container.

Exposure Incidents

Following all infection control policies and procedures may not prevent an occasional exposure to blood or body fluids. OSHA defines an exposure as "specific eye, mouth, or other mucous membrane, non-intact skin, or injection contact with blood or OPIM that results from the employee's duties." In health care, exposure does sometimes occur, either by accident or through negligence. The infection control coordinator of the facility has protocols to follow in the case of an exposure. Some healthcare workers may fear repercussions for not following procedures and may not report an incident. Others report incidents immediately. All exposures should be reported without fear of punishment. Procedures must be followed when an incident occurs. It is important to remain calm and follow the facility's exposure control plan. The protocols found in the plan guide the employee to complete the necessary paperwork, which includes a detailed description of the exposure. The physician evaluates the risk of disease transmission associated with the exposure. The employee receives evaluation, counseling, and baseline blood work if there is potential risk for disease. The employer is responsible for any costs associated with this process. Follow-up testing is done at the direction of the CDC, but is usually done within 6 months of the exposure.

Summary

It is our responsibility as healthcare professionals to prevent the spread of infections. We must always be mindful of the importance of washing our hands and using personal protective equipment when necessary. Proper disposal of sharps and biohazardous waste will also help prevent exposure to potentially infectious materials. Remember to do your part!

Practice Exercises

Multiple Choice

1. A pathogen is an organism:
   a. That can exist only in an oxygen-rich environment
   b. That can cause disease
   c. Has a flagellum
   d. That is not harmful to the body

2. Viral diseases are more difficult to treat because:

   a.   The virus can mutate during reproduction.

   b.   There are very few antiviral drugs available.

   c.   The virus reproduces at a very rapid rate.

   d.   All of the above

3. A common fungal disease is:

   a.   Strep throat

   b.   Pinworms

   c.   Athlete's foot

   d.   Influenza

4. Objects may be sterilized by all of the following methods, except:

   a.   Steam

   b.   Chemical

   c.   Radiation

   d.   Disinfection

5. An example of engineering controls is:

   a.   Hand washing

   b.   Sanitizing solutions

   c.   Fume hoods

   d.   Wearing PPEs

6. Which governmental agency created standards for the use of personal protective equipment?

   a.   Centers for Disease Control and Prevention (CDC)

   b.   Occupational Safety and Health Administration (OSHA)

   c.   Environmental Protection Agency (EPA)

   d.   Governmental Protection Agency (GPA)

Fill in the Blank

1. The most effective physical barrier to blood and body fluids is
   _____.

2. Hand sanitizers must have an alcohol content that is at least
   _____.

3. A sharps container should be _____, leak-proof, and red in color.

Short Answer

1. **What makes a vaccine for the common cold unlikely?**

2. **How are normal flora good for your body?**

INTERNET RESOURCES		
Agency/Organization	Web Address	Resources/Functions
Centers for Disease Control and Prevention (CDC)	www.cdc.gov	Monitors the outbreak and spread of diseases worldwide and provides research for prevention.
MSDS Solution Center	www.msds.com	Material safety data sheets from manufacturers of chemicals and other substances.
Occupational Safety and Health Administration (OSHA)	www.osha.gov	Provides education, training, and enforcement of safety in the workplace.
American Medical Association	www.ama-assn.org	Provides guidelines on hand-washing techniques and other medical practices.

COMMUNICABLE DISEASES 11

Learning Outcomes

11.1 Describe the characteristics of a communicable disease

11.2 Discuss the etiology, transmission, signs and symptoms, and treatment of childhood diseases

11.3 Differentiate between the forms of meningitis

11.4 List and discuss all forms of hepatitis

11.5 Identify diseases classified as sexually transmitted and discuss treatment for each

11.6 Discuss HIV infection in relation to AIDS

11.7 Defend the importance of immunizations

Competencies

CAAHEP
- Describe implications for treatment related to pathology. (CAAHEP I.C.9)
- List major types of infectious agents. (CAAHEP III.C.5)

ABHES
- Recognize and understand various treatment protocols. (ABHES 9.d)

Key Terms

acquired immunodeficiency syndrome (AIDS) A disease caused by the human immunodeficiency virus, which destroys a person's immune system, opening the way for opportunistic infections

attenuated A term used to describe a disease-causing organism that has been weakened and used in a vaccine to protect against that disease

Continued

Communicable diseases are caused by microorganisms, and they are transmitted by people, animals, foods, surfaces, and through the air, as discussed in Chapter 10. This chapter discusses the communicable diseases that remain a threat today. Healthcare workers are exposed on a daily basis to diseases as simple as a common cold to more serious diseases such as hepatitis. Understanding these diseases and how to protect yourself is an important part of your training to become a healthcare professional.

Flashpoint

Healthcare professionals must never become complacent in protecting themselves from communicable diseases.

Childhood Diseases

Some diseases that typically occur during childhood, but may develop later in life in nonimmunized adults, are not as prevalent in today's society due to a rigorous *immunization* schedule, discussed later in this chapter. The diseases that are discussed are contagious, and all infection control principles should be followed when caring for a patient who has contracted the disease.

Measles (Rubeola)

The number of *measles* cases, also known as *rubeola* or red measles, has greatly decreased in our country due to extensive immunizations; however,

Key Terms—cont'd

chickenpox A highly contagious viral illness caused by the varicella virus, which produces flu-like symptoms followed by a rash that progresses to blister lesions

chlamydia The most commonly reported sexually transmitted disease; it may cause damage to the female reproductive system

Flashpoint

Most physicians recommend acetaminophen or ibuprofen for children with a fever.

there are as many as 20 million cases each year worldwide. Measles is a viral illness that is spread through the respiratory tract by direct contact with airborne respiratory secretions as the result of coughing and sneezing. These airborne droplets may be directly inhaled into the lungs or there can be direct contact with secretions on used tissues. The incubation period, which is the time from exposure to first symptoms, is 8 to 13 days. Stage I symptoms include fever, nasal congestion, coughing, sneezing, and conjunctivitis. The classic stage II sign that distinguishes measles from other viral rashes is the red rash that appears first around the hairline and behind the ears and slowly spreads toward the feet (Fig. 11-1). This rash appears about the third or fourth day of the virus and begins to fade after 3 to 4 days. The presence of Koplik spots, small red spots with a bluish center appearing in the mouth, is often the determining factor in a diagnosis of rubeola. Measles is usually a self-limiting disease of about 2 weeks, and treatment is symptomatic. Those at a higher risk of complications are children under 5 years of age and adults over age 20 years. Most physicians advise rest, an increase in the amount of fluids that a person takes, and an antipyretic, such as acetaminophen or ibuprofen if the fever makes the person uncomfortable. A child with a viral illness such as measles must not be given aspirin or aspirin products as there is a risk of developing Reye syndrome, an encephalopathy that follows an acute illness in children that has been linked to the use of aspirin and aspirin-like products during the course of a viral illness.

An untreated fever can lead to febrile seizures. Other complications from measles may include diarrhea leading to dehydration, middle ear infections, pneumonia, and less likely, encephalitis, which is an acute inflammation of the brain. Encephalitis often leads to coma and brain damage. A pregnant woman who contracts measles during her first trimester is at higher risk for miscarriage, premature delivery, and a low birth weight baby. Because it is so easily transmitted, anyone who is not vaccinated will more than likely get the disease when exposed.

Measles is a preventable disease. Having children immunized according to the CDC (Centers for Disease Control and Prevention) immunization schedule should prevent them from contracting measles. The **vaccine** for measles is included in the combination MMR (measles, mumps, and rubella) injection. The vaccine contains a live, weakened **(attenuated)** virus in the safest form possible and provides an immunity that is effective for life in 95% of children. A second dose of

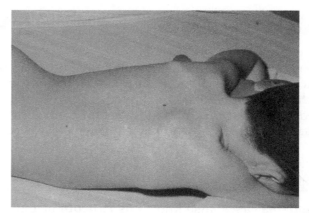

FIGURE 11-1 **Measles rash from rubeola infection in the back of a boy.** (Courtesy of the CDC Public Health Image Library.)

the vaccine is recommended to immunize the other 5% of children as well as to provide a booster to those who are immune. It is important for healthcare workers to determine their immunity, as some early vaccines are ineffective. A blood test called a titer can determine immunity status. (The Healthcare Personnel Vaccination Recommendation chart is in Appendix D).

German Measles (Rubella)

German measles often goes by the name **rubella,** or 3-day measles, and it is also caused by a virus. The virus is spread through the respiratory tract, therefore considered an airborne disease, and has an incubation period of 14 to 23 days. German measles begins with symptoms including a low-grade fever (99°–100°F) and tender, swollen lymph nodes behind the ears and on the back of the neck. An itchy **rash** develops on the face and slowly spreads down the body. The rash is not as well defined as the spots caused by rubeola as some spots join to form reddened patches (Fig. 11-2). As the rash progresses downward, it clears from the face. This rash often lasts no more than 3 days and can leave the skin scaly with flaking of dead skin cells. Symptoms that occur in older children and adults include swollen lymph nodes over the entire body, conjunctivitis, fatigue, and joint pain. Some patients have no symptoms. Children tend to recover within a week, whereas adults tend to recuperate at a slower rate. Like rubeola, treatment for rubella is symptomatic, with acetaminophen or ibuprofen for fever or general malaise, rest, and increased fluids.

Women must be aware of their rubella **immunity** status as exposure to rubella in early pregnancy can result in serious birth defects for the fetus, such as mental retardation, blindness, deafness, or heart defects. Pregnant women cannot be immunized during pregnancy because the vaccine contains the live, although weakened, virus. Nonpregnant women cannot be immunized within 1 month of getting pregnant as the risks of birth defects are significant.

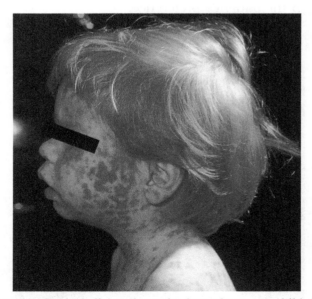

FIGURE 11-2 **German measles (rubella) rash on the face of a young child.** (Courtesy of the CDC Public Health Image Library.)

Flashpoint

Before a measles vaccine was developed, children with the disease were quarantined at home in a dark room until the rash disappeared.

Key Terms—cont'd

communicable Diseases caused by microorganisms that are transmitted by people, animals, foods, surfaces, and through the air

contagious Able to be passed from one person to another by direct or indirect contact

declination statement A statement signed by someone who chooses not to get vaccinated against certain diseases

directly observed therapy (DOT) A type of therapy that reminds patients to take their medication by meeting with a healthcare professional daily or several times per week

Epstein-Barr virus The organism that causes infectious mononucleosis

fifth disease The common name for erythema infectiosum, a common childhood virus that causes a "slapped cheek" rash; caused by the human parvovirus B19

German measles The common name for rubella, a form of 3-day measles caused by a virus; this disease can cause birth defects if contracted by a woman in her first trimester of pregnancy

Continued

Key Terms—cont'd

gonorrhea A commonly reported sexually transmitted bacterial disease that can also be spread from mother to baby during birth

hepatitis A viral illness that affects the liver; there are currently five forms of the disease, each transmitted by a specific mechanism

herpes simplex virus (HSV) A virus that causes infections of the skin and mucous membranes

HSV-1 The form of HSV that causes infections in the oral cavity, often called "fever blisters" or "cold sores"

HSV-2 The form of HSV that causes infections in the genital tract

human immunodeficiency virus (HIV) A virus that attacks a person's immune system and destroys the white blood cells necessary to fight diseases

human papillomavirus (HPV) A sexually transmitted virus that has over 40 different strains causing genital skin infections and cancers; genital warts are an example of this virus

immunity The body's ability to resist a disease; immunity may be natural or the result of a vaccination or previous infection

immunization An injection that will make a person resistant to a particular disease

influenza An acute respiratory disease caused by one of many viruses that can affect children and adults

The vaccine for rubella is included in the **MMR** injection and given according to the CDC recommendations. The risks for developing the disease or other side effects are minimal.

Mumps

Mumps is an acute viral illness spread through respiratory droplets or saliva. Persons who have the disease are contagious from 2 days before their symptoms appear until about 6 days after the symptoms are gone, with an incubation period of 12 to 26 days. Mumps usually starts with a fever as high as 103°F, headache, and loss of appetite. The classic sign of mumps is swelling of the parotid, or salivary glands, toward the back of the cheek between the ear and the jaw (Fig. 11-3). Over the course of 1 to 3 days, the person begins to complain of pain in these swollen glands, making eating, drinking, and talking more difficult. Swelling is usually bilateral but may appear on one side before developing fully on both sides. Mumps in adolescent males may produce a complication called ***orchitis,*** or inflammation of the testicles. Pain and swelling in one or both testicles begins approximately 1 week after the initial fever and swelling of the parotid glands. A high fever may return with chills, headache, nausea, and vomiting. In cases of right testicular swelling, these symptoms may resemble those of appendicitis. Sterility is unlikely, even when the orchitis is bilateral. In female patients, swelling of the ovaries is possible, causing pain and generalized abdominal tenderness. The patient history helps clarify the diagnosis. Other rare complications may include meningitis, encephalitis, and deafness. Research indicates that one in three patients with mumps does not display any symptoms and goes undiagnosed.

Treatment for mumps includes nonaspirin pain relievers, rest, and increased fluid intake. Many patients with mumps find it painful to swallow, so a soft, bland diet may be easier to tolerate. Foods such as mashed potatoes, milkshakes, and soups are good choices, and acidic fruit juices and carbonated beverages may cause unnecessary pain. Warm packs or cold packs may offer some pain relief, based on the patient's preference.

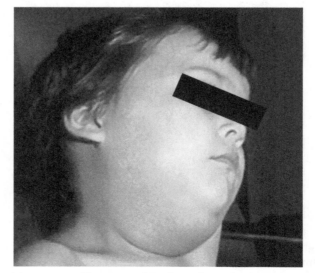

FIGURE 11-3 **Child with mumps.** (Courtesy of Barbara Rice, CDC Public Health Image Library.)

The mumps vaccine is the third component of the MMR vaccine and is administered according to the CDC immunization schedule. Side effects of the vaccine are rare but may include a slight fever, rash, or slight swelling of the parotid glands. These symptoms subside within a week.

Chickenpox (Varicella-Zoster)

Transmitted through respiratory droplets, **chickenpox** begins with a fever and flu-like symptoms, then is followed by a rash that begins as small red bumps resembling an insect bite and progresses to blisters on the skin (Fig. 11-4). The **varicella-zoster virus** is highly **contagious** with an incubation period of 10 to 21 days, but the disease is usually self-limiting. A person with chickenpox is contagious from 2 days prior to the rash until all of the lesions have crusted. During this contagious period when the lesions are developing, which is about 1 week, children should stay home from school. The lesions can cause extreme itching, and children must be persuaded against scratching as doing so can cause a secondary bacterial skin infection. Cool compresses, oatmeal baths, calamine lotion, and some over-the-counter anti-itch medications may be suggested to relieve the itching.

Pregnant women must avoid contact with anyone suspected of having the chickenpox to prevent possible birth defects in the fetus and a risk of more complications for herself. Having chickenpox prior to becoming pregnant offers the baby immunity to the disease for the first few months of its life through the placenta and through breastfeeding.

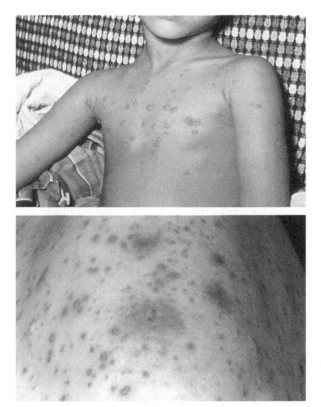

FIGURE 11-4 Rash from chickenpox (varicella-zoster virus). (Courtesy of the CDC Public Health Image Library.)

Flashpoint

Side effects of vaccinations are still safer than the diseases themselves.

Key Terms—cont'd

measles A viral illness that produces respiratory symptoms and a "spotty" rash

meningitis Inflammation of the membranes surrounding the brain and spinal cord; the bacterial form is contagious and often fatal, whereas the viral form is less common and has few lasting effects

MMR The vaccine that provides immunity to measles, mumps, and rubella

mononucleosis An infectious disease caused by the Epstein-Barr virus

mumps A viral illness that presents with respiratory symptoms and swelling of the salivary glands

orchitis Inflammation of the testicles as a possible complication of the mumps

proof of vaccinations Documentation of vaccinations often needed by schools and employers

rash An outbreak on the surface of the skin that appears "spotty" and often reddish and itchy

rubella A form of 3-day measles, often called German measles

Continued

Secondary bacterial skin infections are the most common complications of chickenpox, especially in children who scratch the lesions and open them to bacteria. Antibiotics may be prescribed for this infection, but they have no effect on the varicella virus. Other bacterial infections that can result from chickenpox are arthritis, encephalitis, and pneumonia.

As with other viral diseases, treatment is symptomatic. Although it does not cure the illness, physicians can prescribe the antiviral medication, acyclovir, for people who are at high risk for complications. The medication must be given within 24 hours of the first sign of the rash, and each patient must be evaluated carefully as there are some significant side effects, including anaphylaxis, coma, dizziness, and anemia.

The vaccine for varicella-zoster, Varivax, is also made from a live, attenuated virus, and it is expected to provide lifelong immunity. It provides immunity for up to 90% of those who take it and reduces the severity of the breakthrough cases in 95% of those who develop the disease. The varicella vaccine is also available in a combination form with the MMR, allowing children to receive the maximum vaccinations with fewer injections.

Meningitis

Meningitis is an infection of the fluid and membranes that surround and protect the brain and spinal cord. Often called "spinal meningitis," there are two forms of the disease, viral and bacterial, each with a unique set of symptoms and treatment. It is important to establish early in the disease if the cause is from a bacteria or virus. If it is determined to be bacterial, the specific bacteria must be identified.

A group of viruses called enteroviruses typically cause viral or aseptic meningitis, the less severe of the diseases. Other childhood disease viruses, such as the mumps or chickenpox, have also caused cases of viral meningitis. Bacteria that are responsible for the more serious form of meningitis include *Streptococcus pneumoniae* and *Neisseria meningitidis* (meningococcal meningitis). Prior to the 1990s, the bacteria *Haemophilus influenzae* (Hib) was the cause of most cases of bacterial meningitis. A vaccine to protect children from this form of meningitis became part of the routine immunization schedule and greatly reduced the number of meningitis cases related to the bacteria.

Symptoms include headache, blurred vision, fever, and classically, a stiff neck. Other symptoms that may occur within hours or over the course of 1 to 2 days include nausea, photophobia, confusion, and extreme sleepiness. Complaints of a headache and stiff neck are hard to elicit in infants and young children, so the physician must rely on symptoms such as irritability, poor feeding, or listlessness. In extreme cases, seizures may occur. Healthcare facilities see more cases of meningitis in the summer and fall.

To differentiate between viral and bacterial meningitis, the physician must obtain a sample of the cerebrospinal fluid through a lumbar puncture or spinal tap. This is a sterile procedure accomplished by the insertion of a small needle through the vertebral column and into the meningeal space. The physician may measure the pressure within the meningeal space to determine if there is excess pressure on the brain and spinal cord. Fluid is not withdrawn; rather, it is allowed to drip into a sterile collection container. The fluid is processed in the laboratory to determine the causative organism.

Once the organism is identified, appropriate antibiotics can be prescribed for those with the bacterial form of the disease. Early detection and treatment with effective antibiotics is important for such a dangerous disease. Bacterial meningitis

---

Flashpoint

Telling a child not to scratch an itchy rash is usually not effective.

Key Terms—cont'd

rubeola Often called "red measles," this viral illness produces a rash that begins around the hairline and behind the ears and then progresses toward the feet

shingles The result of the varicella-zoster virus that lays dormant in the body until the adult years; it causes a painful, blister-like rash along the pathway of one nerve

syphilis A bacterial sexually transmitted disease that develops in three phases, from acute to latent

"Take Three" challenge A CDC directive for the prevention of influenza: "Take a flu shot; take everyday precautions; and take antiviral medications when ordered by the physician."

tuberculosis (TB) A bacterial infection that typically attacks the lungs by destroying the healthy tissue and creating holes in the lungs

vaccine A preparation containing weakened or dead microbes of the kind that cause a disease administered to stimulate the immune system to produce antibodies against that disease and provide immunity

varicella-zoster virus The virus that causes chickenpox or shingles

caused by *N. meningitidis* is contagious for those who have extended close contact with the patient, such as family members or those in day-care centers and schools. Transmission is primarily through direct contact with the infected patient's throat and respiratory secretions, but bacterial meningitis is not as easily transmitted as the virus for colds or flu. In most cases, those considered to have close contact with the patient are given prophylactic antibiotics to prevent possible transmission of the disease. Viral forms of the disease have no specific treatment other than rest, increased fluids, and over-the-counter medications for fever and headache.

Vaccines are available to protect against several forms of meningitis. The Hib vaccine is now a part of the childhood vaccination schedule, which helps protect children in day-care centers and schools. Two additional meningitis vaccines protect against most forms of the disease. All of these vaccines have been proved safe and effective. Young adults moving into college dormitories are advised to take the meningitis vaccine in the event of exposure in close living quarters, as are world travelers, those entering military service, and laboratory technicians who are routinely exposed to communicable diseases.

Fifth Disease (Erythema Infectiosum)

Caused by the human parvovirus B19, *fifth disease* is an illness that primarily affects children, causing a low-grade fever, upper respiratory symptoms, and generalized malaise followed by the outbreak of a classic "slapped cheek" rash on the face and a lacy rash on the body and limbs (Fig. 11-5). The child is contagious early on when the fever begins. When the rash appears, the child is no longer contagious and may return to school or other activities. Fifth disease is easily spread because the early symptoms during the contagious period are similar to the common cold. The incubation period is typically 1 to 2 weeks. The rash subsides within a week to 10 days. It is important to understand that this virus is contagious only among humans and is not the same form of parvovirus that dogs and cats are vaccinated against. The two are not transferrable between humans and pets.

Fifth disease is diagnosed by the classic appearance of the rash and confirmed with a blood test to identify the human parvovirus B19. As many as 20% of patients with fifth disease are unaware that they have or have had the

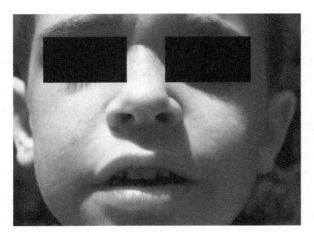

FIGURE 11-5 **"Slapped cheek" appearance associated with fifth disease.** (Courtesy of the CDC Public Health Image Library.)

disease because they have no symptoms but are still contagious. One case of fifth disease provides lifelong immunity. Patients with sickle cell and other forms of anemia may have a more acute illness if they contract fifth disease. These patients do not show the classic signs of the disease, but the anemia becomes more acute, and the patient develops overwhelming weakness. Once the disease has run its course, the anemia begins to correct itself. Treatment is symptomatic, with over-the-counter medications for fever, itching, and occasional joint pain.

Mononucleosis

Infectious **mononucleosis** is caused by the **Epstein-Barr virus** and affects almost everyone at some point. Epstein-Barr is a member of the herpes virus group and is one of the most common viruses to affect humans. Up to 95% of the adult population between the ages of 35 and 50 years in the United States contracts the virus, but many never develop infectious mononucleosis. About half of infected adolescents develop mononucleosis, or "mono," through an infected person's saliva, thus the name "kissing disease."

Symptoms of mononucleosis resemble those of other viral illnesses: low-grade fever, fatigue, sore throat, and swollen lymph glands. In more severe cases, a patient may develop an enlarged spleen and be at a slight risk for rupture of the spleen. For this reason, physicians advise a longer convalescence period, especially for active youth and teenagers.

Adult Viral Diseases

Shingles (Herpes Zoster)

Although **shingles** does not occur in children, there is another condition caused by the varicella-zoster virus (VZV). After exposure, the virus can lie dormant in the body for many years and return later in life as a similar condition known as shingles. Shingles are not transmitted from one person to another. People exposed to VZV do not develop shingles, but if they have never had chickenpox or been vaccinated against it, they could develop chickenpox. Shingles does not usually appear until after age 50 years, and there are about a million cases each year in the United States.

Shingles begins with pain, itching, and tingling along a single nerve pathway where a rash starts and develops into blisters similar to chickenpox. Shingles follows a single nerve and rarely crosses the midline of the body (Fig. 11-6). The blisters scab over in about 5 days and fade away in 2 to 4 weeks. Rarely do shingles have long-lasting effects, but about one in five people with shingles develops severe pain along the path of the rash known as "post-herpetic neuralgia." This complication develops in older adults and tends to be more severe in advanced-aged patients. Patients do not typically have more than one case of shingles in their lifetime, but there are documented cases of patients having a second or third episode.

Antiviral drugs including acyclovir, valacyclovir, and famciclovir given early in the course of the disease can reduce the symptoms and shorten the duration, but the drugs do not cure the virus. Pain relief is also an important part of the treatment for shingles.

Flashpoint

Even though the virus is called herpes zoster, it is not related to the virus that causes genital herpes, the sexually transmitted disease (STD).

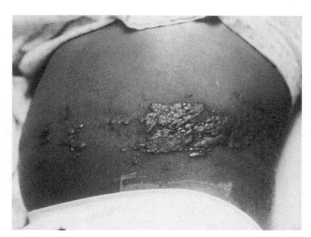

FIGURE 11-6 **Shingles (varicella-zoster infection).** (Courtesy of the CDC Public Health Image Library.)

Herpes Simplex

Herpes simplex virus (HSV) is a common cause of infections of the skin and mucous membranes. HSV has plagued the world for many years because it is one of the most difficult viruses to control. There are two specific strains of the virus: herpes simplex virus 1 (HSV-1), which infects the oral cavity (Fig. 11-7), and herpes simplex virus 2 (HSV-2), which usually attacks the genital area. Both HSV-1 and HSV-2 produce similar signs and symptoms, but they can vary greatly in severity in the areas of the body that they attack. Many people have little or no symptoms of the infection, but what typically occurs is an outbreak of blisters. Although those on the mouth and lips are called "fever blisters" or "cold sores," they are not due to fevers or colds.

HSV-1 can be transmitted by kissing and by casual contact because the virus can live on inanimate objects for up to 4 hours. For this reason, it is advisable not to drink from the same glass after someone with an active fever blister. The first topical antiviral medication for cold sores, penciclovir (Denavir), heals the lesion an average of 1 day quicker than without treatment, and it provides pain relief. There are over-the-counter medications that advertise cold sore healing, but they do not contain antiviral properties. HSV-2 is discussed later in this chapter.

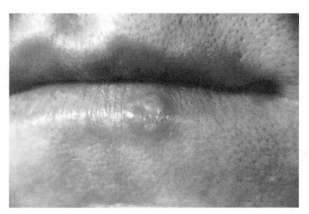

FIGURE 11-7 **Fever blister or cold sore caused by infection with herpes simplex virus 1.** (Courtesy of Dr. Herrmann, the CDC Public Health Image Library.)

Influenza

Influenza, or flu, is an acute respiratory disease caused by one of many viruses that can affect both children and adults. An influenza infection may be mild or severe enough to cause death. Annually, an average 35,000 people die of influenza in the United States. Each year, an influenza vaccine is made available for those who may be at high risk for developing influenza, such as the elderly, the very young, and those with a compromised immune system. Even people who are not considered high risk may choose to take the vaccine in order to avoid an illness that may lead to complications, hospitalization, and possibly life-threatening illnesses. Symptoms of influenza usually appear rapidly, unlike similar cold symptoms that appear gradually, and influenza symptoms include fever, headache, sore throat, cough, and generalized weakness. Digestive symptoms such as nausea, vomiting, and diarrhea may also affect those with influenza. Although influenza is a viral illness, complications may include secondary bacterial infections such as pneumonia and ear or sinus infections, and it may also complicate the person's chronic diseases, such as diabetes, congestive heart failure, and asthma. Dehydration is a common complication of influenza in children and adults.

STOP, THINK, AND LEARN.
Have you had a "flu shot" in the past 5 years? What are the advantages of getting the shot? Are there disadvantages?

Transmission of influenza is by droplet contamination from the coughs and sneezes of those infected as well as from direct contact with these secretions. Many people are contagious as much as a day before they have symptoms, which may increase the transmission of the disease to others unknowingly. This contagious period lasts for up to a week after the first symptoms appear. Anyone who develops influenza should stay home from school or work until he or she is no longer contagious to prevent transmission to others. Infection control practices should include covering your mouth and nose when sneezing or coughing, frequent hand washing with soap, water, and friction, as well as not touching your mouth, eyes, or nose. Alcohol-based hand sanitizers are effective in decreasing transmission when used frequently and properly. Influenza is a viral illness, and it is not treatable with antibiotics unless a secondary bacterial infection develops. There are antiviral drugs that may reduce the symptoms and prevent transmission if they are started within the first 48 hours of the illness. The best method to avoid influenza is by taking the flu vaccine that is offered yearly beginning in the fall (Fig. 11-8). Despite the fact that there are many strains of the influenza virus, the vaccine that is offered each year protects against the three most common strains that cause most cases. The CDC offers the ***"Take Three" challenge*** for prevention of influenza: (1) Take time to get a flu vaccine, (2) take daily preventive actions, and (3) take antiviral flu medications if ordered by your physician. Influenza is a serious contagious disease and should never be taken lightly.

Flashpoint

Protecting yourself by taking an influenza vaccine each year is especially important for healthcare workers.

Hepatitis

Hepatitis is a viral inflammation of the liver caused by toxins, some drugs, heavy alcohol usage, and other bacterial and viral illnesses. Although there are five types of hepatitis, healthcare workers should be most concerned about

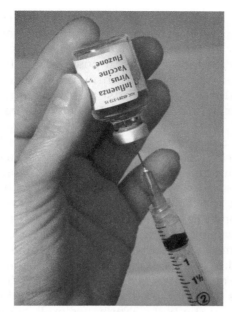

FIGURE 11-8 **Influenza vaccine being withdrawn from a vial.** (Courtesy of Jim Gathany, CDC Public Health Image Library.)

types A, B, and C. Contracting hepatitis in the workplace is a much larger threat to healthcare workers than is contracting HIV. Many of the transmission modes, symptoms, and treatments are the same for all types of hepatitis. Symptoms of all types of acute hepatitis include fever, fatigue, joint pain, loss of appetite, nausea, vomiting, and diarrhea. Because these symptoms are vague and not specific to hepatitis, more classic signs to look for are jaundice and clay-colored bowel movements.

Hepatitis A (HAV) is a form of the disease that is transmitted through fecal matter from close personal contact with an infected person, including sexual contact or the ingestion of contaminated food and drink. Those at risk of developing hepatitis A are those who travel to high-risk areas or have contact with infected persons. The incubation period averages 28 days, but symptoms may show up as early as 2 weeks after exposure or as late as 6 weeks later. People who develop hepatitis A typically recover with supportive care and suffer no long-term liver damage. A vaccination for hepatitis A is available for those at high risk.

Hepatitis B (HBV) remains a major threat to healthcare workers. Transmission is by needlesticks or other sharps injuries, sexual contact with an infected person, sharing needles with a known infected person, and by birth to an infected mother. Any contact with infectious blood or body fluids may put someone at risk for infection. The incubation period for hepatitis B is much longer than for other forms of the disease. The average time from exposure to infection is 4 months, with a minimum of 6 weeks to a maximum of 5 months. The acute phase of hepatitis B is treated symptomatically, and most patients recover without liver damage; however, approximately 2000 to 4000 people die annually from HBV-related illnesses. There are close to a million people who suffer from the chronic form of HBV, and they are monitored closely for signs of liver damage. Many of these patients are treated with antiviral drugs in an effort to lessen the chronic damage to the liver. Vaccinations for HBV are now included in the standard childhood immunization schedule, and those people who did not receive it as an infant are encouraged to obtain the series of three injections over a 6-month period. All healthcare students are strongly encouraged to be vaccinated prior to any clinical experiences and to follow up with post-vaccination testing to confirm immune status. Vaccination is not currently mandatory; however, those not wishing to receive the injections must sign a declination statement (included in the *Instructor Resource* guide). Accidents happen, and it is best to be prepared.

Hepatitis C (HCV) is transmitted through contact with blood from an infected person through sharing contaminated needles or, less commonly, through sexual contact, birth from an infected mother, or needle and other sharps injuries. HCV rarely presents as an acute illness, but rather it develops in the form of cirrhosis or liver cancer in 75% to 85% of patients diagnosed. From exposure to any symptoms, the incubation period may be 2 weeks up to 6 months, averaging 6 weeks. Patients with HCV often demonstrate little or no distinguishable symptoms in the early stages. Symptomatic treatment is recommended for those who develop symptoms. There is currently no HCV vaccine.

Two additional forms of hepatitis are hepatitis D (HDV) and hepatitis E (HEV). HDV is a serious form of liver disease, but it requires the presence of HBV to become active in the body. Transmission is similar to HBV by exposure to infected blood and body fluids. HDV is relatively uncommon in the United States, and there is no vaccination for this form. HEV usually produces an acute illness but no chronic disease. There are very few cases of HEV in the United States, but it is a common problem in countries with poor sanitation and contaminated food and water supplies. HEV is transmitted through fecal matter in the water supply. There is no vaccine available for HEV.

Flashpoint

As a healthcare worker, the average risk of contracting hepatitis B from a needlestick is 6%–30%. The risk of contracting HIV from a needlestick is 0.3%.

Tuberculosis

Caused by the bacteria *Mycobacterium tuberculosis*, **tuberculosis (TB)** typically affects the lungs, but it can attack the brain, the spinal cord, and the kidneys. The infecting organism attacks the body and slowly destroys the healthy tissues, even creating holes in the lungs. Tuberculosis is spread when an infected person coughs, sneezes, or speaks in close proximity to another person. The bacteria can stay in the air for hours, depending on the environment. Once inhaled, the bacteria settle into the lungs and start to grow and multiply, making this newly infected person capable of spreading the disease as well. In a healthy person, the body can stop the *M. tuberculosis* from growing; however, it will remain in the body and can become active later in life. This is known as latent TB infection (Table 11-1). A person who has latent TB infection does not exhibit the usual signs and symptoms of the active disease—coughing, fatigue, chest pain, and night sweats—and cannot spread the disease to others. These people may never develop a full case of TB, but they will always have a reaction to a PPD (purified protein derivative) skin test. TB in organs such as the kidneys and brain is not contagious. The people at high risk of contracting TB from an infected person are those that live, go to school, and work with that person. Diagnosis of TB includes a chest x-ray to look for the appearance of lesions within the lungs and a sputum smear or culture to isolate the *M. tuberculosis* organism.

There is treatment available for TB that includes a medication regimen of several different drugs to combat the bacteria. It is necessary to use a

TABLE 11-1
ACTIVE VERSUS LATENT TUBERCULOSIS

A Person with Latent TB Infection	A Person with Active TB Disease
Does not feel sick	Usually feels sick
Has no symptoms	Has symptoms that may include: • a bad cough that lasts 3 weeks or longer • pain in the chest • coughing up blood or sputum • weakness or fatigue • weight loss • no appetite • chills • fever • sweating at night
Cannot spread TB bacteria to others	May spread TB bacteria to others
Usually has a positive skin test or positive TB blood test	Usually has a positive skin test or positive TB blood test
Has a normal chest x-ray and a negative sputum smear	May have an abnormal chest x-ray or positive sputum smear or culture
Should consider treatment for latent TB infection to prevent active TB disease	Needs treatment for active TB disease

From: Division of Tuberculosis Elimination. Questions and Answers About TB, 2009. CDC website. http://www.cdc.gov/tb/faqs/qa_introduction.htm#Intro4. Modified Feb 10, 2009. Accessed May 12, 2009.

combination of drugs to destroy the bacteria and prevent a recurrence of the disease or a mutation of the bacteria. Failure to complete a prescribed course of therapy can result in an organism that is resistant to the currently available medications. Strains of drug-resistant TB have surfaced in recent years, which have put patients at risk for an untreatable disease that is often fatal. A minimum of 6 months of treatment is necessary to kill the TB bacteria, even though patients often feel better after only a few weeks. A type of treatment known as ***directly observed therapy (DOT)*** can help patients remember to take their medication by meeting with a health professional daily or several times per week.

Each state in the United States has a TB control office charged with the responsibility of monitoring active cases of tuberculosis in an effort to control the number of new cases diagnosed. In the late 1940s, the treatment for TB was discovered, and patients with active disease were often quarantined for the 6 to 9 months of treatment. This led to a decrease in the number of active cases in the United States. According to the CDC, many states "let their guard down and TB control efforts were neglected," which led to a resurgence in the number of active TB cases during the 1980s and 1990s. Once again, there is a significant amount of work toward TB treatment and prevention and a steady decline in the number of new cases. Strains of TB that have become resistant to the primary treatment medications include multidrug-resistant (MDR TB) and extensively drug-resistant (XDR TB) and are monitored closely by the CDC to prevent outbreaks of the more deadly forms of this disease.

Sexually Transmitted Diseases

Herpes Simplex-2

Herpes simplex-2 *(HSV-2)* is transmitted through sexual contact, often without either partner being aware of the infection. When a patient contracts HSV-2, blisters appear on the genital region that break open and leave painful ulcers or sores that can take up to 4 weeks to heal. This primary outbreak is more severe than any recurring episodes, which may occur weeks or months after the initial outbreak. HSV can live dormant in the body indefinitely, and acute outbreaks tend to decrease over time.

Research indicates that genital herpes affects about 45 million or 1 in 5 people ages 12 and over in the United States. It is more common in women, possibly due to the male-to-female transmission rather than female-to-male.

Transmission of the disease results from the release of the virus from the open sores of an outbreak during sexual contact; however, it is still possible to transmit the disease through the skin when there are no blister lesions present. It is possible that a person is unaware that he or she has HSV-2. There is about a 2-week window after exposure in which no signs appear, followed by the possibility of flu-like symptoms, blisters, fever, and swollen lymph glands. Others may mistake the disease for insect bites and be unaware of the infection. When blisters break out, they last about 2 weeks. HSV-2 reoccurs more often than HSV-1, and 90% of those with HSV-2 have a reoccurrence within the first year of the primary outbreak. Many patients experience pre-outbreak symptoms, including flu-like discomfort, nerve pain, itching or tingling, lower abdominal pain, and urinary difficulties. Women often develop a yeast infection prior to or with the eruption of the blisters. These pre-outbreak symptoms are known as a prodrome and may last from several hours to several days and end with the blister formation.

People infected with HSV often suffer psychological distress in addition to the painful outbreaks. In one study, 82% of patients with HSV-2 had symptoms of depression and worried about rejection. It is a very humiliating experience for those diagnosed with HSV-2 to notify all past and present sexual partners. Pregnant women who develop a new infection of HSV during late pregnancy risk transmission of the disease to their unborn child. Most physicians deliver the infant by cesarean section if the mother has an active outbreak of HSV at full term.

HSV is diagnosed by visual exam if there is an active outbreak; otherwise, the physician must rely on the results of a blood test that detects antibodies to the HSV infection.

There is no cure for HSV, but treatment can relieve many of the symptoms. Over-the-counter pain medicines can provide some symptomatic relief, and antiviral medications can shorten the duration and severity of an outbreak. These antiviral medications include acyclovir (Zovirax), famciclovir (Famvir), and valacyclovir (Valtrex), all of which are available in oral form. Famvir and Valtrex are more easily absorbed by the stomach and can be taken less often than Zovirax. There is an intravenous form of these medications that can be given in severe cases of genital herpes or for infants with the virus.

Chlamydia

Chlamydia is the most commonly reported sexually transmitted disease (STD). It is caused by the bacteria *Chlamydia trachamotis*. The danger of this STD is the damage that it can cause to a woman's reproductive organs, possibly resulting in infertility. Because there may be no symptoms, the damage can be done before the woman is aware of the disease. A moderate estimate of the number of chlamydia cases in the United States is over 2 million. Chlamydia is transmitted during sexual contact, and unless all partners are treated, the disease can be passed back and forth, each time increasing the chance for internal organ damage. Chlamydia can be transmitted to a newborn from the mother during childbirth.

In 75% of infected women and 50% of infected men, symptoms do not appear, giving the disease the title of the "silent STD." Symptoms that do appear are typically 1 to 3 weeks after exposure and include an abnormal discharge and urinary difficulties. As the disease progresses in women, abdominal and lower back pain develops, along with abnormal bleeding between menstrual periods.

Treatment for chlamydia must include all exposed sexual partners and includes a single dose of azithromycin or a week of twice-daily doxycycline. To prevent a reinfection, it is imperative to abstain from sexual intercourse until both partners have completed treatment. Latex condoms, used consistently and correctly, can reduce the transmission of chlamydia; however, the only unquestionable method to prevent the disease is abstinence or commitment to a long-term monogamous relationship with an unaffected partner.

Gonorrhea

Caused by the bacterium *Neisseria gonorrhoeae*, this STD thrives in the warm, moist reproductive tract of men and women. **Gonorrhea** is spread through sexual contact and from mother to baby during birth. Gonorrhea can also survive in the eyes, mouth, and throat. It is a common sexually transmitted disease, with reports of over 700,000 new cases reported each year, primarily in sexually active teenagers, young adults, and African Americans. It is possible to contract gonorrhea after completing treatment by having unprotected sexual relations with an infected person.

As with chlamydia, many people who contract gonorrhea have no symptoms. Those who do have symptoms usually develop those that resemble a urinary tract infection, such as painful urination, itching, and a yellowish discharge. These symptoms can appear from 2 to 30 days after exposure. Untreated gonorrhea can spread through the body and lead to conjunctivitis (Fig. 11-9) and other problems, such as reproductive organ damage and pelvic inflammatory disease (PID). Women with PID are at higher risk for ectopic or tubal pregnancies. An ectopic pregnancy develops when a fertilized egg begins to grow outside the uterus, usually in the fallopian tube. As the egg grows, it becomes larger than the circumference of the fallopian tube and may rupture and become a life-threatening condition for the mother. Ectopic pregnancies cannot develop into a normal pregnancy.

Treatment of gonorrhea includes a full course of one of several antibiotics. A recent outbreak of drug-resistant strains of gonorrhea has made treatment of gonorrhea more challenging for physicians and patients. Important patient teaching tips should include instructing the patient to take the entire course of antibiotics to assure effectiveness but that even a cure may not reverse any damage caused by the disease. Additionally, many who suffer from gonorrhea also have chlamydia, which requires the addition of another antibiotic. Both partners should complete the entire course of antibiotics to prevent recurrence of both conditions, and they should be tested for other STDs. Prevention of STDs such as gonorrhea is important. Latex condoms, when used correctly and consistently, can provide some level of protection against these diseases.

Flashpoint

The only guaranteed method to prevent any sexually transmitted disease is a monogamous sexual relationship with a partner who is known to be disease-free.

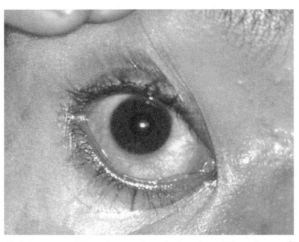

FIGURE 11-9 **Conjunctivitis caused by gonorrhea infection.** (Courtesy of Joe Miller, VD, CDC Public Health Image Library.)

Syphilis

Syphilis is a bacterial sexually transmitted disease caused by the *Treponema pallidum* bacterium. Despite folklore, syphilis is not transmitted from toilet seats, sharing eating utensils, hot tubs, or swimming pools. Transmission of the disease is through direct contact with an open sore, known as a chancre, on the mouth, lips, vagina, anus, or external genital organs, typically during sexual intercourse. Infected pregnant women can pass the disease to their unborn child, which may result in a stillborn infant or one who dies shortly after birth.

Syphilis has three distinct phases, although symptoms are vague and may resemble those of other diseases. For this reason, the CDC has dubbed syphilis as "the great imitator."

The first phase of syphilis, or the primary stage, begins with one or more visible chancre sores at the spot where the syphilis entered the body. The lesion is round, firm, and painless and lasts from 3 to 6 weeks. The chancre fades away without treatment; however, if the disease is untreated, advancement to the secondary phase is likely.

The secondary stage of syphilis may begin with lesions on the mucous membranes or a skin rash. The skin rash may appear on any area of the body, similar to many other disease rashes, or appear as rough, reddish brown spots on the palms and the bottom of the feet (Fig. 11-10). The rash does not itch, and it may be so faint that it is not obvious. The patient may experience swollen lymph nodes, headaches, hair loss, weight loss, and generalized fatigue, which can also be the symptoms of many other diseases. A thorough patient history and physical exam may help the physician correctly diagnose the patient. These symptoms, too, can disappear without treatment, but the disease will continue to damage the body and will progress to the latent phase.

A patient with untreated syphilis can progress into the latent phase of the disease after all signs and symptoms have disappeared. The disease remains in the body, and the patient is contagious. Without treatment, syphilis progresses to the late stage, and damage begins to occur in the internal organs. Most organ systems in latent syphilis are affected, including the nervous system, cardiovascular system, and the musculoskeletal system. Brain damage robs the

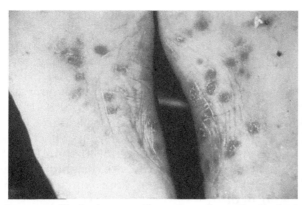

FIGURE 11-10 **Secondary syphilis lesions on the soles of a patient's feet.** (Courtesy of Dr. Gavin Hart, CDC Public Health Image Library.)

infected person of the ability to move and communicate effectively and diminishes his or her sight. The damage from syphilis can be deadly.

The ulcers produced by syphilis in the genital areas can spread the disease when exposed during sexual activity. The risk can be reduced with the correct and diligent use of a latex condom. Latex condoms that contain spermicidal creams are no more effective than plain condoms. Douching, urinating, and washing the genitals after sexual activity do not prevent the transmission of syphilis.

Syphilis is easily diagnosed with a blood test to determine if antibodies are present. Because syphilis is dangerous to the developing fetus, pregnant women should be tested at the first prenatal visit. Once a person has had syphilis, the antibodies may remain in the blood for months or years even after the disease is cured.

Someone who has been diagnosed with syphilis and who has had it for less than a year can be cured with a single injection of penicillin, and multiple doses are given those who have had the disease longer. Those allergic to penicillin can be treated with another antibiotic. Curing syphilis cannot reverse any damage caused by the disease prior to diagnosis. Persons who are at risk for sexually transmitted diseases must be tested often to prevent recurrent episodes of syphilis.

 STOP, THINK, AND LEARN.
Do you think that STD education should be taught in public and private schools (K–12)? If so, in which grade level should it be taught? If not, where do you think children should learn about STDs?

Human Papillomavirus

Human papillomavirus (HPV) is the most commonly transmitted sexual infection. It is likely that someone infected with one of the 40 or more strains of HPV may not know that he or she has the disease, as there are no outward symptoms in the early stages of the disease. HPV infects the skin and mucous membranes in the genital regions of men and women. Some forms of the HPV cause genital warts to appear whereas other forms cause genital cancers, including cervical cancer. The forms of the virus can be termed "low risk" for those causing warts or "high risk" for those causing cancers. The strains of HPV that cause the warts are not the same as the cancer-causing strains. Interestingly enough, according to the CDC, in 90% of cases, a healthy person's immune system can rid the body of both "low risk" and "high risk" HPV within 2 years.

In people who develop symptoms, wart-like growths appear in and around their genital regions. The lesions appear as flat or rounded bumps, and they may be single lesions or in groups of wart-like projections. These warts may appear within weeks or months after exposure to an infected person, and they may continue to enlarge or decrease in size and, in some instances, may disappear completely. Regardless of the number, size, or shape of these warts, they do not develop into an HPV-related cancer. Approximately 10% of women who develop the high-risk form of HPV harbor the virus for many years and are more susceptible to developing cervical cancer.

Prevention of the four types of HPV that cause warts and cervical cancer is available now through a series of vaccinations. There are two licensed HPV vaccines, Gardasil and Cervarix, available to protect against the types of HPV infection that cause most cervical cancers. Gardasil was licensed for use in females, age 9 to 26 years, in June 2006 and for males, age 9 to 26 years, in October 2009. Cervarix was licensed for use in females, age 10 to 25 years, in October 2009.

The vaccine is recommended for girls aged 11 and 12 and older girls through age 26 who did not receive the vaccination series when they were younger. The vaccine series is given over a 6-month period, with the second vaccine 2 months after the initial dose and the third at 6 months. Currently, the vaccine is thought to last for a minimum of 5 years, with the possibility of a booster near the end of that time.

While there is no standard treatment for HPV, if warts appear, they can be treated at home with topical medications prescribed by a physician or through procedures in the physician's office, including cryosurgery (freezing), electrocautery (burning), or the application of an acid solution. Many people affected with the warts forego treatment to see if they disappear spontaneously. Treatment for cervical cancer caused by HPV may include surgery, radiation, or chemotherapy as soon as possible after diagnosis. Regular Pap smear examinations may help prevent HPV cancers.

Human Immunodeficiency Virus

The **human immunodeficiency virus (HIV)** is unlike most viruses because rather than attack the body itself, it attacks a person's immune system and destroys the white blood cells the body uses to fight infections. HIV is the virus that causes acquired immunodeficiency syndrome (AIDS). Through extensive research, the first known case of HIV in a human was discovered in a man from the Republic of Congo in 1959. Theory suggests that the virus was present in a type of chimpanzee in the African jungles and was possibly spread to humans through hunting and exposure to the infected blood. The virus spread slowly through the African continent and then to other parts of the world. The discovery of this virus in the United States in 1981 revealed a significant number of cases in a population of homosexual men who developed a unique cancer known as Kaposi sarcoma. Researchers worked for several years to identify the virus and understand its transmission and methods of prevention. The development of a blood test for HIV led to prevention education for high-risk people. The CDC closely monitored the infection rate and focused much of their attention on high-risk groups. Work continued on diagnosis and treatment for patients infected with HIV. By 1996, there was a decrease in the number of newly diagnosed cases of HIV likely due to the development of medications to control the progression of the virus.

Recent statistics from the CDC indicate that newly diagnosed cases of HIV infection average 55,000 per year. More than 1 million patients in the United States are infected with HIV or have developed *acquired immunodeficiency syndrome (AIDS)*, with as many as 250,000 of those unaware of the infection. Those who do not know they are infected put themselves and others at high risk of contracting and transmitting the disease.

HIV cannot survive for a long period outside the body and is therefore transmitted only through three primary activities: sex (oral, vaginal, anal) with an infected person, sharing needles or syringes with an infected person, and through the delivery or breastfeeding of an infant from an infected mother. Although HIV is transmitted through blood, Red Cross and other donations in the United States have been tested thoroughly since 1985 and are considered safe for transfusion.

Acquired Immunodeficiency Syndrome

AIDS is the end stage of an HIV infection and occurs whether or not a person receives treatment during the course of the infection. There are AIDS-specific diseases and cancers that indicate the body has entered the final stages of the disease. Laboratory testing reveals a very low number of CD4 cells, the white blood cells that play the most important part in a person's immunity. Many variables determine the amount of time from HIV infection to AIDS. Early treatment allows many people infected with HIV to live for years without the development of AIDS and related illnesses while some have a more rapid progression from the virus to the disease.

The only absolute way to determine if you are infected with HIV is to be tested at a legitimate laboratory. It is possible to be tested anonymously at some locations where you receive a number or code with which to get your results. Prior to testing, a health professional is available to provide you with counseling regarding the confidential test and results.

Advanced treatment modalities have added years to the lives of those who are infected with HIV or who have developed AIDS. It is extremely important that those affected find a physician who is well versed in the care of HIV/AIDS patients and follow his or her specific guidelines. Keeping appointments and taking medications as directed are central to a healthier life. Adopting a healthy lifestyle by eating nourishing foods to keep up strength and weight, exercising, and getting enough rest increases both the quality and length of life for patients.

Immunizations

Are They Safe?

Eradication of many deadly diseases in our country is the result of stringent vaccination practices that make continued comprehensive immunization programs a high priority. There are no longer the outbreaks of pertussis (whooping cough),

Flashpoint
HIV is a very fragile virus and is not transmitted through casual contact such as shaking hands, hugging, sitting on a toilet seat, or drinking from a water fountain.

Flashpoint
Every 9½ minutes, someone in the United States is infected with HIV.

Flashpoint
Donating blood is a safe, simple, and life-saving procedure.

diphtheria, or smallpox that once plagued our nation. Measles and mumps are no longer common childhood diseases. Polio no longer threatens children in our country.

While most parents routinely take their children for immunizations, there are those who no longer take vaccinations simply on the recommendation of his or her physician. The decision not to have children immunized can be the result of a parent's religious or philosophical beliefs. Why should children be vaccinated against diseases that are no longer a threat? Some parents do not believe that the government should interfere with raising their children by mandating regular immunizations. Many parents are frightened by recent studies that appeared to erroneously link vaccinations with autism and other diseases. The CDC attempts to demystify many myths associated with vaccinations. Many people think that diseases began to disappear before vaccinations were developed because of better sanitation practices, discovery of antibiotics, and a healthier lifestyle. Living conditions have improved, which may diminish the spread of some diseases, but research shows a clear decrease in these diseases after the development of vaccines. The fact that many people developed the disease after vaccination is another reason some question the integrity of vaccines. No vaccine is 100% effective, and there will always be some people who do not convert to immune status, which is fully expected in any vaccination series. Adverse side effects and tragic conditions, including sudden infant death syndrome and neurological catastrophes, weigh heavy on the minds of parents with healthy children.

In recent years, the CDC has worked closely with vaccine manufacturers to improve the quality of the medications. Today's vaccines meet the highest standards of quality and are closely monitored to maintain the safety of those receiving the injections. Thimerosal, which is a mercury-based preservative, was included in most vaccines until research found a possible link to mercury and many vaccination-related complications. In 2001, the American Academy of Pediatrics, together with the vaccine manufacturers, agreed that thimerosal should be eliminated as a preservative in the vaccines. Today, with the exception of some of the influenza vaccines, it has been removed from all routine childhood vaccines. Those still containing thimerosal contain only trace amounts. The manufacturers continually monitor the quality and safety of the vaccines to decrease the potential for adverse reactions or harmful side effects.

Some people believe increased exposure to thimerosal (from the addition of important new vaccines recommended for children) explains the higher prevalence of autism in children in recent years. However, evidence from several studies examining trends in vaccine use and changes in autism frequency does not support such an association. Furthermore, a scientific review by the Institute of Medicine (IOM) concluded that there is no causal relationship between thimerosal-containing vaccines and autism. The CDC supports the IOM conclusion.

As a healthcare professional, you must provide parents with all of the information available concerning vaccinations so that they may make an informed decision about vaccinating their children. According to the CDC, the risks of not routinely vaccinating children against deadly diseases are much greater than the side effects that may result from the vaccines.

Documentation

Also important in the vaccination process is the documentation of vaccination. Most schools require **proof of vaccinations** or a **declination statement** from parents prior to admission. International travelers may find it necessary to receive and provide documentation of certain immunizations prior to entering countries where specific diseases are prevalent. The CDC provides a comprehensive list of vaccinations recommended before traveling.

Many states are developing or have developed computerized documentation systems to provide a confidential but comprehensive reporting mechanism. At a minimum, such a system should include the date given, the vaccine, manufacturer and lot number, the site of administration, patient/parent education sheets given, and the signature of the person administering the vaccination. Whether computerized or manual, all of the information is crucial to effective monitoring of the vaccinations. Records may be maintained at the physician's office or at local health departments. Some schools maintain the records but only for a specified time period after the child graduates. Parents of children should be encouraged to maintain a secure copy of these and other health documents as most facilities do not keep the documentation for an indefinite period of time. With the evolvement of electronic health records, documentation can be maintained indefinitely. The vaccination schedules located in Appendix D describe each recommended vaccination and the associated time line.

Flashpoint

Many clinical facilities require proof of your immunizations prior to any clinical experiences in your program of study.

Summary

Communicable diseases will remain a threat to the healthcare industry every day. It is up to healthcare workers to protect themselves as well as their patients from transmission of these diseases. Your daily activities in the healthcare setting will include caring for patients with communicable diseases. Understanding the transmission of these diseases and how to protect yourself are paramount in your education and training. Healthcare workers are the first line of defense in preventing the spread of communicable diseases. We should never become complacent in following infection control practices to protect our patients and ourselves.

Practice Exercises

Multiple Choice

1. Which of the following diseases is caused by a virus?

   a. Measles

   b. Strep throat

   c. Mononucleosis

   d. Both a and c

2. A distinguishing sign of rubeola is:

   a. Vesicle-like lesions on the back

   b. Homan sign

   c. Koplik spots

   d. Kalpick spots

3. The classic sign of mumps is:

   a. Swelling of the parotid glands

   b. Orchitis

   c. Swelling of the axillary lymph nodes

   d. A fine red rash over the trunk

4. The most commonly reported sexually transmitted disease is:

   a. Syphilis

   b. Gonorrhea

   c. Herpes simplex I

   d. Chlamydia

5. When the dormant varicella virus appears in adults, it is known as:

   a. Shingles

   b. Syphilis

   c. Herpes simplex II

   d. Rubella

6. The form of hepatitis that is the greatest risk for healthcare providers is:

   a. Hepatitis A

   b. Hepatitis B

   c. Hepatitis C

   d. Hepatitis D

Fill in the Blank

1. The cause of a fever blister is _____.

2. The MMR vaccine offers immunity to measles, mumps, and _____.

3. An untreated fever can lead to _____.

Short Answer

1. **Why is DOT (directly observed therapy) important in the treatment of tuberculosis?**

2. **What makes some parents uneasy about routine vaccinations for their children?**

3. **What is the CDC's "Take Three" challenge as related to influenza?**

INTERNET RESOURCES

Resource	Web Address
Immunization information	http://immunize.org
CDC immunization abbreviations	http://cdc.gov/vaccines/about/terms/vacc-abbrev.htm
Immunization information for travelers	http://cdc.gov/travel/content/vaccinations.aspx
American Academy of Pediatrics	www.aap.org
Institute of Medicine of the National Academies	www.iom.edu

12 HEALTH CARE–ASSOCIATED INFECTIONS

Key Terms

antibiotic-resistant organisms Organisms that cannot be destroyed by antibiotic medications

aspiration Inhaling liquids or other foreign materials into the lungs

broad-spectrum antibiotics Antibiotics that are nontoxic, relatively inexpensive, and able to kill a wide range of bacteria

catheterization Insertion of a plastic tube into a body cavity to drain off or inject liquid

central line An intravenous catheter inserted into the thoracic portion of one of the body's largest veins for delivery of concentrated or long-term medication or intravenous fluids

clean Surgical procedures that do not involve the respiratory, gastrointestinal, or genitourinary systems, such as an orthopedic procedure, and have no break in sterile technique

clean-contaminated Surgical procedures that enter the respiratory, gastrointestinal, or genitourinary systems with no obvious lapses in sterile technique

Learning Outcomes

12.1 Define healthcare-associated infections (HAIs)

12.2 Identify the four major categories of HAIs

12.3 Describe patients who are at a higher risk for developing HAIs

12.4 Discuss costs associated with HAIs

12.5 Identify methods to reduce the number of HAIs

Competencies

CAAHEP
- Define asepsis. (CAAHEP III.C.2)
- Discuss infection control procedures. (CAAHEP III.C.3)
- Compare different methods of controlling the growth of microorganisms. (CAAHEP III.C.6)

ABHES
- Apply principles of aseptic techniques and infection control. (ABHES 9.b)
- Use standard precautions. (ABHES 9.i)
- Practice quality control. (ABHES 10.a)

Patients entering a healthcare facility do so for treatment of a current condition and do not expect to become sick with an infection acquired during the encounter. However, as many as 1.7 million patients—equivalent to 4.5 out of 100 patients in healthcare facilities—acquire such an infection each year, with a mortality rate of 99,000 patients, or 5.8%. Once called a "hospital-acquired" or **nosocomial** infection, terminology has changed to include all other healthcare venues because infections have been diagnosed after encounters at nursing homes, dialysis clinics, outpatient surgery centers, and home health visits. The term **health care–associated infection (HAI)** addresses all infections and all facilities. Studies have suggested that as many as 5% of hospitalized patients developed an infection during their stay, and up to 8% of those undergoing invasive procedures are affected.

The definition of HAI is an infection that a patient develops within 48 to 72 hours of admission to a healthcare facility that was not present or incubating on admission. Infections occurring later in a lengthy hospital stay may also be considered HAIs if they meet criteria described.

The costs associated with HAIs in the United States are $28.4–$33.8 billion per year, with the cost of an average stay for a patient with an HAI of $185,000 compared with $32,000 for a patient without such an infection (Fig. 12-1). Prevention of these infections can cost $5.7–$21.5 billion, an amount that although large is still a significant savings to the healthcare industry and result in an improvement in patient care, as well (Fig. 12-2). Research indicates that 70% of these infections are preventable with proper care and treatment.

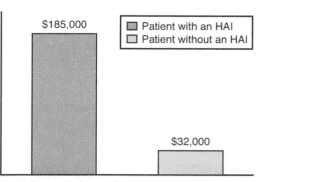

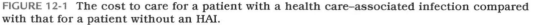

FIGURE 12-1 The cost to care for a patient with a health care–associated infection compared with that for a patient without an HAI.

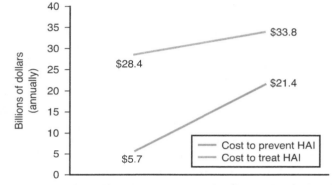

FIGURE 12-2 The cost to treat versus the cost to prevent HAIs.

STOP, THINK, AND LEARN.

What is the impact of increased patient care costs due to HAIs on the healthcare facility? On the patient? On a patient's insurance company? On the healthcare consumer?

HAIs are the result of many factors, such as compromised immune systems in patients, newly discovered microorganisms, and increasing **resistance** to antibiotics. Resistance is a person's natural ability to resist microorganisms or toxins that are produced in disease. A person can also build up a resistance to antibiotics, which makes the antibiotics ineffective in fighting disease. The bacteria that often cause a healthcare-associated infection come from the patient's own body. Other bacteria are introduced to the patient through **cross-contamination** from healthcare personnel, instruments, or the environment. As hospital stays are shorter now, many patients do not realize they have an infection until they are at home. HAIs lengthen hospital stays and costs and can increase a patient's emotional distress because they must deal with the acquired infection as well as the initial illness.

Patients with **compromised immune systems,** or immune systems that do not function at full capacity due to illness or disease, are at higher risk of developing an HAI. Healthcare factors that increase the possibility of HAIs are invasive techniques and medical devices that are inserted through the patient's first

Key Terms—cont'd

closed drainage system A catheterization system that does not have a continuous opening, such as a Foley catheter system

colonized Overgrown with foreign organisms that have settled into a body area without causing disease

compromised immune system The weakening of resistance to disease that occurs when the body's protective system is not functioning at full capacity due to illness or medication

contaminated Surgical procedures that include gross spillage from the gastrointestinal tract, entry into the biliary or urinary systems when there is infected bile or urine, and major breaks in sterile technique

cross-contamination Spreading germs by reusing dirty equipment or supplies and not washing your hands between procedures with different patients

E. coli Escherichia coli is a normal flora organism in the gastrointestinal system, but it is the primary cause of urinary tract infections

Continued

Flashpoint

You can play a significant role in the prevention of HAIs by following all infection control guidelines set by your healthcare facility.

line of defense, the skin. Other devices include tubes inserted through orifices such as the airway or the bladder. Each of these devices allows bacteria to enter the body and the bloodstream, which can potentially cause an infection. The possibility of an infection increases each day the device is in place. Healthcare workers must be cognizant of this possibility and take all measures to prevent an infection. Prevention includes sufficient hand washing or alcohol-based sanitization and general attention to detail when inserting devices into the skin or a body orifice. This chapter discusses the four most common HAIs.

Flashpoint

Washing your hands often and well is the best way to prevent healthcare-associated infections.

Catheter-Associated Urinary Tract Infections

The most common HAI is a *urinary tract infection (UTI),* which accounts for 32% of all infections. The origins of 65% to 85% of these infections are from the actual *catheterization* procedure, and the development of an infection may depend on how long the catheter remains in place in the patient. Catheterization is the process of placing a urinary catheter, a plastic tube, into a patient's bladder through the urethra, which connects the urinary bladder to the genitals for the removal of urine. The urinary catheter tube is slid gently through the urethral tube to drain urine freely from the bladder for collection or to inject liquids used for treatment or diagnosis of bladder conditions. Urinary catheters are needed when the patient's bladder muscle has lost the ability to contract enough to completely empty the bladder, when bladder function is compromised after surgery, and when patients are born with a disease that affects the function of their bladder. Daily manipulations in cleaning and draining the catheter increase the chance of bacterial invasion into the body. Most urinary catheters have a *closed drainage system* in which the catheter remains in the patient for a few days to a few months and continually drains into a collection bag. The catheter attaches to a collection bag, which is emptied by opening a valve found at the bottom of the bag. Infection occurs with the improper drainage of this closed system when microorganisms enter the drainage system and make their way to the patient. In an *open drainage system,* the catheter is inserted into the patient for just a few minutes to drain the bladder when the bladder is full. When the bladder is empty, the catheter is removed and is not inserted again until the bladder is full. The urine drains into a collection device that is then emptied into the toilet for disposal. The infection rate soars to 100% after the fourth continuous day of catheterization. Elderly, debilitated, and postpartum patients are the most susceptible to HAIs of the urinary tract.

Bacteria can enter the bladder on the outside of the catheter, suggesting non-sterile supplies or procedure. Bacteria can also migrate along the outside of the catheter once inserted or through the inner lumen, or inner passageway, of the catheter after the tract has been contaminated during the drainage process (Fig. 12-3).

Key Terms—cont'd

half-life The amount of time that the body takes to metabolize or eliminate one-half of a medication dosage

health care–associated infection (HAI) An infection that a patient develops within 48 to 72 hours of admission to a healthcare facility that was not present or incubating when he or she entered the facility

Flashpoint

All patients who have catheters with open drainage systems for more than 4 days straight get a urinary tract infection!

 STOP, THINK, AND LEARN.
What signs and symptoms would you expect in a patient who has developed a urinary tract infection?

The organisms that are primarily responsible for UTIs are those that reside as normal flora in the gastrointestinal system—*Escherichia coli* **(E. coli)** and

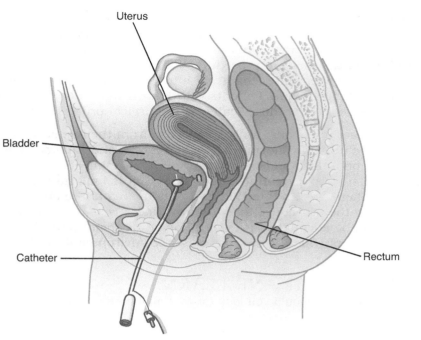

Uterus

Bladder

Catheter

Rectum

FIGURE 12-3 **A urinary catheter in place in a female.**

Enterococcus—or other microorganisms, including *Proteus, Klebsiella,* and *Pseudomonas.* An infection due to these organisms suggests **cross-contamination** by healthcare personnel or exposure to contaminated equipment or nonsterile technique and supplies. UTIs due to bacteria other than those found in the gastrointestinal tract suggest contamination from an outside source. In otherwise healthy patients, the UTI may resolve with the removal of the catheter, but those who are in a compromised state of health can develop significant secondary infections in the urogenital tract such as kidney disease or pelvic inflammatory disease (PID).

Surgical Site Infections

A **surgical site infection (SSI)** is classified as "incisional," indicating the infection has developed in the superficial layers of the skin and subcutaneous tissue, or as organ or body cavity manipulation, a deeper and much more dangerous infection. Morbidity increases significantly in these deeper infections. Patients are classified prior to surgery as clean, clean-contaminated, contaminated, or infected, which alerts operating room personnel to any preexisting conditions that increase the possibility of an SSI.

- **Clean** cases are those that do not involve the respiratory, gastrointestinal, or genitourinary systems, such as an orthopedic procedure, and have no break in sterile technique.
- **Clean-contaminated** are those procedures that enter the respiratory, gastrointestinal, or genitourinary systems, but there are no obvious lapses in sterile technique.

- **Contaminated** are those cases that involve spillage of gastrointestinal contents into the wound, entry into the biliary or urinary systems in the presence of infected bile or urine, and major breaks in sterile technique.
- **Infected or dirty** cases are procedures for major traumatic injuries, excess leakage from the gastrointestinal tract into the wound, and significant breaks in sterile technique. Patients with known wound or other infections are also classified in the "dirty" category of surgical procedures.

Like urinary tract infections, an SSI can arise from the bacteria on the patient's skin, including two forms of *Staphylococcus* and *Enterococcus*. SSIs caused by other organisms indicate that bacteria were introduced from an external source, such as personnel or equipment. It is important to note before a surgery if a patient has an infection in a remote area of the body that may proliferate during the procedure to involve the operative site. It is essential that the surgical team be adequately prepared, including themselves, the equipment, and the patient, to provide the cleanest possible environment for the procedure.

STOP, THINK, AND LEARN.
What symptoms would you look for that might indicate an SSI? What would you expect the incision to look like?

Patients at risk for SSIs are those with chronic medical conditions, preoperative steroid use, obesity, or malnutrition. Nonsterile technique or using nonsterile instruments before, during, or immediately after a surgical procedure can put a patient at high risk for an SSI. Not as common but equally dangerous is an object left in a body cavity after surgery. Items used in surgery such as needles, sponges, and instruments may sometimes be left in the patient after the surgical procedure. Infection may occur quickly after surgery or may not show up for years. Surgical team members perform what is called a "count" at the beginning of a surgical procedure and at the end to ensure that all of the surgical instruments and supplies are accounted for. The goal of this process is to decrease the risk of infection to patients. Hospital stays have become shorter, and many procedures are being performed on an outpatient basis. This expediency may be the cause of increasing rates of SSIs.

Before some surgical procedures, a physician may order prophylactic or preventive antibiotics. Although effective in most cases, it is possible for an SSI to develop if the infecting organism is not sensitive to that antibiotic. It is advantageous to provide optimal antibiotic coverage for patients undergoing complicated or lengthy procedures as these risk factors increase the possibility of an SSI. **Broad-spectrum antibiotics** are effective against a wide range of infectious organisms, are relatively inexpensive but effective, have a low toxicity level, and should be given initially within 30 minutes of the initial incision and again during the procedure if the procedure lasts longer than the **half-life** of the antibiotic. Half-life is the time it takes for one-half of the medication to be excreted from the body. If a medication is said to have a half-life of 4 hours, then it takes the body 4 hours to process one-half of the dose of the medication and excrete it from the body. For this same medication, it would take the body 8 hours to metabolize and excrete the full dose of medication.

Antibiotic use after surgery is not always necessary. In an effort to prevent the further development of **antibiotic-resistant organisms,** organisms that become resistant to antibiotics over time, the antibiotics should be discontinued within 24 hours of the end of the procedure. When administered according to the guidelines of Centers for Disease Control and Prevention (CDC) and the

Flashpoint

The half-life of a medication is the amount of time that the body takes to metabolize or eliminate one-half of the dose of medication.

Center for Medicare and Medicaid Services (CMS), prophylactic antibiotics may decrease the incidence of SSIs by 40% to 80%.

Patients with chronic medical conditions, such as diabetes, present an additional risk for the development of an SSI. Close monitoring and control of the patient's blood glucose levels during the procedure may decrease their increased risk. Providing supplemental oxygen during the procedure may also be beneficial.

Central Line–Associated Bloodstream Infections

A *central line* is an extended-length intravenous catheter passed into a large vein, usually the subclavian or jugular vein (Fig. 12-4). A central line is used to deliver concentrated medications short term when venous access is limited or long term when a patient requires extended medication therapy. Central lines are also used for specialized blood pressure and cardiac output monitoring. Patients requiring this monitoring are typically hospitalized in an intensive care unit, and the monitoring also presents special risk factors for the development of an HAI. These risk factors include the underlying condition, compromised immune system, and the use of other invasive devices.

Similar to the way bacteria enter the urinary bladder on and through a catheter, bacteria can enter the bloodstream directly via the central line catheter. Insertion of the catheter requires sterile technique and requires care for the insertion site for the length of time the catheter remains in place. Patients may go home with the central line in place, which makes patient education on proper care of the line an important issue.

Ventilator-Associated Pneumonia

A patient requiring artificial respiration with the aid of a *ventilator* is at risk for developing an HAI. A ventilator is a machine that mechanically helps patients breathe by assisting with the exchange of oxygen and carbon dioxide, a

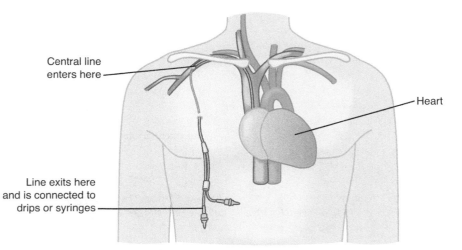

FIGURE 12-4 **Placement of a central line.**

basic component of breathing. The patient is connected to the ventilator through tubing. An endotracheal tube is a flexible plastic tube that is passed through the patient's mouth into the trachea. An inflatable bulb on the lower portion of the tube prevents air from escaping back through the patient's mouth or nose (Fig. 12-5). The endotracheal tube is attached to other tubing that connects to the ventilator. As with the central line–associated bloodstream infections, a patient on a ventilator has underlying chronic diseases or respiratory failure that makes him or her susceptible to development of an infection. There is a correlation between the development of an infection and the length of time a patient is on the ventilator.

Aspiration of gastric contents, inability to clear pulmonary secretions, and immobility are causes of pneumonia in a ventilated patient. Aspiration may occur when stomach contents move into the respiratory tract when the patient inhales, or breathes in. Measures to prevent pneumonia include keeping the patient in a semireclining position; pulmonary hygiene, such as cleaning the patient's mouth; changing the pulmonary tubing at regular intervals; keeping the pulmonary equipment clean and functioning; and changing the patient's position as frequently as possible. Patients who must remain immobile present a special risk for an infection. When intubating the patient, an oral approach is preferable over the nasal route, as the nose may be ***colonized,*** or overgrown, with bacteria.

Control and Prevention

Control and prevention of HAIs must be an integrated part of everyone's daily activities in the healthcare setting. The CDC has issued specific measures for preventing healthcare-associated infections (Table 12-1). It is important that healthcare workers consistently use methods that lessen a patient's chance of developing an infection. Proper hand washing is the most effective means of preventing and controlling the spread of HAIs. This simple means of controlling the spread of organisms is often ignored or thought to be insignificant; however, past and current research continues to promote the practice of hand washing before and after any contact with a patient.

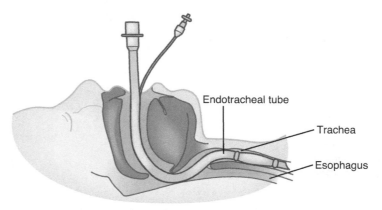

FIGURE 12-5 **An endotracheal tube in the lungs.**

TABLE 12-1

SPECIFIC MEASURES FOR PREVENTION OF HEALTHCARE-ASSOCIATED INFECTIONS RECOMMENDED BY THE CDC

Healthcare-Associated Infection	Preventive Measure	Definition
All HAIs	Hand hygiene	Washing hands before and after each patient contact
Central venous catheter–related bloodstream infections	Maximal sterile barrier precautions	Use aseptic technique, including the use of a cap, mask, sterile gown, sterile gloves, and a large sterile sheet for the insertion of all central venous catheters (CVCs)
	Chlorhexidine skin antisepsis	Use 2% chlorhexidine gluconate solution for skin sterilization at the CVC insertion site
	Appropriate insertion site selection	Avoid femoral site for nonemergency CVC insertion
	Prompt removal of unnecessary catheters	Removal of CVC that is no longer essential for care
Surgical site infection	Appropriate use of perioperative antibiotics	Administration of appropriate prophylactic antibiotic, generally begun within 1 hour before skin incision and discontinued within 24 hours
	Avoidance of shaving of the operative site	Use clippers or other methods for hair removal in the area of skin incision(s)
	Perioperative glucose control	Maintenance of blood glucose less than 150 mg/dL during postoperative period (tighter control may be more beneficial in specific patient populations)
Ventilator-associated pneumonia	Semirecumbent positioning	Elevation of the head of the bed to more than 30 degrees for all mechanically ventilated patients
	Daily assessment of readiness for weaning	Minimize duration of mechanical ventilation by minimizing sedative administration (including daily "sedation holidays") and/or using protocolized weaning
Catheter-associated urinary tract infection	Aseptic insertion and catheter care	Use of skin antisepsis at insertion and proper aseptic technique for maintenance of catheter and drainage bag; use of closed urinary drainage system
	Prompt removal of unnecessary catheters	Removal of urinary catheter when no longer essential for care

(From: Ranji, S.R., Shetty, K., Posley, K.A., et al. Prevention of healthcare-associated infections. In: Shojania, K.G., McDonald, K.M., et al., Eds. *Closing the Quality Gap: A Critical Analysis of Quality Improvement Strategies.* Technical Review 9. AHRQ Publication No. 04-0051-6. Rockville, MD: Agency for Healthcare Research and Quality, 2007. Used with permission.)

Using gloves is important, but it does not replace hand washing. Hands must be washed before and after wearing gloves. Chapter 10 discusses hand washing, gloves, and alcohol-based hand sanitizers in detail.

The administration in a healthcare facility must be supportive of efforts to reduce the risks of HAIs by providing adequate personnel, supplies, and training.

Flashpoint
Wearing gloves is no substitute for washing your hands!

Flashpoint
Every healthcare practitioner should be provided an annual training session in infection control.

Quality control is a process that ensures that every healthcare facility has sufficient sterile supplies and sterilization equipment for procedures. In addition to hand washing, sterile supplies can help reduce the risk of HAIs. Sterile supplies are only as good as the technique used with them. Practitioners should be trained in the use of sterile technique and supplies at least annually or with the addition of new supplies or techniques. No one working in health care should become complacent in his or her use of proper infection control techniques.

It takes the combined effort of all healthcare team members to reduce the numbers of health care–associated infections that occur each year in our nation's healthcare facilities.

Summary

HAIs are an increasing problem facing health care today. All healthcare professionals must be vigilant in their infection control procedures to help prevent the spread of infection and avoid contributing to the resistance of organisms.

Practice Exercises

Multiple Choice

1. It is estimated that what percent of hospitalized patients develop an HAI?
   a.   1%
   b.   5%
   c.   10%
   d.   15%

2. An HAI develops within _____ hours of admission to a facility.
   a.   12–24
   b.   24–48
   c.   48–72
   d.   72–96

3. The organism that causes most urinary tract infection is:
   a.   *Staphylococcus*
   b.   *Streptococcus*
   c.   *E. coli*
   d.   *Proteus*

4. Cases that involve spillage of gastrointestinal contents into the wound are known as:

   a. Clean

   b. Clean-contaminated

   c. Contaminated

   d. Dirty

5. The most effective method of preventing and controlling HAIs is:

   a. Stronger antibiotics

   b. Alcohol-based sanitizers

   c. Using only prepackaged supplies

   d. Hand washing

6. Which of the following patients would be at higher risk of developing an HAI?

   a. A healthy teenager having a tonsillectomy

   b. A brittle diabetic undergoing an appendectomy for a ruptured appendix

   c. A child having tubes in her ears

   d. A new mother having a tubal ligation after delivery

Fill in the Blank

1. Most catheters use a _____ drainage system.

2. To help prevent a respiratory infection, you should keep the patient in a _____ position.

3. A surgical procedure in which there is no break in sterile technique is known as _____.

Short Answer

1. **Why was the term "hospital-acquired infection" changed to health care–associated infection?**

2. **What quality control measures can be used to prevent or reduce HAIs?**

INTERNET RESOURCES

Agency/Organization	Web Address	Resources/Functions
Centers for Disease Control and Prevention	www.cdc.gov	Outlines methods of preventing healthcare-acquired infections
World Health Organization	http://apps.who.int/medicinedocs/documents/s16355e/s16355e.pdf	A guide to the prevention of HAIs presented by the World Health Organization
Safe Patient Project	http://safepatientproject.org/topic/hospital_acquired_infections	A Consumers Union clearinghouse site for articles related to HAIs.
Drug Reference	www.rxlist.com	Comprehensive drug information

RESISTANT ORGANISMS 13

Learning Outcomes

13.1 Discuss the discovery of penicillin

13.2 Define resistance and how some organisms become resistant

13.3 Describe the characteristics of methicillin-resistant *Staphylococcus*

aureus (MRSA) and other resistant bacteria

13.4 Define "necrotizing fasciitis" and the risks associated with the disease

13.5 Explain infection control as it relates to resistant organisms

Competencies

CAAHEP
- Discuss infection control procedures. (CAAHEP III.C.3)
- Identify personal safety precautions as established by the Occupational Safety and Health Administration (OSHA). (CAAHEP III.C.4)
- Compare different methods of controlling the growth of microorganisms. (CAAHEP III.C.6)

ABHES
- Apply principles of aseptic techniques and infection control. (ABHES 9.b)
- Use standard precautions. (ABHES 9.i)

The world has always been home to bacteria, viruses, and other organisms that cause disease, and most existed long before humans populated the earth. As the human race has evolved, so have these organisms, which have caused many diseases and **epidemics.** The bubonic plague, or "black death," caused by the *Yersinia pestis* bacteria, killed millions of people in Europe in the early 1300s. This bacterium was transmitted through the bite of an infected flea and claimed the lives of more than half its victims within 3 to 7 days. Other diseases present as an **endemic,** a slow but steady progression of a disease, such as malaria in Africa, which is spread by infected mosquitoes. Many soldiers in World War I died from overwhelming infections that complicated the wounds suffered during combat. Death due to infection was common during these early years because there were no definitive treatments to prevent or cure these infections.

The discovery of **penicillin** by Scottish biologist and pharmacologist Alexander Fleming changed the course of medicine and began to reduce the numbers of people who succumbed to infections. In the 1928 accident that paved the way for modern antibiotic therapy, spores blew into Fleming's laboratory through an open window and landed on Petri dishes in which he was culturing *Staphylococcus.*

Observing the cultures, Fleming noticed that *Staphylococcus* grew rapidly except in the area of the mold. He discovered that this mold, which at first he called "mould juice" and later named penicillin, had properties that prevented the growth of bacteria such as *Staphylococcus.* Fleming continued his research and determined that this penicillin was effective in killing other bacteria with

Key Terms

antibiotics A medication that destroys most bacterial organisms

broad-spectrum Antibiotics that are nontoxic, relatively inexpensive, and able to kill a wide range of bacteria

CA-MRSA Community-associated methicillin-resistant *Staphylococcus aureus* (MRSA); this strain of MRSA affects a community, usually surrounding athletic venues and players

culture and sensitivity test A test done to identify an infectious bacteria and the antibiotic that is effective against it

endemic A slow but steady progression of a particular disease

Continued

Flashpoint
Fleming's mold was much like the greenish mold spores that attach to bread, then use the moisture and nutrients in the bread to multiply, appearing as green fuzz.

gram-positive properties, but not those with *gram-negative traits.* Fleming published his discovery in the *British Journal of Experimental Pathology* in 1929, but very few paid attention. He grew weary of the research and believed it would be too difficult to produce the mold in quantities sufficient to treat an infection. After extensive research using the mold as a surface antiseptic, his penicillin did not appear to be as effective as he thought. He eventually deserted his research and attempts to refine the mold when no one came forward.

Not long after Fleming stopped his research in 1940, scientists Ernst Chain, Norman Heatley, and Howard Florey resumed the isolation and purification of the penicillin into a form that, after clinical trials, was mass-produced with financial support of the U.S. and British governments. Enough of the penicillin was refined and produced by D-Day, June 6, 1944, to treat most of the wounded Allied soldiers.

The accidental discovery of penicillin in 1928 revolutionized the treatment of infectious diseases by using *antibiotics.* In his research, Fleming also discovered another very important aspect of antibiotics. When too little of the penicillin was used or not used long enough to kill the organism, the medicine proved ineffective. Fleming urged the medical community to use penicillin in sufficient quantities and for an extended period to prevent the organism from developing a resistance.

The term *resistant organism* indicates that a strain of bacteria is no longer affected by treatment with antibiotic agents that had previously been effective in killing the organism. Resistance can be compared with slowly easing into an icy cold lake on a warm day. First, you dip your big toe and then gently ease your entire foot into the icy water. In contrast to the sun beating down on your back, the water feels extremely cold, so you hesitate before moving further into the lake. You are allowing your body to become resistant to the cold lake water. As your body adjusts to the environment change, you slowly work your entire body into the water, allowing the cold to engulf your legs, trunk, and neck. Once you are used to the cold water, you submerge your head under the surface. After a few minutes, the water no longer feels cold due to your resistance to the temperature, and you are able to swim in the water without being aware of the water's temperature.

Organisms develop resistance to antibiotics for several reasons, some of which are the result of today's practice of medicine. The overprescribing of antibiotics have contributed to this resistance. Many bacteria have the ability to quickly become resistant to antibiotics through *mutation* or by chemical changes within the organism to resist the destructive properties of the antibiotics. Resistant organisms can lead to serious illnesses, extended hospital stays, and even death. Research and development of stronger antibiotics is an expensive and lengthy process, creating higher costs for patients when the new medications become available on the market.

Physicians must be careful when prescribing antibiotics for an infection. It is extremely important to determine the causative organism prior to treatment. Antibiotics are ineffective in treating a viral illness and should not be prescribed for illnesses such as a cold or the flu. There are few antiviral medications on the market today. Some antibiotics are effective against a large number of infections caused by bacteria with gram-positive characteristics as well as those with gram-negative traits. Gram-positive and gram-negative refer to the staining properties of an organism and thus its ability to cause disease. Examples of gram-positive organisms include *Staphylococcus* and *Streptococcus,* which cause illnesses such as impetigo and strep throat. Gram-negative bacteria include *Escherichia coli* and *Salmonella,* which cause many gastrointestinal and urinary tract infections. Gram-negative organisms are responsible for most sexually transmitted diseases.

Flashpoint

Fleming noted, "When I woke up just after dawn on September 28, 1928, I certainly didn't plan to revolutionize all medicine by discovering the world's first antibiotic, or bacteria killer, but I guess that is exactly what I did."

Flashpoint

Many people stop taking their antibiotics once they feel better, which gives the bacteria a chance to develop resistance.

Key Terms—cont'd

epidemic An outbreak of a disease that affects a large group of people in a geographic region or defined population group; an example is the bubonic plague

gram-negative The staining properties of bacterial organisms; this type does not retain the stain applied in the Gram stain process, so the organisms appear pink or red under the microscope

gram-positive The staining properties of bacterial organisms; this type retains the stain applied in the Gram stain process, so the organisms appear purple under the microscope

Treating organisms based on their staining properties can be effective, but it is a broad approach; and the more specific the treatment, the less likely it is that an organism will become resistant. Ideally, a **culture and sensitivity test** (C&S) is performed to identify the bacteria and which antibiotics are effective against it. Once the physician knows exactly what bacteria are causing the illness, the physician can prescribe the antibiotic that is most effective. Once the correct antibiotic has been determined and prescribed, it is important to educate the patient on the proper way to take the medications.

In the picture of the culture plate (Fig. 13-1), the gold area covering the entire plate is the bacteria that are actively growing. The small, dark disks are pads saturated with specific antibiotics. Notice how some areas around the disks are completely cleared of the bacteria, and others show minimal or partial destruction. The disks with the largest area of antibacterial properties are the most effective in treating this disease.

Careless prescribing of antibiotics and failure on the patient's part to complete the therapy are two major causes of concern for resistant organisms. Many times patients will not leave a physician's office without a prescription for an antibiotic, regardless of the diagnosis, because they think, in error, that antibiotics can cure anything. Also, many patients believe that a visit to the physician's office should automatically result in a prescription for medication. Some patients have difficulty understanding that there are often other ways to treat illness. Taking unnecessary antibiotics contributes to the development of resistant organisms; however, the overuse of antibiotics is starting to decline as the public learns more about these resistant organisms.

STOP, THINK, AND LEARN.

Do you use antibacterial soap every time you wash your hands? What do you think is happening to the bacteria that normally reside on and protect your skin? List at least three times that you should use antibacterial soap on your hands. What are the three things necessary for washing your hands? (See Chapter 10.)

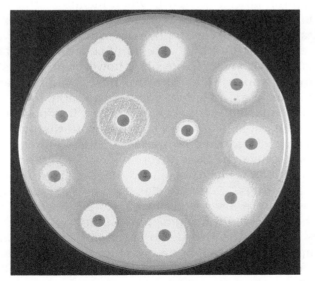

FIGURE 13-1 **Culture plate showing actively growing bacteria (gold areas) and areas that are cleared of bacteria around small, dark disks saturated with antibiotics.** (Courtesy of Gilda L. Jones, CDC Public Health Image Library.)

Flashpoint

Many times an antibiotic can destroy the body's normal bacteria, causing a yeast infection to appear. Eating yogurt each day while taking antibiotics may help prevent this side effect.

Key Terms—cont'd

intravenous immunoglobulin (IVIG) A newer form of treatment for flesh-eating bacteria that involves a direct injection of immunoglobulin—a protein found in blood plasma—into a vein

MRSA Methicillin-resistant *Staphylococcus aureus;* a highly resistant strain of *Staphylococcus* bacteria that does not respond to treatment with most antibiotics

mutation A change in the DNA sequence of a gene that can cause an organism to become resistant to medications

necrotizing fasciitis "Flesh-eating bacteria"; a devastating disease caused by group A *Streptococcus* bacteria that can destroy the skin and fascia
Continued

Patients who are given appropriate antibiotics must be given specific instructions to complete the entire course of treatment regardless of the fact that they may begin to feel better 24 to 48 hours after starting the medication. As Fleming found, short-term use of an antibiotic resulted in inefficient destruction of the bacteria. A standard dose of antibiotics is given for 7 to 10 days, although newer drugs can be effective after fewer than 5 days. Taking a substandard dosage of antibiotics or taking them for less than the prescribed length of time required gives organisms the ability to develop resistance.

The term **superbug** describes organisms that have developed resistance to many antibiotics, especially drugs that have been around for many years, such as penicillin. Many of the older, first-line antibiotics are no longer effective against any bacteria, which has led to the research and development of new, more potent, but more expensive medicines. There are certain groups of people that are more likely to develop resistant organisms through daily contact. The groups most affected are children in a group setting such as day care or school, the elderly in long-term care facilities, and hospitalized patients.

Research is also being conducted on resistant organisms and antibiotics used in agriculture. Antibiotics have been used to treat or prevent infectious diseases in the food chain, and it now appears that some of these antibiotics may be contributing to the increasing number of resistant organisms. Antibiotics and resistant organisms are found in the air, soil, and groundwater on farms as well as in the meat, poultry, and produce that is sold to retail markets. These foodborne organisms are taken into homes, where they contaminate surfaces and are then transferred into the body when the foods that contain them are consumed. Many times, gastric secretions can destroy the harmful bacteria; however, some do survive and thrive in the body. The probability of contracting a form of resistant bacteria during the course of a meal is reasonably low. You can protect yourself by maintaining strict cleaning guidelines in the kitchen.

Methicillin-Resistant *Staphylococcus aureus*

The most common drug-resistant bacteria is *Staphylococcus aureus*, often called "staph" or **MRSA** (pronounced "mersa"), which means methicillin-resistant *S. aureus*. This form of bacteria has become resistant to the **broad-spectrum** antibiotics normally used to treat staph. Years of unnecessary antibiotic use for colds and flu or minor self-limiting bacterial infections has led to the development of MRSA as a superbug. It is possible, however, to have staphylococcal organisms growing on your skin and in your nose, but if you are healthy and not showing any signs of an infection, you are said only to be "colonized" and not "infected" with *Staphylococcus*. It is possible to transmit the *Staphylococcus* to others, so it is important that you wash your hands frequently and always dispose of tissues appropriately. This staphylococcus can be innocuous unless it enters the body through a cut or scrape.

Many MRSA infections occur in hospitals, long-term care facilities, and other ambulatory health settings. These are classified as the health care–associated infections (HAI), which are discussed in Chapter 12. Recently, another classification of MRSA has emerged, known as community-associated MRSA, or **CA-MRSA.** Cases of CA-MRSA have been found in locker rooms, artificial turf, and athletic equipment. Children are more vulnerable because their immune systems are not fully developed. Young adults contract the MRSA during contact sports and by sharing equipment.

Signs and symptoms of MRSA may begin as small lesions that resemble a pimple or insect bite that is warm and tender to the touch and is surrounded

Flashpoint

The longer you live with a little bit of irritation, the more you learn to tolerate it. Eventually, it does not bother you anymore. The same is true for bacteria and antibiotics.

Key Terms—cont'd

penicillin Discovered in 1928, the world's first antibiotic, which paved the way for modern antibiotic therapy

resistant organism An organism that can withstand the effects of a medication that would normally destroy it

superbug Another term for a resistant organism; one that will not respond to most antibiotics

vancomyin An older-generation antibiotic that is effective against MRSA in some situations

VRE Vancomycin-resistant *Enterococcus;* like MRSA, an enterococcal infection is resistant to the antibiotic vancomycin

Flashpoint

Children need to be reminded frequently to wash their hands.

by reddened skin. The lesion may be filled with pus (Fig. 13-2), and the patient may develop a fever. These papules can develop into larger, deeper abscesses that must be removed surgically. People with these lesions should not try to drain them with a sharp object or by mashing them. Doing so may cause MRSA to penetrate the deeper tissues, causing life-threatening infections in the bones and joints, or even more dangerous, the heart valves and the lungs. There is a very dangerous form of pneumonia caused by MRSA that children and young adults can develop after contact with the organism. Crowded and unsanitary living conditions such as prisons, military camps, and homeless shelters may promote the development of MRSA. Healthcare workers must be very careful when working with patients suffering from a MRSA infection. Isolation protocol must be followed diligently to prevent the spread of MRSA to other patients and the healthcare worker's own family.

Those who are at high risk of developing MRSA are people who have recently been hospitalized, especially those with a weak immune system, with severe burns, or who have had major surgery. Patients in long-term care facilities, mental health institutions, or ambulatory care clinics such as hemodialysis centers are also at high risk. Another group of high-risk patients includes those with indwelling devices such as catheters, feeding tubes, dialysis shunts, or central venous lines. An implanted device gives the bacteria an opening into the body.

A diagnosis of MRSA is made by evaluating the drainage in a culture plate. A normal culture requires 48 hours to "grow," but there are new tests that detect the staph DNA within hours, which is extremely helpful in preventing the spread of the bacteria. It is important to know conclusively if the organism is MRSA so that it can be treated appropriately. Some physicians may choose to drain a wound that is infected with MRSA rather than treat the patient with medications. Physicians may use the antibiotic **vancomycin** in the treatment of MRSA, as in most cases it is still effective, although it is becoming less effective with some strains of these bacteria.

Hospitals and other healthcare facilities are trying to combat MRSA through comprehensive programs aimed at prevention. Many pediatric wards test all infants and children being admitted in an effort to reduce the risk of

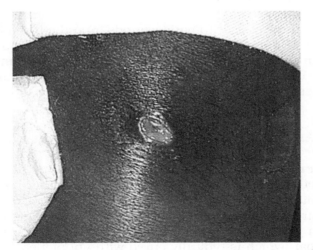

FIGURE 13-2 **Abscess on the knee caused by methicillin-resistant _Staphylococcus aureus_ bacteria, or MRSA.** (Courtesy of Bruno Coignard, MD, and Jeff Hageman, MHS, CDC Public Health Image Library.)

transmission to other hospitalized children. All shared equipment throughout the facility is cleaned thoroughly after each use, and isolation protocols are followed for those diagnosed with MRSA. Strict hand-washing policies are enforced. The use of a hand sanitizer that is at least 60% alcohol is suggested before touching any patient or equipment or when immediate hand washing is not available. Gloves and gowns are used when contact with an infected patient is necessary. Healthcare professionals must make sure to use sterile conditions and equipment when inserting devices such as bladder catheters and intravenous catheters.

In the community, the best protection against CA-MRSA is by consistent hand washing and being cautious with personal belongings. Proper hand washing cannot be stressed enough to prevent the spread of MRSA. Sharing towels, brushes or combs, or clothing may increase risk of contracting MRSA because these objects can carry the organism. Washing any shared items in hot water with bleach and drying them on a hot setting may help destroy any bacteria prior to contact. In case of a cut or scrape, keep it covered, and do not participate in group activities until it is healed. Drainage from these wounds can contaminate surfaces, making transmission to others possible. After engaging in sports activities, a thorough shower with soap also decreases possibility of infection. When a physician does prescribe an antibiotic, take the entire prescription as ordered, never skipping a dose or sharing the medication with others.

Vancomycin-Resistant Enterococci

Enterococcus is another bacterium that has become a superbug. Normally, enterococci live in the intestines and the female genital tract. Exposure to *Enterococcus* in the environment is also made through contaminated water and animal feces. The Environmental Protection Agency (EPA), along with local governments, monitors the cleanliness of beaches and the environment. For many years, enterococcal infections were treated with the antibiotic vancomycin. Today, many strains of *Enterococcus* are resistant to this antibiotic. They are called vancomycin-resistant *Enterococcus* **(VRE).**

As with MRSA, the enterococcal organisms can live in and on our body without causing infections, which is known as colonization. Most VRE infections develop while patients are hospitalized. VRE can cause infections primarily in the urinary tract, surgical or traumatic wounds, and the bloodstream. People at risk of developing VRE are those who have received long-term antibiotic therapy or previous treatment with vancomycin and those with weak immune systems.

Treatment of VRE is similar to that of MRSA, including vigilant hand washing, isolation when necessary, and use of sterile technique and equipment.

Necrotizing Fasciitis

Necrotizing fasciitis (NF), also known as the "flesh-eating bacteria," destroys fascia, the protective covering on muscles, bones, and other body structures. This form of fasciitis is caused by the group A *Streptococcus* organism that is transmitted by direct contact or through respiratory droplets. Individuals can be colonized with group A strep without being ill. This same organism also causes strep throat, which is typically cured with antibiotics. There is a stronger strain, however, that is resistant to antibiotics and causes the necrotizing fasciitis. This disease destroys subcutaneous tissue and can be fatal. When muscle tissue is destroyed, the term "necrotizing myositis" is used. The bacteria often enter the body through a small opening in the skin or through skin that is weak due to an abrasion, bruise, or blister. In many cases, the point of entry is unknown.

Prevention is not always possible, but using proper precautions can reduce chances of contracting this dangerous disease. Because the bacteria can be spread through coughing and sneezing, it is imperative that, when doing so, you cover your mouth and nose and dispose of used tissues to prevent the possible spread of the streptococcal germs. Immediate hand washing after someone coughs or sneezes on you is also important. Research indicates that 15% to 30% of the population carries group A *Streptococcus* and has no warning symptoms. Careful precautions around anyone complaining of a sore throat are necessary. Teaching people to cough into their elbow as opposed to their hands may help prevent the spread of infection as contaminants on the hands are more easily spread. Keeping a container of alcohol-based hand sanitizer is always a good idea. Caring for nicks and scrapes in the skin with proper cleaning and antibiotic ointments is important. Healthcare workers who have a break in the skin on their hands should always wear a bandage over the break and gloves when involved in patient care.

Within 24 hours of exposure, there may be pain in the general area that begins to exceed what would be expected for that type of wound. Flu-like symptoms follow and may lead to dehydration, dizziness, weakness, and confusion. This combination and intensity of these symptoms should cause the person to seek medical care. Later symptoms may include massive swelling of the affected area and marked discoloration of the area. A dark purple rash may appear, followed by blisters with a blackened fluid. This is the beginning stage of the tissue necrosis. By the fourth or fifth day, the patient may become critically ill with hypotension and possible toxic shock syndrome.

Many cases of NF are misdiagnosed. When early symptoms are detected, it is important that NF be ruled out to prevent the dangerous progression of the disease. The early, vague symptoms can be attributed to many other diseases, making the diagnosis difficult.

Although not totally resistant to antibiotics, NF can be difficult to treat when diagnosed in later stages of the disease. Débridement, or cutting away of the affected tissue, can slow the progression of the disease, along with intravenous antibiotics and other medications to treat the symptoms of shock. Physicians have begun to use a new therapy for NF in the form of **intravenous immunoglobulin (IVIG),** a protein found in blood plasma. Patients may also receive oxygen-under-pressure therapy in a closed hyperbaric chamber. A closed hyperbaric chamber delivers oxygen to the patient at a level higher than at atmospheric pressure. Certain diseases, such as diabetes or anemia, do not allow blood cells to become supersaturated with oxygen at normal atmospheric pressure. By placing the patient in a hyperbaric chamber and administering pure oxygen, doctors can increase the amount of oxygen cells carry through the bloodstream. Patients suffering from gas gangrene or flesh-eating bacterial infections can also benefit from the hyperbaric chamber's increased atmospheric pressure.

As discussed in Chapter 10, infection control should be a top priority at all times. Stringent hand washing tops the list of infection control activities along with careful attention to open wounds and methods of transmission. Infection control practices are only as good as the consistency with which they are used. The Centers for Disease Control and Prevention (CDC) advise the use of

Flashpoint

It is best to keep wounds covered, but remember to change the dressing frequently and properly dispose of old bandages.

antibacterial soap when hands are noticeably dirty or if there is a chance of contact with a contaminated surface. Using warm water, soap, and friction on all surfaces of the hands for a minimum of 20 seconds should be sufficient to destroy pathogens. In today's world, actual hand washing compliance is about 50%. The addition of alcohol-based hand sanitizers has significantly improved the percentage of healthcare workers cleaning their hands due to the ease of use. These sanitizers use isopropanol, ethanol, and n-propanol, or a combination of these substances, as the active ingredient. The alcohol has the ability to destroy the protein in the bacteria, thus rendering them inactive. This is true even with resistant organisms such as MRSA and VRE. Alcohol-based sanitizers cannot retain the antibacterial properties for an extended period of time, so it is important to use it frequently and always before and after patient contact.

Summary

Healthcare professionals are responsible for reporting exposures to infectious diseases, including needlesticks or direct contact with infectious materials, in an effort to decrease transmission of these diseases. The information in this chapter is presented to make you aware of the diseases that exist in society. Individuals must be sensible when given a prescription for medication, and healthcare professionals should take the time to make sure that patients understand the importance of taking antibiotics as prescribed. Education is a key factor.

Practice Exercises

Multiple Choice

1. Which of these scientists is credited with the discovery of penicillin?

   a. Galen

   b. Hippocrates

   c. Fleming

   d. Heatley

2. An outbreak of a disease that affects a large group of people in a geographic region or defined population group is known as a(n):

   a. Endemic

   b. Epidemic

   c. Wave

   d. Plague

3. A strain of bacteria that has become unaffected by treatment with antibiotic agents that have previously been effective is called:

   a. Resistant

   b. Mutant

   c. Sensitive

   d. Intermediate

4. Some organisms become resistant to antibiotics due to:

   a. Gram staining

   b. Sensitivity

   c. Culturing

   d. Mutation

5. A major reason that organisms have become resistant is:

   a. Overuse of antibiotics

   b. Failure of patients to complete therapy

   c. The increasing costs to produce new antibiotics

   d. Both a and b

6. In the event of an exposure to infectious blood and body fluids, healthcare professionals should:

   a. Report the incident immediately

   b. Check the patient's medical record for laboratory reports

   c. Clean the wound with alcohol

   d. Be tested for HIV

Fill in the Blank

1. The term _____ describes organisms that have developed resistance to many antibiotics.

2. Antibiotics and resistant organisms are found in the _____, _____, and _____ on farms as well as in the meat, poultry, and produce that is sold to retail markets.

3. To identify the organism and the most effective antibiotic, a physician would order a _____ and _____ test.

Short Answer

1. **What factors may increase the development and transmission of MRSA?**

2. **What is CA-MRSA?**

3. **When hand-washing equipment is not readily available, what can you do?**

INTERNET RESOURCES	
Resource/Organization	**Web Address**
Alexander Fleming	http://time.com/time/time100/scientist/profile/fleming.html http://nobelprize.org/nobel_prizes/medicine/laureates/1945/fleming-bio.html
National Necrotizing Fasciitis Foundation	http://nnff.org (Warning: Graphic images)
United States Department of Agriculture Organic Foods Information	http://fnic.nal.usda.gov
MRSA	http://staph-infection-resources.com/mrsa-pictures.html
Clean Beaches	http://water.epa.gov/type/oceb/beaches/
Environmental Protection Agency	www.epa.gov

PATIENT ASSESSMENT

14

Learning Outcomes

14.1 Describe the role of the healthcare professional in obtaining the patient history

14.2 Explain the importance of privacy during the patient interview

14.3 List effective methods of both verbal and nonverbal communication

14.4 Define the review of systems and the physical examination

14.5 Recognize the need for accurate and professional documentation

Competencies

CAAHEP

- Identify styles and types of verbal communication. (CAAHEP IV.C.1)
- Identify nonverbal communication. (CAAHEP IV.C.2)
- Recognize communication barriers. (CAAHEP IV.C.3)
- Identify techniques for overcoming communication barriers. (CAAHEP IV.C.4)
- Recognize the elements of oral communication using a sender-receiver process. (CAAHEP IV.C.5)
- Differentiate between subjective and objective information. (CAAHEP IV.C.6)
- Identify resources and adaptations that are required based on individual needs, i.e., culture and environment, developmental life stage, language, and physical threats to communication. (CAAHEP IV.C.7)

ABHES

- Obtain chief complaint, recording patient history. (ABHES 9.a)

Key Terms

allergic reactions Signs and symptoms, such as itching, hives, nausea, or difficulty breathing, that may indicate the patient cannot tolerate a medication

auscultation The act of listening to body sounds, typically done with a stethoscope placed over body organs to hear both normal and abnormal sounds

current medications A list of all medicines a patient is presently taking, including the dosage and schedule for each one

demographics The patient's full name, date of birth, social security number, current address, telephone numbers, e-mail address, insurance information, and emergency contact names and phone numbers

Continued

Demographics and Background Information

When a patient schedules an appointment at a physician's office or visits a healthcare facility, a **medical record** must be created. This chapter details the

Key Terms—cont'd

family history A thorough investigation of the patient's family background related to disease, including, but not limited to, grandparents and their descendants

inspection Observation of the patient to note changes in skin color, swelling, respiratory distress, and other signs of problems

legal documents Paperwork, including medical records, that is admissible in a court of law

medical history The patient's background related to diseases, medications, and surgical procedures

medical record A complete and accurate account (recorded on paper or electronically) of all patient visits to the facility

nonverbal clues An unspoken sign that may indicate the patient is uncomfortable with a question or does not understand what you are asking

obstetrical history A woman's background related to pregnancies, noted with outcomes and reproductive status

palpation Using the fingertips to lightly press on the patient's body to determine the size of a mass or the amount of tenderness in a certain part of the body

patient interview The initial contact with the patient to determine medical history, current medications, and chief complaint

purpose and content of the patient history and assessment that are included in the patient's medical record.

Before the medical history is taken, the patient or a family member is asked to complete a form that collects demographic information. **Demographics** include the patient's full name, date of birth, social security number, address, telephone numbers, current e-mail address, insurance information, and emergency contact information. Complete information is essential to prevent confusion in case patients with the same name visit the practice. This form may be sent to patients prior to the visit or given to them when they arrive. Once the information is collected, an update should be requested at least annually.

Many offices provide each patient with a copy of the physician's financial policies and ask that patients sign a receipt. These policies include copay billing, insurance filing, and any finance charges for unpaid balances. This disclosure complies with the Truth in Lending Act, a part of the Consumer Credit Protection Act. Patients with private insurance are asked for a copy of their identification card and are asked to sign the Assignment of Benefits form, which allows the insurance company to pay directly to the physician. Additionally, to protect the patient's privacy, a Health Insurance Portability and Accountability Act (HIPAA) form is signed by the patient. All these documents become a part of the patient's medical record. In an electronic setting, the forms are scanned into the computer system for inclusion in the patient record.

Patient Interview

Once demographic information is collected, the **patient interview** begins. Care of any patient begins with a thorough assessment, including a complete medical history. Because some disease processes can be genetic, it is important to gather data about a patient's parents, grandparents, and other blood relatives, a process known as the **family history.** The **medical history** is the basis for the physician's plan of treatment for the patient and provides a reminder to the physician of the patient's status each time he or she visits. It also contains information about preexisting conditions that can be useful to the patient's insurance company or to the legal system if the patient makes a claim against the physician or another party. Many healthcare facilities have a questionnaire that patients are asked to complete prior to the visit. This form may ask for basic information such as childhood diseases, previous surgical procedures, and current health concerns, and more details are gathered when the patient is seen in the office (Fig. 14-1). A thorough medical history is better accomplished by interviewing the patient. Specialty offices may gather only information that is pertinent to the type of care the patient receives, whereas a family physician or general practitioner requires overall health information.

 STOP, THINK, AND LEARN.
What was your first impression when you last visited a physician's office? What, if anything, would you change about a patient's first encounter if you were employed at that office?

Medical History

The medical information you provide at this time is important to our understanding of your health and treatment of your problems. Please take the time to fully and completely fill out this information.

Last name:_____ First name: _____

Social History

Do you smoke?	No_____	Yes_____	Packs per day:_____
Did you ever use tobacco?	No_____	Yes_____	When did you quit?_____
Do you drink alcohol?	No_____	Yes_____	When did you quit?_____
Do you exercise?	No_____	Yes_____	Hours per week:_____

Type of exercise:_____

Personal History of Illness or Injury *(Please check all that apply)*

High blood pressure	_____	Yellow jaundice	_____
Diabetes	_____	Thyroid problems	_____
Peptic ulcers	_____	Lung problems	_____
Hepatitis	_____	Cancer	_____
Gallstone	_____	Heart disease	_____
Kidney stones	_____	Stroke	_____
Abnormal bleeding	_____	Arthritis	_____
Diverticulosis	_____		

Other (list)_____

Family History of Illness *(Please check all that apply)*

Cancer	_____	Family member:_____
Heart disease	_____	Family member:_____
Stroke	_____	Family member:_____
Arthritis	_____	Family member:_____

Personal History of Previous Surgery *(Please give names and dates of operations)*

Type of Surgery   Year

_____   _____

_____   _____

_____   _____

_____   _____

Please indicate any hospital admissions of medical conditions not covered above.

_____

_____

_____

_____

Females only

Are you pregnant?   Yes_____   No_____

The above information is true and correct to the best of my belief.

_____   _____

Patient signature (or parent if patient is a minor)   Date

FIGURE 14-1 **Sample of a medical history that a patient might be asked to complete before being interviewed.**

Key Terms—cont'd

percussion A method of tapping with the fingers over body organs to determine their size and whether there is fluid collection or gas accumulation

physical assessment Includes the patient interview, a thorough review of all body systems, and a physical examination

physical examination The process of using the four techniques, inspection, auscultation, palpation, and percussion, to evaluate a patient's health status and determine a diagnosis

review of systems (ROS) A portion of the patient assessment that includes questions about each body system; notes are made if a symptom may need further investigation

social history A record of the patient's marital status, occupation, sexual habits, and use of alcohol, tobacco, or other recreational drugs

vital signs An accounting of the patient's temperature, pulse, respiratory rate, blood pressure, and sometimes height and weight

Approach to the Patient

In a physician's office, a nurse, a medical assistant, or the physician may **interview** the patient extensively on the initial visit and more briefly on subsequent visits. Patient interviews are more successful if the interviewer follows standard guidelines. Ensure a private, tidy space in which to interview the patient and that you have properly introduced yourself, including statement of your job title. Note on the outside of the door that the room is in use and request that there be no interruptions. Make your patient feel as if he or she is the only one in the office at that time. A private interview room is important because many items in the medical history can be embarrassing, and patients may feel uncomfortable answering the questions in an open space or one in which there are constant interruptions. Do not stop to take telephone calls or leave the room during the interview.

It is best to start with a simple comment, such as, "Please come in and make yourself comfortable." A pleasant voice and possibly a simple touch on the arm may help put a nervous patient at ease. Address the patient using his or her title and last name: Mr. Smith, Mrs. Jones, or Ms. Turner, if you are unsure of a woman's marital status. Do not ask questions such as "How are you today?" as many patients have come to the physician because they already do not feel well. Also, they may have had a frustrating experience finding the office or they had to wait longer than expected. Maintain focus on the patient and not issues that are irrelevant. Always leave personal issues outside so the patient does not feel as if he or she is bothering you.

You may want to tell patients about the confidentiality of their medical records. With electronic health records, you can describe the security system used. For offices using hard copy medical records, you can describe the filing procedures that keep their information safe. Once the medical history is complete, it becomes a part of the legal medical record. This may help allay any apprehension the patients may have about who may see their medical records.

Before you begin taking the history, make sure that you are at eye level with the patient and that you respect their personal space. **Personal space** is defined as the perimeter around you that you consider your own comfort zone, or the distance you prefer others to keep (Fig. 14-2). In this professional setting, your personal space may be significantly different from the space you need when you are with your friends or family. Patients may have a different definition of their own personal space, which varies due to a patient's culture. In the United States, most people prefer a personal space of 1.5 to 4 feet. To learn more about personal space preferences of people from different cultures, see Table 14-1. Most people do not invite others into their personal space until trust and rapport are established. If you lean in to ask a question and the patient leans away, it is advisable to increase the distance between you. Treat each patient with respect and sensitivity. Make sure to take care of personal hygiene matters if you have just returned from a spicy lunch or a coffee break. This first interview with the patient sets the stage for the patient's comfort level with the facility and its staff.

Be sensitive to the questions you are asking and the information that the patient is giving. Do not hesitate to ask a patient for clarification if you do not hear or understand an answer. It is better to ask twice than to record incorrect information. Speak clearly in a normal voice. Do not assume that an elderly patient is hard of hearing. If a patient cannot understand you, he or she will ask you to speak louder. Avoid using terms such as "sweetie" or "honey," as these words can be insulting or condescending to many patients.

Some patients are overly talkative and may try to monopolize the conversation. You are responsible for keeping the conversation on track because many people want to share stories and unimportant details. Using the office-approved format helps you keep the interview moving forward. Anxiety or hostility may be a factor in the patient's inability to focus on your questions. Without being patronizing, make the patient as comfortable as possible to minimize distractions. There must

---

Flashpoint

It is true that you don't often get a second chance to make a good first impression.

Flashpoint

Always keep in mind that there may be cultural differences that are a factor in gathering the medical history and be sensitive to these issues.

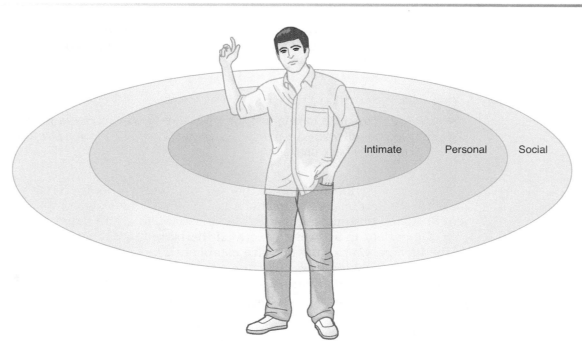

FIGURE 14-2 Personal space is the area around you that you consider your own comfort zone or the distance that you prefer others to keep. It can vary by gender and race or ethnicity.

TABLE 14-1
CULTURAL DIFFERENCES IN HEALTH CARE

Culture or Religion	Personal Space Preference	Communication Style	Reaction to Health Care
American, European (Caucasian)	Close	Direct eye contact, therapeutic touch, loud speech	May challenge medical opinions
African American	Close	Direct eye contact, therapeutic touch, loud speech	May challenge medical opinions, may distrust medical professionals
African or Caribbean	Close	Direct eye contact, therapeutic touch, loud speech	Highly emotional
Arabic	Distant	Females avoid direct eye contact, men engage in direct eye contact, no touching between men and women, loud speech	Do not discuss sexual dysfunction, contraception, mental illness, birth defects; women not permitted to be examined by male medical professional; combine folk medicine, religious beliefs, and Western medicine
Asian	Close but no touching	Indirect or avoid eye contact, avoid therapeutic touch, soft speech	Little emotion, may agree with medical professional even when don't understand information
Hispanic and Latin	Close but not touching	Direct eye contact, possible indirect eye contact with authority figures, soft speech	Combine folk medicine and religious beliefs with Western medicine
Native American	Distant	Avoid eye contact, soft speech	Combine folk medicine and natural elements with Western medicine
West Indian	Distant	Avoid eye contact	Modest regarding body; Western medicine

be a careful balance during the interview. You should not appear disinterested in the patient's details, but it is important to move forward in order to collect all the necessary information.

STOP, THINK, AND LEARN.
Your patient is talking nonstop. Your time for the interview is limited, but you do not want the patient to feel rushed. What can you say to get the interview back on track?

Try not to use medical words that the patient may not understand. Be prepared to explain terms or questions if the patient does not completely understand. Giving examples or asking the questions in a different form may better help the patient to answer correctly. If there are intimate or personal questions in the history, wait until you have established a comfortable rapport with the patient before asking those. The interview process should be informative and completed in a timely manner. Be aware of any **nonverbal cues** that may indicate the patient is uncomfortable with a question or does not understand what you are asking, such as looking away, crossing the arms across the chest, or frowning. Nonverbal communication involves the use of facial expressions, body language, gestures, eye contact, and touch to convey meaning. It is important that you not only hear what the patient is telling you but also assess his or her nonverbal communication for any cues that are not consistent with the patient's verbal communication. If the patient gets upset during the history, perhaps remembering an ill or deceased relative, it is acceptable to gently touch the patient's arm and give him or her time to regain composure. In addition to personal space, you must maintain a professional boundary with the patient.

As a healthcare worker, a key part of your job entails touching people. When patients seek medical care, they expect some degree of touching to be involved. However, this does not automatically make patients comfortable with being touched. To earn and maintain the patient's trust that all touching is appropriate and professional, protect the patient's privacy and dignity at all times. Prior to conducting any medical patient-centered task, whether it's merely taking a patient's pulse or assisting with a pelvic examination, always explain the task or procedure to the patient. If the patient refuses to be touched, honor this request and explore further with the patient why he or she is hesitant to be touched.

Medical History

The medical history, which is completed in its entirety on the first visit and updated on subsequent visits, includes all the patient's health issues, including childhood diseases, hospitalizations, major illnesses (e.g., hypertension, diabetes, and heart disease), and any previous surgeries. A woman's record should include **obstetrical history,** including number of pregnancies, live births, and other outcomes. **Current medications** are listed along with dosage and schedule. Remind the patient that other medications such as over-the-counter (OTC) pain relievers, vitamins, or herbal supplements should be included in this history because some may interact with medications prescribed by the physician. **Allergic reactions** to any medications, foods, or environmental substances should be noted in detail to alert the physician to medication allergies. Many offices note allergies in bold red print on the record cover or with an alert in the electronic system. All patients should have an updated immunization record on file. Additionally, any alternative medical treatments in which the patient engages must be recorded.

Medical records become **legal documents** and must be complete and accurate. When you are documenting a patient's history, it is sometimes best to put direct patient quotes in the record. A well-documented record can be a good defense if there is a legal case surrounding the patient's treatment. Poorly documented records indicate questionable care. The best practice is to document everything that involves a patient's care, including laboratory and radiology reports from other practitioners, telephone calls, prescription requests, and referrals to other physicians with the utmost care and attention to detail.

Family History

A family history determines the presence of certain conditions that have been diagnosed in the patient's blood relatives. This information is important because some diagnoses, such as heart disease, diabetes, and hypertension, are hereditary. Knowing that a disease is prevalent in a patient's family prompts the physician to look for signs or symptoms in the patient that may indicate the early signs of that disease so that preventive care may be provided. Advances in medical technology today allow physicians to make medical diagnoses much more quickly and efficiently.

Social History

A **social history** consists of the patient's marital status, occupation, sexual habits, use of alcohol and tobacco, and other recreational drugs. Although very personal, this information is necessary so that the physician may know the patient as thoroughly as possible. Patients may be reluctant to divulge this information to you, but they may feel more comfortable discussing it with the physician. A quick reminder to the patient that all information is kept in strict confidence may be necessary. You can defer these questions to the physician if the patient feels uncomfortable discussing it with you.

It is important to be especially sensitive to questions of social history when interviewing an adolescent in the presence of a parent or an elderly patient with a caregiver. A teenager may not admit to being sexually active with a parent in the room even when it may have an impact on the diagnosis or treatment. Elderly patients may likewise not feel comfortable discussing issues with a non-family member present. Occasionally, a situation of elder abuse may be discovered when a caregiver is not present. Discussing these questions may be more appropriate once the parent or caregiver has left the room. It may also be necessary to interview the parent or the caregiver separately to ensure that you have all the necessary information.

Be aware of clues that give you insight about the home situation when you are interviewing an elderly patient, adolescent, or the parent of a young child. Facial expressions or interactions between the caregiver and the patient may indicate a need for further investigation. Other indications that may alert you to problems are poor hygiene, unexplained lesions, and malnutrition.

Flashpoint
If it isn't documented, it wasn't done.

Completing the Interview

You may want to note on the patient history form any information that you were unable to obtain or that needs further definition so the physician can acquire it during the exam.

Once the initial interview is completed, *vital signs* are taken and recorded in the patient record.

Once you have completed your portion of the record, if the interview has taken place elsewhere, escort the patient to the exam room and prepare him or her for the physical examination.

Review of Systems

A complete history and physical examination includes a thorough review of all body systems to rule out asymptomatic conditions or future health concerns for the patient. This is a very systematic interview of the patient from head to toe, asking for any symptoms related to each of the body systems. The *review of systems (ROS)* provides the healthcare facility with a wealth of information about the patient, and it is a vital part of the patient assessment. As the physician progresses through the interview, he or she makes a notation of items that need further investigation. The review of systems, when merged with the patient history and the physical assessment, provides the physician with all of the information necessary to provide a diagnosis and treatment plan for the patient.

General

A physician gets an idea of the patient's overall health, including height, weight, vital signs, age-appropriate movements such as reflexes, and aptitude, during time spent with the patient and from the medical record. Vital signs, including temperature, pulse rate, respiratory rate, and blood pressure are key elements of the physical examination. Vital signs are discussed at length in Chapter 15.

Flashpoint

If you will listen, the patient will tell you the diagnosis.

Skin

Color, texture, and turgor (moisture content) of the skin and the presence of lesions or nodules are important factors for the physician to consider when he or she begins the examination. A bluish tint to the skin (cyanosis) may indicate a lack of oxygen, and very pale skin or mucous membranes may be a sign of anemia. These clues help the physician when making the clinical diagnosis.

Eyes, Ears, Nose, and Throat

Often abbreviated EENT, or HEENT to include the head, the eyes, ears, nose, and throat are examined by the physician to determine the patient's ability to breathe freely and see appropriately and to determine any signs or symptoms of upper respiratory conditions, dental disease, or thyroid conditions. During the EENT exam, the patient is asked about headaches, neck stiffness, vision difficulties, hearing difficulties, and dizziness.

STOP, THINK, AND LEARN.
As people age, some are reluctant to admit to hearing or vision difficulties. What are some clues that may indicate that a person may be having trouble hearing you or seeing something that you are showing him or her?

Cardiovascular

Listening to the patient's pulse with a stethoscope over the heart (apical pulse), the physician listens for abnormal pulse rate or rhythm and a swooshing sound that may indicate a heart murmur. The patient is asked about chest discomfort, shortness of breath after exercise, fainting, swelling of the feet, and any heart palpitations. The presence of varicose veins may also indicate early cardiovascular diseases.

Respiratory

The lungs and airways are assessed by listening with the stethoscope (auscultation) to determine any wheezes or other abnormal sounds. The physician asks the patient about shortness of breath or other breathing difficulties. Other symptoms that lead to further investigation are coughing up blood (hemoptysis), a productive cough, or any exposure to tuberculosis.

Gastrointestinal

Patients often disregard or discount symptoms of this body system because they seem insignificant; however, they are still important to the complete assessment. Physicians often have to ask very specific questions such as how often a patient has indigestion, if the patient has noticed a change in appetite, or if vomiting and diarrhea are present.

Genitourinary

This portion of the review includes both the urinary and reproductive systems. To assess the urinary system, the physician should question the patient about symptoms such as frequency and urgency or retention of urination, painful urination, or change in the color or clarity of the urine. The reproductive system can be evaluated with a woman's menstrual and obstetrical history. A man's reproductive history should include number of children, libido, and exposure to sexually transmitted diseases.

Musculoskeletal

Swelling, pain, or inability to move joints may indicate problems with both the muscular and skeletal systems. Conditions such as arthritis, sprains, and strains are often found during review of these body systems.

Neurological/Psychiatric

A patient's neurological history should include any episodes of convulsions, paralysis, forgetfulness, and depression and anxiety. Certain psychiatric diagnoses or emotional issues may mean that the physician has to alter the original treatment plan.

Endocrine and Immune

Symptoms such as palpitations, increased thirst, hunger, and urination are indications of certain endocrine diseases, such as diabetes mellitus, and require laboratory testing. Any allergies are also determined during this review, including medication, food, and environmental reactions.

Physical Assessment

The physician is the primary healthcare provider that performs the ***physical assessment*** of the patient, but a nurse practitioner or physician's assistant can also do it. The nurse or medical assistant chaperones the physician during the examination and should be prepared to assist the physician at any time during the examination. The ***physical examination*** can be a complete physical in which all body systems are examined or, in the case of a specialist or a patient with a specific need, an examination is limited to the area of concern. Healthcare professionals learn to use sight, sound, and touch to thoroughly evaluate a patient. Four tools are used in the physical assessment, as detailed below.

Inspection

Just by looking at the patient, or performing an ***inspection,*** many healthcare professionals can quickly assess the patient's well-being. Observation of skin color changes, swelling, or respiratory distress leads the physician to make an immediate decision about care for the patient.

Auscultation

The act of listening to body sounds, ***auscultation*** is performed with a stethoscope placed over body organs. Physicians can hear both normal and abnormal sounds in the heart, lungs, and abdomen. Specialized stethoscopes are used to hear fetal heart tones inside the mother's womb, and electronic stethoscopes are used to hear blood flow in major arteries and veins. Any abnormal sounds detected through auscultation can be evaluated with further testing.

Palpation

Using the fingertips to lightly press on the patient's body, or ***palpation,*** a physician can determine the size of a mass or the amount of tenderness in a certain part of the body. Palpation also allows the physician to determine whether a mass is moveable or if a joint is displaced. Making a diagnosis of appendicitis depends on palpation of the patient's lower abdomen and how much pain the patient feels.

Percussion

If you think of drumming when you hear the word *percussion,* you are correct. Using a finger, the physician can tap over certain organs of the body to determine organ size, fluid collection, or gas accumulation. Tapping over the lungs of a patient with pneumonia determines the amount of fluid within the lungs, giving the physician the information needed to treat the patient.

Summary

All information gathered in the history, the review of systems, and the physical assessment becomes a part of the patient record and is available for any healthcare provider treating the patient or for payment of an insurance claim. This comprehensive collection of data is the patient's story and establishes a baseline for the patient's care throughout his or her life.

As a healthcare professional, understanding the history and physical process helps you anticipate the needs of both the physician and the patient during the office visit. Follow-up care is easier when you know and understand the patient's history.

Practice Exercises

Multiple Choice

1. A patient medical record begins with collecting the:
   a. Patient's medical history
   b. Demographic information
   c. Family history
   d. Insurance information

2. The Truth in Lending Act requires that an office provide each patient with:
   a. The physician's weekly schedule
   b. The physician's malpractice carrier
   c. The physician's policies on financial practices
   d. The physician's annual patient volume

3. Which of the following would be found in the patient's family history?

   a.   Patient had a tonsillectomy as a child

   b.   Grandfather died of heart failure at age 67

   c.   Husband's cousin has uncontrolled diabetes

   d.   Patient has had three pregnancies with three live births

4. The best possible place for the patient interview to take place is:

   a.   In the laboratory so that you can take vital signs while interviewing

   b.   In the reception area

   c.   In the physician's private office

   d.   In a private area away from the general flow of the office

5. Which of the following would be determined during the HEENT exam?

   a.   Possible sinus infection

   b.   Hypertension

   c.   Irregular heart beat

   d.   Shortness of breath

6. A patient's complaint of test anxiety would be covered under which system?

   a.   Musculoskeletal

   b.   Neurological

   c.   Endocrine

   d.   Cardiovascular

Fill in the Blank

1. The act of listening to body sounds is known as _____.

2. Using the fingertips to lightly press on the patient's body is known as _____, whereas _____ is using a finger to tap over certain organs of the body to determine organ size, fluid collection, or gas accumulation.

3. A systematic interview of the patient from head to toe is the _____.

Short Answer

1. **When interviewing teenagers, questions about their social history may make them uncomfortable if a parent is in the room. How can you handle this situation?**

2. **What is personal space, and why is it important during an interview?**

INTERNET RESOURCES		
Agency/Organization	Web Address	Resources/Functions
Truth in Lending Act	http://fdic.gov/regulations/laws/rules/6500-1400.html	Consumer protection information as it relates to payment for medical services
American Association of Orthopaedic Surgeons	http://aaos.org/education/csmp/InitialMedEncounter.cfm	Although this site is dedicated to orthopedic surgeons, it contains an excellent patient interview/assessment.
National Institutes of Health	http://ncbi.nlm.nih.gov/bookshelf/br.fcgi?book=cm&part=A245	Interview skills and techniques.

15 VITAL SIGNS

Key Terms

afebrile Not having a fever

aneroid A device that uses air pressure to measure a patient's blood pressure

antecubital space The portion of the forearm commonly known as the bend of the elbow

apical pulse Another method for assessing pulse rate by placing a stethoscope over the apex of the heart and counting heartbeats for 1 minute

bradycardia A very slow heart rate of less than 60 beats per minute

circadian rhythm A 24-hour human clock that is synchronized with the normal lightness of day and darkness of night

cyanosis A bluish discoloration of the skin usually indicating a lack of oxygen

diastolic The bottom number on a blood pressure reading that indicates the pressure during cardiac relaxation

effort The energy a patient uses to breathe

febrile With fever

homeostasis The body's ability to maintain a stable internal environment regardless of external changes

Learning Outcomes

15.1 Identify the role of the healthcare professional in taking and recording vital signs

15.2 Define circadian rhythm and how it affects vital signs and homeostasis

15.3 Discuss the importance of accurately measuring and recording a patient's height and weight

15.4 Describe the methods of assessing the patient's temperature, pulse, respirations, and blood pressure

Competencies

CAAHEP
- Describe the normal function of each body system. (CAAHEP I.C.5)
- Obtain vital signs. (CAAHEP I.P.1)
- Apply critical thinking skills in performing patient assessment and care. (CAAHEP I.A.1)

ABHES
- Take vital signs. (ABHES 9.c)

The Role of Vital Signs in Health Care

To function properly, the body must maintain a stable internal environment regardless of changes that may occur outside it. The term **homeostasis** means that the body can adjust to an unstable environment with minimal noticeable changes. The body must maintain a normal heart rate (pulse), respiratory rate, blood pressure, and temperature to sustain life. Many changes occur within the body at a constant rate, such as the secretion of digestive enzymes to break down food into usable chemicals, insulin excretion from the pancreas to move the sugar consumed into the cells to be used for energy, and the exchange of the waste product carbon dioxide for oxygen to supply the tissues. These actions and reactions occur constantly. When an expected change does not occur or an unexpected change happens, the body may indicate a problem. For example, if the body does not get sufficient oxygen to replace the carbon dioxide, the heart rate increases to compensate for the low oxygen levels. A rise in the pulse rate alerts the healthcare professional to investigate. When a person develops an infection, body heat increases and is reflected in a person's temperature.

These basic life functions, called **vital signs,** can be measured easily, and they provide physicians with valuable information about the patient's overall condition. Vital signs are the first measurements taken when a person enters a healthcare facility. The term **mensuration** means the act or process of measuring, and it is used when referring to vital signs. They are recorded in the narrative form as T (temperature), P (pulse), R (respirations), and BP (blood pressure). A complete set of vital signs may also include the patient's height and weight in the event the physician needs to order medications based on body mass. These measurements are especially important in infants and children. (Chapter 7 discusses growth and development and the need for close monitoring.)

The human body follows a *circadian rhythm,* or a 24-hour human clock that is synchronized with the normal light of day and dark of night (Fig. 15-1). Ideally, people sleep for 8 hours and are awake for 16 hours. During this 24-hour cycle, fluctuations occur in body temperature, blood pressure, reflexes, muscle activity, hormone secretion, and other physiological processes in the body. For example, in a person who awakens early, eats about noon, and sleeps all night, the body temperature is highest at 7 p.m. and lowest at 4:30 a.m. Other significant changes include the sharpest rise in blood pressure just before 7 a.m. and our deepest sleep occurring at 2 a.m. Detailed changes also occur, such as the times at which kidneys filter out specific waste products and reabsorb the most water. Because of this cycle, it is important to document the time that vital signs are taken.

Although vital signs vary from patient to patient and from time to time, establishing baseline vital signs for each patient is important. Each time a patient visits a healthcare facility, vital signs are taken and recorded so the physician is able to identify abnormalities. Vital signs are documented in note form or plotted in graphic format (Fig. 15-2).

Each component of the vital signs follows.

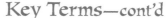

Key Terms—cont'd

hypertension A blood pressure reading that is consistently above normal for a patient

hypotension A blood pressure reading that is lower than normal for a patient

irregularly irregular A pulse rate that is irregular in pattern and rate.

mensuration The act or process of measuring something

Continued

Flashpoint

Travelers can develop jet lag after frequent cross-country or transoceanic trips. This condition of mental and physical fatigue is due to the interruption of the circadian rhythm.

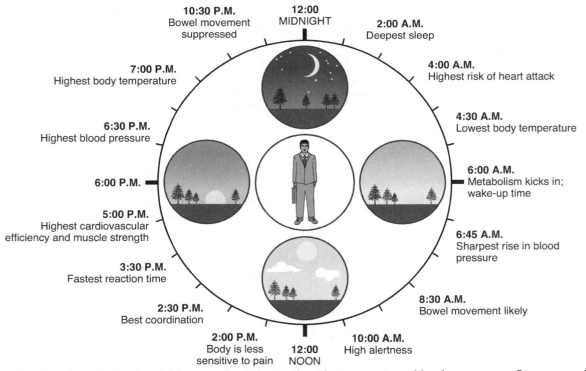

FIGURE 15-1 The circadian rhythm is a 24-hour cycle of fluctuations in temperature, blood pressure, reflexes, muscle activity, hormone secretion, and other physiological processes in the body.

MEDICAL RECORD		VITAL SIGNS RECORD									
HOSPITAL DAY	1	2									
POST- DAY											
MONTH-YEAR DAY	5	6									
JAN 20 12 HOUR	8 12 16	8 12 16	8 12 16								

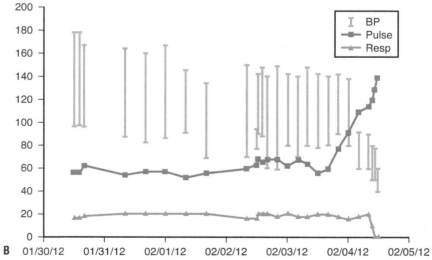

PULSE (0)   TEMP. F (°)   ...   TEMP. C (Centigrade equivalents, for reference only)

180	105°		40.6°	
	104°		40.0°	
170	103°		39.4°	
160	102°		38.9°	
150	101°		38.3°	
140	100°		37.8°	
130	99°		37.2°	
	98.6°		37.0°	
120	98°		36.7°	
110	97°		36.1°	
100	96°		35.6°	
90	95°		35.0°	
80				
70				
60				
50				
40				

RESPIRATION RECORD	20 21 19	19 22 20	18 18 20								
BLOOD PRESSURE	140/98 134/92 130/90	128/94 134/88 134/96	126/96 122/40 130/84								
HEIGHT: 69"	WEIGHT	160									

A

FIGURE 15-2 Vital signs can be recorded in chart form to show changes over time and highs and lows of specific readings. (A) A hospital-based paper form. (B) An office-based chart created from an electronic health record.

Height

Height is measured in feet and inches or in centimeters. Children and adults are measured in an upright position on a standard medical scale, and infants are measured using a flexible measuring tape (Fig. 15-3A). The patient should stand unassisted on the upright scale with his or her back to the tall arm of the scale. The measuring rod should be elevated above the patient's head and slowly lowered to sit lightly and straight on the top of the head. The height is measured at the level of the cross bar (Fig 15-3B). Stand close to patients who are on the scale in the event that they lose their balance. Assist the patient on

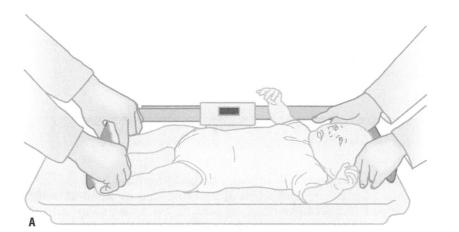

A

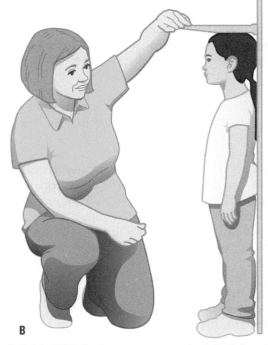

B

FIGURE 15-3 **Measuring height. (A) Infants are measured while lying down on a special table or scale or by using a flexible tape. (B) Children and adults are measured while standing using a special rod found on medical scales.**

Key Terms—cont'd

mm Hg Millimeters of mercury; used when recording blood pressure readings

pulse The number of times a patient's heart beats in 1 minute

pulse oximetry The measurement of the oxygen content in arterial blood using an infrared technology instrument attached to the patient's index finger

respiration A cycle of one inspiration and one exhalation

rhythm The indication that the heart is beating in an even or an uneven pattern

sphygmomanometer Used to measure blood pressure in an artery, an instrument that consists of a pressure gauge, an inflatable cuff placed around the upper arm, and an inflator bulb or pressure pump

strength A term used to describe how the patient's pulse feels

systolic The top number in the blood pressure reading that is the highest and indicates the pressure during cardiac contraction

tachycardia A fast heart rate of more than 100 beats per minute

temporal artery thermometer An electronic thermometer that uses infrared technology to measure the temperature in a major artery

tympanic thermometer An electronic thermometer that uses infrared technology to measure the temperature at the tympanic membrane (eardrum)

Continued

Key Terms—cont'd

vital signs An accounting of the patient's temperature, pulse, respiratory rate, blood pressure, and sometimes his or her height and weight

zero out A scale should be balanced at zero prior to weighing a patient

and off of the scales. Some healthcare practitioners prefer that patients are measured without shoes to obtain an exact height. If you ask the patient to remove his or her shoes, place a protective barrier on the scale prior to them stepping on.

An infant's head and chest circumferences are measured with the flexible tape and recorded to determine growth patterns. Monitoring height is most important in infants and children to determine abnormalities in growth patterns. Failure to increase in height may indicate musculoskeletal or endocrine issues such as dwarfism or a lack of sufficient growth hormone secreted by the pituitary gland. If such a condition is suspected, the height of the parents is measured and recorded, and further studies are conducted to determine the cause of the short stature. Osteoporosis, a condition that affects women primarily, causes weakness in the bones and may lead to fractures or compression of the vertebral column. This compression may cause a patient's height to decrease as aging occurs. Even such a small indicator may be valuable in the patient's overall wellness and treatment. A person's height is primarily genetic, but it can be affected by environmental and cultural conditions such as diet, social class, and access to healthcare.

Weight

Weight is measured in pounds and ounces or kilograms and grams. Regardless of the type of scales used, they should be balanced or **zeroed out** prior to weighing each patient. This is done by sliding both the large and the small weights to the zero position and making sure that the beam is stabilized in the center of the chamber at the end of the crossbar. Infants are weighed in the supine position on a set of medical balance scales, whereas children and adults stand on an upright medical balance scale (Fig. 15-4). The patient must stand unassisted in the center of the scales to achieve an accurate weight. Infants are placed in the center of the platform with the provider's hand just above for safety. It is helpful to ask the patient for his or her usual or previous weight so that you know where to begin. Move the larger weight first on the scale to the patient's approximate weight, and slowly slide the smaller weight across the beam until the bar stabilizes in the chamber. Adding the number of the larger and smaller weights gives you the patient's weight. Some healthcare facilities use digital scales that can be zeroed out electronically.

Infants and children should show a steady increase in weight during the growing years, but they should stabilize when they reach adulthood. In adulthood, a patient's weight may fluctuate based on medical conditions or the patient's diet and activity level. Obesity is a major health issue that many patients are trying to conquer. Attempting to lose weight is accomplished best with the help and advice of a physician. Obese patients may suffer from hypertension or diabetes and need to remain in close contact with the physician when trying to alter their weight. Recording their weight accurately on each visit helps with the patient's course of treatment.

Weight may also fluctuate when a patient's condition becomes unstable. A patient who develops heart failure may start to retain fluid, causing weight to increase overnight. Pregnant women who have a rapid weight gain may be at risk for toxemia. Such changes in weight can alert the healthcare practitioner to the need for medication and treatment evaluation. Likewise, a patient whose weight continues to decline, despite no changes in their eating or exercise

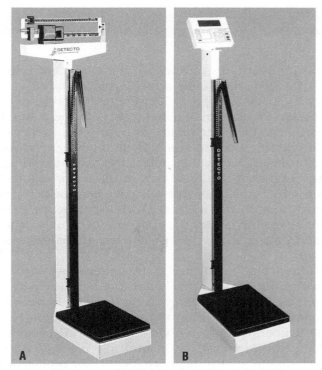

FIGURE 15-4 **Medical balance scales. (A) Mechanical. (B) Digital. (Courtesy of Detecto, a Division of Cardinal Scale Mfg. Co., Webb City, MO.)**

habits, should also be evaluated for medical conditions such as diabetes or hyperthyroidism.

In the event the patient cannot stand alone to be weighed, there are bed or wheelchair scales that are calibrated to exclude the weight of the bed or wheelchair and lift scales that can mechanically lift the patient to be weighed. Make sure there are no objects that add unnecessary weight to the patient.

It is important to know conversion tables to be able to provide information in the system the healthcare provider prefers (Table 15-1).

Flashpoint

Because weight is a sensitive issue with many patients, be sure to weigh them in a private location in the office.

STOP, THINK, AND LEARN.

Convert the following heights and weights:

5 ft, 5 in. = _____cm	8 lb, 4 oz = _____gm
78 lb = _____kg	4,758 gm = _____lb, ____oz
87 cm = _____in.	6 ft = _____in.
68 in. = _____ft ___in.	198 lb = _____kg
54 kg =_____lb	19 in. = _____cm

TABLE 15-1

METRIC/STANDARD CONVERSION TABLE

Metric System	Customary System	Examples
Kilogram (kg)	Pound (lb)	1 kg = 2.2 lb
Gram (gm)	Ounce (oz)	28.35 gm = 1 oz
Centimeter (cm)	Inch (in.) Foot (ft)	2.54 cm = 1 in. 1 ft = 12 in.

Temperature

The body's temperature fluctuates throughout the day, as the circadian rhythm clock indicates, but the body maintains a range that is within a few degrees. Homeostasis allows the body to adjust when the temperature outside is extreme. When the body gets too hot, the small blood vessels in the skin dilate and allow excess heat to escape. The body begins to sweat, and the evaporation allows the temperature to stay within a normal range. Drinking water (rehydrating) helps replace the water lost through sweating. When the body is cold, these small blood vessels narrow and shift the blood flow to the major organs for heat. Shivering is a process that increases muscle movement, which produces heat. An elevated temperature indicates a fever, which is the body's response to the invasion of pathogenic organisms such as bacteria or viruses. The term *febrile* is used to note that a patient has a fever. The term *afebrile* means the patient no longer has a fever.

Temperature readings can be affected if the patient has had a hot or cold drink or smoked within the 30 minutes before the measurement. Ask the patient about these possibilities prior to taking the temperature or in the event you get a measurement higher or lower than normal. Waiting 15 to 20 minutes before retaking the temperature should yield an accurate reading.

Body temperature can be measured in multiple places with different devices. Glass thermometers with mercury have been replaced with electronic devices due to the concern of mercury poisoning. Digital thermometers are the most common type used in households and healthcare facilities today. A home-use digital thermometer is readily available, inexpensive, accurate, and easy to use. Electronic thermometers used in healthcare facilities are much more sophisticated and expensive, but just as easy to use. All electronic thermometers can be used for measuring oral, rectal, and axillary (armpit) temperatures.

An electronic ear thermometer measures the tympanic, or eardrum, temperature. A **tympanic thermometer** measures very quickly, but it is more expensive than other thermometers and is not effective in infants (Fig. 15-5A). A newer technology in rapid temperature measurement is the **temporal artery thermometer** (Fig. 15-5B). A quick swipe of the patient's forehead with this thermometer gives an accurate temperature measurement. Also available on the market today is a pacifier thermometer. This device may indicate an increase in an infant's temperature, but it does not give an accurate measure of the true body temperature.

Plastic strip or chemical dot thermometers are available, but they are not as accurate as most of the methods discussed here.

All electronic thermometers are equipped with a probe that should be enclosed in a disposable probe cover before each use. All external parts of the thermometer should be cleaned thoroughly after each use.

Body temperature can be measured by different methods. Oral, rectal, and axillary are the most common, although tympanic and forehead methods were mentioned above. What most people consider "normal" body temperature is a range from 97.6°F to 99.6°F. A rectal or tympanic temperature may be 1° higher than an oral reading, and an axillary reading may be 1 degree lower than the oral. Temperature is recorded on a Fahrenheit or Celsius scale. Most

Flashpoint

A digital thermometer should be in every home's first aid kit and marked for method of use.

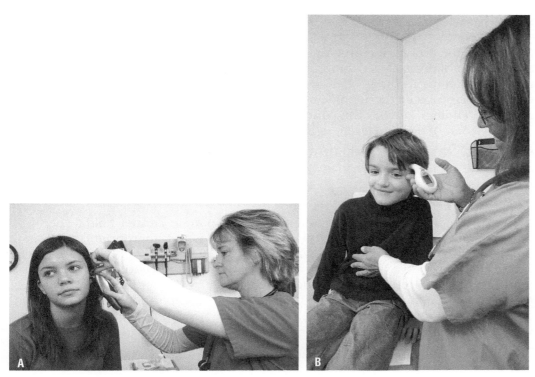

FIGURE 15-5 (A) A tympanic thermometer measures body temperature at the eardrum. (B) A temporal artery thermometer is swiped across the patient's forehead to get a reading. (From: Eagle, S., et al. *The Professional Medical Assistant: An Integrative, Teamwork-Based Approach.* Philadelphia: FA Davis Company, 2009. Used with permission.)

thermometers can be calibrated to either scale. Table 15-2 can be used to convert temperatures from one scale to the other.

STOP, THINK, AND LEARN.

Using Table 15-2, convert the following temperatures:

101.4°F = _____ °C	99.2°F = _____ °C
39.5°C = _____ °F	38.6° C = _____ °F
100.8°F = _____ °C	37°C = _____ °F

TABLE 15-2

CONVERSION OF TEMPERATURE

Fahrenheit	Step 1	Step 2	Step 3	Celsius
98.6°F	Subtract 32 98.6 − 32 = 66.6	Divide by 9 66.6 ÷ 9 = 7.4	Multiply by 5 7.4 × 5 = 37	37°C
Celsius	**Step 1**	**Step 2**	**Step 3**	**Fahrenheit**
37°C	Multiply by 9 37 × 9 = 333	Divide by 5 333 ÷ 5 = 66.6	Add 32 66.6 + 32 = 98.6	98.6°F

Oral Temperature

Measuring the oral temperature is the most straightforward method in conscious adults and children. Cover the probe with a disposable cover and place it directly under the tongue in the pocket on the back side of the mouth. Remember to support the probe or thermometer so that it remains firmly in place and gives an accurate reading. Remind the patient to refrain from biting down on the probe. The electronic thermometer gives a quick reading that can be recorded on the patient record. Discard the probe cover in the appropriate waste container.

Axillary Temperature

An axillary temperature may be taken when the patient cannot hold a thermometer under the tongue and the rectal method is not appropriate, such as in a patient with diarrhea or a child who is not old enough to hold the thermometer under the tongue but is too old for the invasive rectal procedure. Axillary temperature is measured by placing the thermometer in the center of the axilla, or armpit, and holding the arm close to the body. It is important that the axilla is dry prior to taking the temperature, so it may be necessary to pat the area dry with a cloth. Once the temperature is taken, record the value and note that it is an axillary reading with the letter *A*, for example, T 97.9° (A).

Rectal Temperature

The rectal temperature is considered to be the most accurate measure of body temperature. Rectal temperature is 1 degree higher than oral temperature. Taking a rectal temperature, however, is an invasive procedure and not always appropriate. This method is most often used in infants and unconscious patients who cannot participate in the oral method. To properly take an infant's rectal temperature, position the infant on the stomach, lubricate the thermometer or probe, and gently insert it $1/2$ to 1 inch into the anus. For an unconscious patient, it is easier to roll the patient to the left side and pull the right leg slightly upward to expose the anus. Lubricate the thermometer and slowly insert it about 1 to $1^1/_2$ inches. Hold the thermometer during the entire process to avoid movement. Once the temperature has been registered, remove the thermometer, dispose of the sheath and wipe down the thermometer with a disinfectant solution, and remove excess lubricant from the patient. Record the temperature with a notation that it was taken rectally, for example, T 99.8° (R).

Tympanic Temperature

The tympanic, or eardrum, temperature is also considered a core body temperature. It may also be called the "aural" temperature, a term that can be misunderstood as "oral." The electronic tympanic thermometer is one of the fastest methods of taking a temperature, sometimes taking less than 5 seconds. It is important that the patient be cooperative for the procedure, which means that it is not always the best method in young, curious children who may try turning their head to see the procedure. After placing a disposable cover on the thermometer, it must be inserted quickly and firmly to register the correct temperature. The thermometer can then be removed quickly and the value documented.

Regardless of the method of temperature measurement, it is important to remember infection control guidelines. Always wash the hands before beginning the procedure and again after finishing. Explain the procedure to the patient, or parent, before beginning, and document that it occurred according to your facility's guidelines.

Pulse

Each time the heart beats, it forces blood through the arteries and creates a pulsing sensation, or *pulse,* at key points on the body. Counting these pulsations tells how many times the patient's heart is beating in 1 full minute. This measurement is important so the healthcare practitioner can evaluate the patient's cardiac function. There are accepted normal pulse rates that vary depending on age, as depicted in Table 15-3.

Medications and medical conditions can affect the patient's heart rate, which makes the patient history a very important part of the physical examination. Some cardiac medications are known to slow the heart rate whereas others may increase the rate. Dehydration is a condition that may affect the pulse rate. A well-conditioned athlete has, in the process of training, strengthened the heart muscle, allowing it to beat slower and more efficiently to supply the body with oxygen and nutrients.

When taking the pulse rate, take note of three factors. **Rate** is the actual number of times the heart beats in 1 minute. **Rhythm** is the indication that the heart is beating in an even or an uneven pattern. Regular rhythm is the even pattern, and an irregular rhythm is the variable pattern. Within the irregular pattern, the rhythm may be regularly irregular, meaning that while the pattern is irregular, there is a specific pattern to the irregularity. One example is a pattern in which every third beat is missing over the entire course of the measurement. If the pattern misses an occasional beat randomly, it is known as an *irregularly irregular rhythm.*

The third facet of the pulse is the *strength.* You will note the strength when you place your fingers over the pulse point. Terms such as "strong" or "bounding" are used if the pulse feels more forceful than a normal pulse, and "thready" indicates that the pulse is weak or barely felt.

The pulse rate may be taken manually in specific locations on the body where the artery passes close to the skin; however, the radial pulse is most

Flashpoint

"Irregularly irregular" is a very important fact for the healthcare practitioner.

TABLE 15-3	
NORMAL PULSE RATES	
Age	**Pulse Rate**
Newborn to 1 year	100–160 beats per minute
Children 1 to 10 years	70–120 beats per minute
Children over 10 years to adult	60–100 beats per minute
Well-conditioned athletes	40–60 beats per minute

commonly used during a physical examination. The radial pulse can be felt on the thumb side of the wrist in the shallow indention on the underside. Other pulse point locations include the temporal artery, located on either side of the forehead; the carotid on the front side of the neck; the brachial on the inner aspect of the elbow; the femoral in the groin; the popliteal located behind the knee; and the dorsalis pedis, or pedal pulse, located on the top of the foot. Although each of the points has a palpable pulse, the radial pulse remains the most easily accessible.

The standard time for measuring and recording the pulse rate is 1 minute. Designated by the letter *P*, the rate is recorded simply as the correct number of beats per minute, for example, P 84.

To determine the pulse rate, place two fingers over the pulse point and press gently, a process known as palpation. Too much pressure may block the arterial flow and obliterate the pulse. Do not use the thumb to measure pulse rate because the thumb has a palpable pulse that may be mistaken for the patient's pulse. Count for 1 full minute according to your watch to determine the pulse rate. Taking the pulse rate for an entire minute determines any irregularities in the patient's heart rhythm.

Another method of assessing the pulse rate is the ***apical pulse,*** which requires the use of your stethoscope and watch. The apical pulse may be used for cardiac patients, those with irregular rhythms, and most commonly for infants, because their pulse rate cannot be easily palpated. Using the stethoscope, place the bell over the apex of the heart, located in the fifth intercostal space and the midclavicular line or just below the left nipple. The heart beat has two distinct sounds, "lub" and "dub." These are the sounds of the valves opening and closing during one cardiac cycle or heartbeat. The sequence of "lub-dub" is one beat. Once you have established the sequence of the heart beat, you can begin to count the pulse. An apical pulse is always counted for 1 full minute and recorded, noting the apical measurement with the letter *A*, for example, P 76(A). Taking an infant's apical pulse requires practice because of the fast rate at which the heart beats and the inability of the infant to remain still and quiet.

Terms used to describe abnormal pulse rates include ***tachycardia,*** meaning a faster than normal heart rate, and ***bradycardia,*** which indicates a slower than normal rate. Tachycardia indicates a pulse rate of above 100 for an adult, and bradycardia demonstrates a heartbeat of less than 60 beats per minute. These conditions may be the result of medical conditions, medications, fever, and level of physical activity.

Flashpoint

It is important to wear a watch with a second hand or a digital watch with a function that tracks seconds so that you can accurately measure the pulse and respiratory rates for precisely 1 minute.

Respiration

The number of times a person breathes each minute is known as the respiratory rate, or respirations. Each time a person breathes in, it is an inspiration, and the chest cavity expands to take in oxygen. When the person lets the air out of the lungs and the lungs contract back down, it is an exhalation. A cycle of one inspiration and one exhalation is known as a ***respiration.*** The respiratory rate, or respirations, is determined by counting the number of cycles in 1 minute. Respirations are documented using the letter *R* to indicate the number of breaths that a patient takes in 1 minute, for example, R 16.

Counting the respiratory rate can be problematic in that many patients know that you are watching them breathe and unintentionally alter their breathing patterns. By leaving your fingers on the pulse point after counting the pulse, you can shift your attention to counting the respirations, and patients will not realize that you are watching them breathe. Some patients are anxious about the visit to the physician and may exhibit a faster respiratory rate. If you notice this, engage the patient in a conversation that may help him or her relax and breathe normally.

During the respirations, you should observe the patient for three characteristics of their breathing pattern. Determine the rate or number of times the patient completes a respiration cycle in 1 minute. Because the respiratory rate in adults is slow, counting for a full minute may be necessary to get an accurate count. The rhythm of breathing is important. The respiratory cycle should be regular, with even spaces between breaths. Respiratory **effort** is important to note. The patient should be breathing through the nose quietly and not in a labored or distressed fashion. If the patient appears to be working hard to breathe or you hear sounds such as wheezes or crackling sounds, make a note on the patient record. As with other vital signs, there are external causes for rapid, depressed, and noisy respirations. Medications may increase or decrease respirations, as do respiratory illnesses such as asthma, bronchitis, and pneumonia. A significant increase in the number of respirations or noticeable sounds may indicate the patient is not getting enough oxygen into the body. Look at the patient's lips and nail beds to see if they have signs of **cyanosis,** a bluish discoloration of the skin showing the lack of oxygen in the blood. Also helpful is the **pulse oximetry** device that attaches to the patient's index finger and gives you an accurate measurement of the patient's oxygen levels through infrared technology. Normal respiratory rates vary by age, which you can see in Table 15-4.

Flashpoint

Remember that respiration can be consciously altered by the patient, which affects the respiratory rate.

Blood Pressure

The final component of vital signs is the patient's blood pressure. A person's blood pressure indicates how hard the heart is working to supply the body with oxygen and nutrients. The harder the heart has to pump the blood, the higher the blood pressure reading. Blood pressure readings contain two numbers separated by a slash. The top number in the reading is the highest, and it is the **systolic** pressure, which indicates the pressure during cardiac contraction. The bottom number is lower and is the **diastolic** reading, which indicates the pressure during cardiac relaxation. Taken together, the numbers can give the physician valuable information about the patient's cardiovascular system. The American Heart Association recommends a healthy blood pressure of a systolic reading less than 120 and a diastolic reading less than 80. When the diastolic reading is high, the heart is working hard even at rest. Consistently lower

TABLE 15-4	
NORMAL RESPIRATORY RATES	
Age	Normal Respiratory Rate
Newborn to 1 year	40–60 breaths per minute
Children 1 to 6 years	18–30 breaths per minute
Children 7 to adult	12–24 breaths per minute

readings may indicate **hypotension** (low blood pressure), and consistently higher readings may be a sign of **hypertension** (high blood pressure). Untreated hypertension can lead to cardiovascular and cerebrovascular disease, including arteriosclerosis (hardening of the arteries), which may cause a heart attack or stroke. Hypertension is called the "silent killer," as there are often no symptoms associated with high blood pressure. Patients should be educated on the importance of treating their hypertension for life whether they have symptoms or not. It is not uncommon for patients to stop taking their medications because they do not "feel bad" or the medications make them feel sluggish.

Taking a blood pressure requires the use of your stethoscope and a **sphygmomanometer,** or blood pressure cuff. The sphygmomanometers originally contained a column of mercury or a circular **aneroid** dial, and blood pressure was measured in millimeters of mercury, abbreviated **mm Hg.** The column and the dial are calibrated, with each line measuring 2 mm Hg. Because research shows mercury to be toxic, the column type of sphygmomanometers is no longer used. The cuff portion, usually made of cloth or other synthetic material with a hook and loop closure, contains a bladder that is connected to and inflated with a bulb. The bulb is controlled with a small screw that opens and closes the tube that inflates and deflates the bulb. Closing the screw valve allows air to be pumped into the bladder without escaping. Releasing the screw valve with your thumb and forefinger allows the air to escape, producing the sounds that you hear that indicates the reading.

It helps to learn blood pressure measurement by pumping the sphygmomanometer up and then slowly deflating it in order to gain control of the process. Releasing the air must be a smooth process in order to hear the sounds that correspond to the blood pressure reading. When taking a manual blood pressure reading, the cuff should wrap and overlap around the patient's upper arm. The size of the cuff makes a significant difference in the blood pressure reading, and failure to use the correct size results in an erroneous reading. Using a standard-sized cuff on an overweight person may give falsely high blood pressure readings. Likewise, a cuff that is too large for the patient's arm may give falsely low readings. For the healthcare practitioner to adequately treat the patient, accurate blood pressure readings are necessary. Take the necessary time to find the right equipment before you begin taking vital signs.

Place the correct size cuff on the patient's upper arm just below the axilla and about $1^1/_2$ inches above the **antecubital space,** or the inside area of the elbow. Support the patient's arm in your arm or lay it on a flat surface to keep the arm from moving. Feel for the brachial pulse and place the diaphragm (the larger flat disk) of the stethoscope over this area for better volume. Inflate the cuff to just above 160 mm Hg, unless the patient has a history of hypertension, and inflate to just above 180 mm Hg for those patients. Slowly release the valve and listen for the first pulse beat. Note the number on the dial. Continue to deflate the cuff, and listen as the pulse sound diminishes. Remember the number on the dial when you heard the last sound. Knowing that each mark on the dial is an even number, record your blood pressure with the systolic reading over the diastolic reading. In the patient record, the blood pressure is abbreviated BP, for example, BP 142/78. Taking blood pressure is a technically difficult procedure and requires much practice to become proficient. It is important to release the cuff steadily so you do not cause undue discomfort to the patient. If the patient becomes anxious because of the tight cuff, the blood pressure may increase, giving you an inaccurate reading.

Many healthcare facilities now use electronic devices to record blood pressure, in which case the placement of the cuff and the activation of the device is all that is required of the healthcare provider. It is important to remember the

Flashpoint

Remember: "righty-tighty, lefty-loosey."

guidelines for cuff size and placement when using an electronic device. In instances where a functioning stethoscope is unavailable, a blood pressure by palpation may be accomplished by pumping up the cuff and manually palpating the pulse in the antecubital area where the head of the stethoscope typically lays. Once the pressure is released from the cuff, the point at which a pulse is first felt should be recorded as the systolic blood pressure. There is no diastolic pressure recorded in this instance, and the pressure should be recorded as "by palpation." For example, a systolic blood pressure may be reported to the physician as "120 systolic by palpation." This method is often used in noisy environments when hearing the pulse of the blood pressure is difficult.

Patients who are postmastectomy (surgical removal of one or both breasts in the presence of cancer) or who have had vascular and lymphatic surgery, patients with a kidney dialysis shunt, and patients receiving intravenous fluids should never have their blood pressure taken in the affected arm. In the event that neither arm is accessible for blood pressure, it is possible to use a thigh cuff and take the reading using the popliteal artery or to use the forearm and take the reading from the radial artery.

Blood pressure can increase as the result of medications such as decongestants, diseases such as kidney failure, and by emotional factors. A diagnosis of hypertension, or high blood pressure, is not made on one elevated reading. To make a diagnosis of hypertension, the healthcare practitioner monitors blood pressure readings over several days, with readings taken at regularly scheduled times as well as some random times. There are also factors that can decrease a patient's blood pressure. Dehydration, medications, and other conditions can cause an abnormally low blood pressure that may make the patient weak and dizzy. These patients should be warned not to stand up quickly, as the sudden change in posture may cause fainting.

Flashpoint

Some patients suffer from "white coat syndrome" and have an increase in blood pressure simply because they become so anxious while visiting the doctor.

Summary

Taking vital signs is fundamental to any visit to a healthcare facility. As you can see, these four components provide the practitioner with a baseline of the patient's basic physiological functions. By providing the healthcare practitioner with accurate vital signs, multiple body systems can be evaluated quickly, and the values can help guide the practitioner to an accurate diagnosis and treatment plan.

Practice Exercises

Multiple Choice

1. Medications are often ordered based on the patient's:

   a. Height

   b. Weight

   c. Head circumference

   d. Body mass

2. Our body's internal 24-hour "clock" is known as our:

    a. Homeostatic rhythm

    b. Circadian rhythm

    c. Metabolic clock

    d. Rhythm clock

3. You take a patient's temperature and notice that it is elevated. The patient states he drank a cup of coffee while waiting. You should:

    a. Note the patient drank coffee on the patient record

    b. Document 98.6°F as you know it was probably normal before the coffee

    c. Do not document a temperature

    d. Wait for 10 to 15 minutes and retake the temperature

4. The most accurate temperature reading is:

    a. Oral

    b. Rectal

    c. Axillary

    d. Temporal artery

5. When checking a radial pulse, which of the following is not important?

    a. Rate

    b. Rhythm

    c. Strength

    d. Bruit

6. An accurate measurement of the patient's oxygen level through infrared technology is:

    a. Respiration count

    b. Pulse oximetry

    c. Respiratory effort

    d. Oxygen saturation

Fill in the Blank

1. To check an apical pulse, you must place the stethoscope over the _____ of the heart at the 5th _____ space.

2. A fast pulse is known as _____ , and a slow pulse is known as _____.

3. Each respiration includes one _____ and one _____.

Short Answer

1. **What is the best method of counting a patient's respiratory rate?**

2. **What factors may increase a patient's blood pressure?**

3. **When is a patient diagnosed with hypertension?**

INTERNET RESOURCES

Agency/Organization	Web Address	Resources/Functions
National Heart, Lung and Blood Institute of the National Institutes of Health	www.nhlbi.nih.gov/health/ health-topics/topics/hbp	Information on high blood pressure
American Heart Association	http://heart.org	Information on blood pressure readings
MedicineNet	http://medicinenet.com/ aches_pain_fever/article.htm	Consumer information for fever
American Heart Association	http://heart.org	Target heart rates
National Institutes of Health	http://ncbi.nlm.nih.gov/bookshelf/ br.fcgi?book=cm&part=A1308	Information on respiratory rates and measurement

16 PROFESSIONALISM AND ETHICS

Key Terms

attendance Being at work when you are scheduled to be there

attitude A general feeling about something

bioethics The ethical or moral implications of new technologies and advances in health care

character The qualities that make someone unique, including morals and actions

communication The exchange of information between people either verbally or nonverbally

cooperation Working together to accomplish a common goal

dependability Able to be trusted; reliable

ethics The moral compass that allows someone to determine right from wrong

initiative The ability to act and make decisions without the help or advice of other people

organization Having a plan to fully accomplish daily tasks in an orderly fashion

productivity The ability to accomplish a set amount of work within a specified time

Learning Outcomes

16.1 Define professionalism in the health-care arena

16.2 Outline the characteristics of a health-care professional

16.3 Identify methods of effective communication within your profession

16.4 Recognize the importance of a professional image in appearance and conduct

16.5 Differentiate between ethics and bioethics

Competencies

CAAHEP

- Apply ethical behaviors, including honesty/integrity in performance of medical assisting practice. (CAAHEP X.A.1)
- Examine the impact personal ethics and morals may have on the individual's practice. (CAAHEP X.A.2)

ABHES

- Demonstrate professionalism by being cognizant of ethical boundaries. (ABHES 11.b.4)

A career in health care must not be entered into lightly. It is a demanding but rewarding calling for those who are interested in caring for both the physical and emotional needs of people. The hours are long, and the work is taxing, which makes the job one that requires more than just an education. Some healthcare careers pay high wages, but no amount of money makes a job worthwhile if you are not prepared for and passionate about what you do.

Finding the right job will be easier if you are prepared personally and professionally. Employers want to hire professionals who possess higher-order skills, such as critical thinking and the ability to analyze and solve problems. It is important for you to learn theory and technical skills during your training, but you also must learn to apply those skills to situations that you encounter in your job. Most employers terminate employees not because of their lack of technical skills but because of a lack of professional skills. Employers want employees who have a good work ethic and who work productively with a positive attitude. In short, they want employees who display **professionalism,** indicating that they understand and accept the responsibilities of their job and are willing to conduct themselves accordingly.

The Marks of a Professional

Key Terms—cont'd

punctuality Arriving promptly and on time for a job or appointment

respect A feeling of admiration for other people or for their thoughts and ideas

responsibility Accepting a task and following through with it; being accountable for an action or idea

self-confidence The ability to believe in yourself and your potential for success

Attendance and Punctuality

Healthcare facilities depend on their employees to be present when scheduled. Unlike other businesses, health care demands that all members of the team be present to deliver quality patient care. There are certain positions that require licensure, registration, or certification to perform the duties of the job, which means that not just anyone can fill that position when the employee is absent.

In healthcare facilities that operate around the clock, employees must be on time to relieve those who are completing their shifts. Failing to show up for work on time means that someone has to stay late or someone must be called in on his or her day off. There are certainly times when sickness or another emergency prevents you from going to work, and in these situations notify your employer as soon as possible so that a suitable replacement can be found in time to deliver seamless care to the patients.

Your **attendance** and **punctuality** can prove to your employer that you are a valuable employee who takes pride in your job. If the need to change jobs arises, you want to be assured that your employer provides a respectable reference for you. Attendance and punctuality are always an issue when a prospective employer is considering you for an open position.

STOP, THINK, AND LEARN.
Mary Lee, the night supervisor at Mercy Hospital, answers the phone at 6:45 a.m. The nurse scheduled for the shift from 7 a.m. to 3 p.m. tells her that her car will not start, so she will not be in to work. The nursing unit is extremely busy with late admissions and early surgeries. What problems does this create? How will the oncoming and offgoing shifts react?

Character

Your **character** includes a sense of **responsibility,** loyalty to your employer, honesty, trustworthiness, initiative, and self-discipline. These traits are important to an employer because they represent someone who wants to be a productive member of the team and who takes pride in the work. Health care is a field that demands employees who are passionate about patient care. Not everyone can work in this field, especially those who do not enjoy interaction with people.

Honest employees are an asset to any organization. What would happen if a medication error was made and the employee failed to notify anyone? The results could be disastrous, and the patient and family would suffer from someone's dishonesty. Honesty extends to the amount of time you spend at work. If you make a habit of taking additional time at lunch and breaks or sending personal e-mails and viewing the Internet when you are supposed to be performing your job, you are stealing time from your employer. Taking liberties such as making personal long-distance calls from work or taking supplies home in your pockets is also dishonest. These seemingly small elements cost your employer money that could be used to provide better patient care or employee benefits.

A dependable employee is someone who is always present on time and puts in an honest day's work for an honest day's pay. **Dependability** means being reliable to do the job as it should be done—not taking shortcuts, omitting tasks, or leaving work for others. Being dependable means that your coworkers can count on you.

Someone once said, "There are three types of people in this world: those who make it happen, those who watch it happen, and those who say 'what happened?'" A trait of valued employees is that they take the **initiative;** that is, when they see something that needs to be done, they do it or take steps to ensure that it gets done. By taking the initiative, you show that you want to work and want to provide quality patient care.

By demonstrating the traits of honesty and dependability and showing initiative, employers in return put their trust in you as a valuable employee. Your employer, your patients, and your coworkers know that you can be trusted to put forth your best effort when and where it is needed. HIPAA privacy laws require that you keep work-related information confidential, but your own trustworthiness should be the primary reason that you keep such information private.

These character traits—dependability, initiative, honesty, and trustworthiness—are the result of self-discipline. You have so many choices in life. No one says that you have to get up in the morning, that you have to go to school or work, or even tells you when to eat. These are all choices that you make because you accept the responsibility and want to prove that you are a self-disciplined individual who cares about your actions. Besides your actions, you must keep your emotions under control by not engaging in childish behaviors or angry expressions. Control your feelings rather than let them control you. Employers and patients alike will appreciate your professional demeanor.

STOP, THINK, AND LEARN.
How would you complete the following statements?

Making excuses is a way to avoid _____.

After repeatedly making excuses, some people begin to _____ the excuses.

Your employer may _____ if you constantly make excuses.

Appearance

As a healthcare professional, you want to look the part. Your sense of pride in the profession should show in your clothing and your hygiene. Employers and patients expect your appearance to be appropriate for working in the healthcare field. You must also remember that how a patient or employer perceives you creates a lasting impression. It is true that you never get a second chance to make a first impression. Remember that it is your appearance that makes a large part of that impression.

What you wear or how you style your hair may not be appropriate for the job you are doing. Jewelry harbors bacteria and should be limited during working hours. Fingernails, natural and acrylic, that extend beyond the length of the finger can be a haven for bacteria even when you wash your hands frequently. Long fingernails can also be a hazard when working with patients. You would never intentionally scratch a patient, but there are times when close contact may injure the patient. Your hair should be clean and styled neatly so as not to interfere with care of the patient. Make sure that when you lean over the patient your hair does not fall onto him or her. Facial hair on men should be neat and well groomed so that it does not offend the patient or impede care.

Conservative makeup is recommended for healthcare professionals while working. Everyone should want to look nice when working with patients and other members of the healthcare team, and this can be accomplished without overdoing the makeup. Perfume can be offensive to patients and other employees and thus should not be worn in a healthcare setting. A good deodorant is important to prevent offensive body odor. Brushing your teeth helps prevent halitosis, or bad breath, when you are close to the patient's face. Some foods and beverages cause bad breath even after you have brushed your teeth, so having breath mints available may help. Chewing gum while working is never appropriate.

 STOP, THINK, AND LEARN.
You are working in a group setting when someone makes an offensive comment. How do you react? You overhear a group of fellow students laughing and saying they are going to buy a bar of soap and a tube of toothpaste for your birthday. How does that make you feel?

Civility and Courtesy

Patients, families, and other healthcare workers watch your actions and behaviors in the workplace. Interrupting others during a conversation and not paying attention when someone is talking to you are inappropriate behaviors and may be considered unprofessional. You are likely to have coworkers who are not your friends outside of work and whom you may not like very much. Nevertheless, it is a hallmark of professionalism to treat your fellow employees, even those you do not take to on a personal basis, with respect and civility, especially when patients are present. Arguing with someone during working hours causes a disturbance for everyone and does not give others a good impression of you. Disagreements should be handled calmly and behind closed doors, possibly with a supervisor present. Because it always takes two to argue, you can simply walk away. Finally, a genuine "please" and "thank you" is always well received and implies polite behaviors and professionalism.

Attitude

It has been said that we control our ***attitude,*** or it controls us. Negative attitudes can decrease self-esteem and productivity. And when someone calls attention to this negative attitude, it worsens the situation because we realize that others are aware of our problems. The expression, "Smiling's contagious; frowning's outrageous," tells only part of the story, as frowning is also contagious. When you are around people who constantly complain, do you find yourself sinking to their level and voicing your own complaints? Everyone has bad days and encounters events that negatively affect attitude. Recognize that these events are temporary.

Going to work each day with an upbeat outlook and the intention to do the absolute best job that you can and taking pride in your work can help uplift coworkers who are feeling low and inspire them to try harder as well. Working with people who are always upbeat and self-confident can improve your attitude because a good attitude can be as contagious as a bad one. Never underestimate the power of a positive attitude.

A good attitude is developed by making yourself available to learn new information and skills and making the best of all situations. The learning opportunities that you accept help to build your self-confidence in the workplace. It may be a scary experience the first time that you are sent out for a clinical rotation, but having the right attitude helps mold you into the healthcare professional that you want to be.

STOP, THINK, AND LEARN.

Each morning before you leave for school or work, what are your thoughts when you look in the mirror? How do you describe "self-esteem," and why is it important in your life?

Self-Confidence

People who do not have **self-confidence** may appear dull and not interested in being a part of the team. Lack of participation results in no longer being asked to be involved in the work of the team, which may have a negative effect on that person, further lowering his or her self-esteem and attitude. On the other end of the spectrum are the know-it-alls who want to be in charge of all aspects of work because of their inflated self-esteem. These people believe that their opinion is the only one that counts because they know more than anyone else in the group. It can be frustrating to work with someone like this, and we need to keep our own attitude in check to prevent resentment and maintain our own self-confidence. Setting realistic goals for yourself, soliciting feedback so you can improve your performance, and taking a moment to feel a sense of accomplishment when you have achieved goals and have done a good job help you to build and maintain self-worth and to reach your full potential as a healthcare professional.

Productivity and Organization

Good work habits are essential in health care. Most healthcare workers carry a heavy workload that involves patient care, paperwork, and computer tasks. Facilities typically keep staff to a minimum to lower expenses, so **productivity**—focusing, applying yourself, and getting the job done—is a very important quality to employers and vital to being a professional.

Health care is all about attention to detail, whether you are following your instructor's directions or providing a specific treatment for a patient. For example, facilities that deliver patient care have protocols for keeping patients and employees safe. As an employee, it is your responsibility to follow the guidelines set forth to provide safe, quality patient care and to protect your own safety. Each safety guideline is in place for a specific reason and should never be viewed as punitive. In any organization, when an employee is injured on the job, everyone loses. The employee must deal with the physical injury, the other employees must pick up extra duties, and the employer loses money through the worker's compensation payments. Increased workload on the other employees may create a morale problem and decrease overall productivity.

Conserving supplies helps cut down on unnecessary expenses for the facility. It is easy to put small things such as alcohol pads in your pocket to use during your shift and then go home with them still in your pocket. If everyone did that, it would add up to a significant amount of wasted money each year. Be very aware of the type and amount of supplies that you need to perform a procedure and always return unused items to stock. Healthcare facilities often tag single-use items in a supply room or on a supply cart. When you use the items, make sure the tags are placed in the correct place for the patient to be charged. Small losses add up to large losses when employees are careless about supplies and charges.

Your productivity increases if you read all instructions prior to beginning a procedure that you have forgotten or have never performed. Understanding the entire process before you begin eliminates wasted time and supplies. Most important, failure to follow directions can be catastrophic for the patient.

 ## STOP, THINK, AND LEARN.
How well do you follow directions? Do you read or listen to all instructions before you begin a task, or do you scan the directions and start to work immediately?

Organizational skills go hand in hand with productivity. It is hard to be productive when you have to stop frequently to gather supplies, put the chart together, or get the equipment ready for procedures. When you look in your book bag, can you find exactly what you are looking for very quickly, or do you have to search for several minutes? In the mornings when you are getting ready for school or work, are all of your clothes readily available, or do you have to look in your closet, the dresser, under the bed, or in another room to gather everything you need? Imagine how much time you would save if you had everything organized in one place. ***Organization*** is one of the most difficult skills to master, but once you have done so, the skill can save you time and money.

Performing your daily duties in addition to keeping your work area neat may seem like more than you can do, but it is much easier to work in a neat space. You can be more productive if you do not have to stop and move items around to find something specific. Keeping your work area neat is not only essential for being productive but also can be a safety issue. Your work space is your responsibility, even if you share it with others. Make sure that you leave the area neat so that another employee does not have to clean up after you. Be a team player and clean your work area before you leave.

Being organized also means being able to manage your time effectively. Using your time wisely is important in your workplace as well as in your life. We are a "busy" society, and we often use business as an excuse for not completing small or mundane tasks. Often, finishing those tasks allows more time for the things that we want to do. Some people have trouble saying "no" to friends, family, and even employers. Taking on too many responsibilities or activities may result in a stressful lifestyle, leaving you with little time for yourself. It is acceptable to say no when you know that you will not be able to complete the task. Many people are more frustrated when they accept a responsibility and are not able to complete the task efficiently or to their standards than they would be if they had just said no. It usually is not wise to overextend yourself in an attempt to prove something to your employer or your coworkers.

When you find yourself with a list of activities or responsibilities, you must prioritize them in order to get them all done in a reasonable amount of time and thereby be productive. If you have several patients who all need laboratory work or other tests, how do you decide who gets treated first? Taking a moment to prioritize the patients' needs makes it easier for you to complete the tasks, and the patients will be satisfied. The patients would rather know that when you get to them you are committed to their care and not preoccupied with how you will take care of the rest of the patients. When you have many tasks to complete, setting timetables also helps you organize your schedule. Make sure that when you set these timetables they are realistic so you do not set yourself up for failure.

Communication

Communicating effectively is important in health care and life in general. Professional communication is essential to ensure that patients receive the quality care they deserve. Verbal communication is the spoken or written word, and we would like to believe that every verbal communication is interpreted as we mean it. That is not always the case, however, and we should make efforts to prevent misinterpretation or be ready to clarify any mistaken meaning. Using the correct terminology and making sure that your body language reinforces your message help to convey the correct meaning.

Communication should always be a two-way exchange that includes a message and response or feedback. In health care, there are barriers that prevent effective communication. Many medical terms are unfamiliar, strange, and even frightening to laypeople, so use language that the patient understands. This grows harder when a common language is not shared. Language barriers prevent a healthcare professional from comprehending what is wrong with a patient and prevents the patient from understanding the details of treatments or procedures.

To be fully effective, communication must go both ways; that is, poor listening skills impede productive communication. When a patient is talking, listen intently so that you can correctly assess his or her condition. If you are constantly talking and asking questions but do not allow the patient to answer or do not attend closely to the answer, you will never get the information you need to process the patient's information. The patient also feels this rush and thinks that you are not interested in what he or she has to say. Never interrupt a patient or finish his or her sentences, but do not let the patient ramble until you fail to get the necessary information for the encounter.

STOP, THINK, AND LEARN.
Have you ever noticed someone making multiple hand gestures and facial expressions while talking on the telephone? Can you tell the general idea of their conversation? Role-play with another member of your class as someone who is experiencing an angry phone call, a good news phone call, and a sad phone call.

Written communication must be very clear and concise to be effective, or it may be misunderstood. For instance, did you know that using all caps in an e-mail implies that you are yelling at the recipient? Choose your words carefully so that your message is clear and the receiver fully understands what you are saying. Never leave the recipient wondering what you meant. But more importantly, documentation in a medical record is part of a legal document and should describe the patient's condition and care so there are no questions as to what happened during the encounter. When you begin to write, it becomes a document that can be saved, so you want to make sure that you do not incriminate yourself in a volatile situation or agree to do something with which you do not intend to follow through. In the healthcare arena, making an error when you write down a laboratory result or in patient instructions can have detrimental effects on the patient's care.

Nonverbal communication is just as important as what you say or write, however. If you speak to a patient as you are leaving the room and do not stop to turn and be sure he or she is hearing you, it implies that you do not care to take the time to ensure understanding. Or, you may be trying to communicate with a difficult patient or family member by speaking slowly and calmly, but your clenched hands and gritted teeth indicate that you are frustrated and angry. This contradiction prevents useful communication. It follows that you should stay attuned to a patient's nonverbal cues because they may tell you what he or she is not saying or cannot say.

In many patient care situations, you will find yourself faced with unpleasant sights, sounds, and smells. You must be careful to avoid facial expressions or comments that indicate your inability to control your reaction. Patients and their family members may be offended at such behavior. Such reactions may disrupt the lines of communication between you and the patient and family.

Body language and appearance enhance or weaken the process of communication. Healthcare workers who dress professionally and carry themselves in a confident manner are often able to communicate more effectively with the patient simply because the patient is more likely to believe what these people say. A healthcare worker who is sloppily dressed and looks uninterested is not as successful in communicating with the patient.

Another important aspect of nonverbal communication is personal space, as described in Chapters 3 and 14 of this text. Invasion of personal space often appears threatening. Moving too far into a patient's personal space may be intimidating and make the patient uncomfortable and unable to communicate effectively.

Telephone communication is essential in health care. Answering the phone quickly and with a smile on your face helps the person on the other end of the line, whether a patient or another healthcare professional, know that you are ready and willing to listen. Answering the phone and immediately asking the person to hold without waiting for an answer communicates disinterest or the feeling that you are too busy to help. You should always try to assist the caller, but if you cannot, tell them who can, what the correct extension is, and transfer them to that person. When talking to a patient on the telephone, refrain from using medical terminology that he or she will not understand. When talking with another healthcare professional, don't use slang terms such as "yeah" or "uh-huh." Your telephone communication should be as professional as if you were standing face to face with the other person. If you are asked to take a telephone message, it is imperative that you get the necessary information. Repeat the call-back number and name to the caller before hanging up. Write clearly so your information is easily read by the person receiving the message.

Communicating with angry patients and family members presents a challenge to the healthcare worker. When communicating with an angry person, allow him or her to verbalize his or her frustrations before you try to resolve the issue. Offer positive reinforcement in a calm, quiet tone with phrases such as "I understand," "I hear what you're saying," "I can hear that you are frustrated," or "I'd like to hear your complaint." Do not tell an angry or upset person to "calm down" because this does nothing to calm the person, and it may anger him or her further. Once the person has an opportunity to voice his or her complaint, tell the person that your priority is to help resolve the issue and then do so. If you need the assistance of another staff member to do this, call for help. If the patient or family member does not calm down and is verbally abusive or threatening, you have the right to walk away from the situation and alert your supervisor. If your safety is threatened, do not hesitate to call security.

When dealing with grieving patients and family members, mentally challenged persons, and those with communication barriers, speak slowly and softly. The hearing impaired or patients who do not understand English may require the assistance of a language interpreter. Grieving persons and those with mental disorders deserve respect and empathy just as your other patients do. If you find it difficult to communicate with these groups, ask your supervisor for assistance.

Communication, whether written, spoken, or nonverbal, is an important part of professional healthcare behavior. Make sure that your part in the transmission and receipt of information is clear before acting or relaying it further.

Cooperation

Health care requires teamwork. Teamwork requires **cooperation.** To take the best possible care of the patient, all healthcare workers must do their part in making sure that happens. Considering the traits that have been discussed in this chapter, if one person does not communicate effectively or another does not manage his or her time well, the patient is likely to suffer. The team must work as a unit with someone directing the activities.

STOP, THINK, AND LEARN.
You are placed in a group with two other students. Your instructor gives your group $1.75 in quarters. The instructions are that the group must divide the money between only two of the group members. There can be no drawings or other games of chance. How does your group decide which two members will get the money? How do you try to convince the others that you should get part of the money? Are you willing to listen to the others as to why they should receive part of the money?

You are not born with leadership skills. These skills are developed as you work in school or at your job or even find your place within your family. You do not need the title of supervisor to be an effective leader. You can develop leadership skills when working as part of a group to accomplish a task. If everyone has his or her own idea, it may take just one person to make a suggestion that pulls the group together or to combine several ideas into one that works and avoids conflict. The group then finds out that a group that acts with a spirit of cooperation accomplishes more than a group that is splintered. Suggestions to the group that accommodate as many ideas as possible also have a calming effect on the group. There may not be one single answer to how to make team members cooperate, but making small steps with these suggestions may help develop the best care for the patient, which is the ultimate goal.

Respect

Respect is a merit that is earned and not demanded. As a healthcare professional, you should desire to be respected by your patients, your employer, and your coworkers. You must give respect to get respect in both your professional and personal life. The Golden Rule, which says that we should treat others as we wish to be treated, is a major component of respect. In any situation, you should put yourself in the other person's shoes and ask yourself if you would like to be treated in the same manner. We are a diverse population, and each person has the right to be accepted for who he or she is regardless of culture or beliefs. When you display the traits that have been discussed in this chapter, you are on your way to earning respect.

STOP, THINK, AND LEARN.
Look at the following words and determine if they are socially acceptable terms, and if not, what term could you use to show respect? Chairman, nerd, fireman, congressman, "girly-man," tomboy, jerk.

You have heard of the harassment laws that protect workers from hostile work environments. These laws were developed as the result of workers who would disregard the feelings of others in the workplace with unwanted touching, jokes, or intimidation. Harassment includes coercion or other behavior in an effort to control the employee's career, off-color jokes or statements, unsolicited print material, and intimidation. Any statement that is offensive to you, regardless of how it was intended, is considered harassment. Likewise, any statement that you make to another student or employee that offends him or her is harassment.

You deserve to learn and work in a safe and comfortable environment, just as patients deserve the same in a healthcare facility environment.

STOP, THINK, AND LEARN.
Another student in your class asks to copy your homework assignment. You say no, but the student keeps asking. The following day, the student tells you that you will be reported for cheating if you do not hand over the homework. What do you do?

Respect can be summed up by the following: do the right thing, treat others as you want to be treated, and report any instances of harassment. Help to make your school or your workplace a pleasant environment by respecting those with whom you work.

Accepting and Providing Feedback

As a healthcare worker, you most likely have superiors to whom you report as well as subordinates whom you manage. Within this hierarchy there is the need to accept and provide feedback regarding one's performance in order to provide the best care possible to patients. Not only are you subjected to a formal job review at pre-determined intervals in which you are given a written synopsis of your job performance, but your supervisor also provides verbal feedback to you at his or her discretion. You may be responsible for providing verbal feedback to workers you manage or to whom you delegate tasks.

When receiving positive feedback, it is important that you acknowledge the praise and thank the person who offers it. It is not easy for some people to offer praise, whereas other people are generous with positive feedback. When managing others, give praise where praise is due. When we do a good job, it feels nice to be recognized for our efforts.

On the other hand, when receiving constructive criticism, criticism that is not meant to be a personal attack but rather suggestions to help you improve your job performance, accept this information with maturity and professionalism. If you don't understand the constructive criticism, ask for more information. Thank the person for giving you the feedback and vow to incorporate it into your job in order to improve yourself and your department. When you find yourself in the position of having to offer constructive criticism, be sure to focus on the person's job performance and not his or her personal traits. For example, saying "You do a great job with dispensing the lunch trays. However, I've noticed that sometimes the trays aren't picked up from the patients' rooms until 4 p.m. Is there some way we can resolve this?" is preferable to saying "You are so lazy and it is inexcusable. Why does it take you so long to pick up the lunch trays?"

There are always opportunities to improve one's job performance. The willingness to recognize possible improvements and the belief that they can be accomplished, at the same time supporting the work of others in a team framework, is in the best interest of the patient and the facility.

Balance

While working in health care, maintain a professional balance between caring for patients in a professional manner and crossing over the line of professionalism. When caring for patients, it is easy to become too involved in the details of their personal lives or overly friendly with their family members. This extensive emotional investment on the part of the healthcare worker can lead to burnout.

It is important to maintain an emotionally healthy distance with your patients not only to promote professionalism but also to protect you from becoming overly burdened with your patients' problems. For instance, imagine that a young female patient tells you about the problems she is experiencing with her boyfriend. An unprofessional response to this is something like, "Oh, that sounds terrible. What are you going to do? If that were my boyfriend, I'd tell him to take a hike." An appropriate response to the situation is "I'm sorry to hear that. Relationship issues are always a challenge. I hope it works out the way you want it to." This statement lets the patient know that you've heard her complaint, you've validated her feelings, and you've offered encouragement without becoming overly involved in her personal problems.

Maintaining a healthy professional distance with patients does not mean that you do not care about them or what they are experiencing, but it does mean that you are able to do your job effectively without experiencing emotional burnout.

Ethics and Bioethics

A healthcare professional encounters many situations that require an ethical judgment or decision. **Ethics** are your moral compass and help you determine right from wrong. Many decisions in health care are controversial and often do not have a right or wrong answer. In such situations, you can ask yourself the following questions to help you make your decisions.

Is it legal?
Is it fair to all of those involved?
How will it make me feel about myself?
How will it look in the newspaper or on the evening news?

Ethical decisions are hard to make, but if you answer the questions above, you should be able to come to an acceptable answer. Patients or families may ask your opinion about an issue. Be careful that you do not sway their decision by voicing your own feelings. Suggest that they make a list of the pros and cons of the decision. Seeing the information in writing is often a better way to look at the whole picture to make the best decision.

STOP, THINK, AND LEARN.
The physician that you work for sees "special" patients on Wednesday afternoon after office hours. You are not asked to set up appointments or pull records for these patients, but the physician asks if you will stay over to make sure the patients are seen in the order they arrive. You are offered double pay for each Wednesday afternoon. You agree, and after several weeks, one of the patients becomes irate because he cannot be seen before 5:00 to "get my fix." You become suspicious of the physician's activities on Wednesday afternoons but continue to work. One Thursday morning, the police show up at the office with arrest warrants for you and the physician on drug distribution charges. How do you defend yourself? What could you have done differently? What red flags should have alerted you to possible trouble?

When you are placed in a questionable situation, do not rationalize that the end is worth the means or that no one will ever find out. In the Stop, Think, and Learn scenario, the extra money would help you out of a financial crisis, and as long as the "special" patients were happy and the physician was making money, who would know? Did you do anything that was illegal?

Health care is a field of advancing technology and the subsequent bioethical decisions. **Bioethics** are the ethical or moral implications of these new technologies and advances in health care. Genetic engineering and drug research are areas of recent controversy. Genetic engineering is a process that scientists are using to alter a person's phenotype, or genetic makeup, to cure a disease or prevent a congenital condition in a newborn. The research is as intense as the controversy. Many healthcare professionals have taken a definite stand on what they believe is right or wrong with the testing and findings. Until you understand the full intent of the research, it is hard to decide how you feel. Other issues that stir controversy in health care are gender selection, which allows prospective parents to choose the sex of their baby, selective reduction of multiple embryos with assisted reproductive technology, and stem cell research.

STOP, THINK, AND LEARN.

Choose one of the bioethical issues listed above and do your own research. Were you able to gather enough information to make an informed decision about your position? What information could you use to convince your friends or family that your decision is correct?

You may find yourself in an ethical or bioethical dilemma while working in health care. Asking yourself the questions in the beginning of this section will help you to make most of your decisions. Always do your research to make sure you fully understand the topic and the implications for your career. Understanding the topic means that you have read not only the published research but also the contradictory information as well.

Summary

Professionalism and ethics go hand in hand in a medical career. You are entrusted with patients' health and lives, and thus you should present yourself as a consummate professional. Many patients are embarrassed or scared when they have an encounter in a healthcare facility. As a professional, you can make them as comfortable as possible in the situation so they can receive the benefits available to them. Failure of the healthcare worker to act in a professional manner may cause the patient to avoid further care. Every patient has the right to be treated with courtesy and respect, as do you when you need health care.

Practice Exercises

Multiple Choice

1. Many employers terminate employees due to their lack of:
   a. Social skills
   b. Technical skills
   c. Professional skills
   d. Experience

2. Making yourself available to learn new information and skills and making the best of all situations will help you to develop:

   a.   A good attitude

   b.   A bad attitude

   c.   Organizational skills

   d.   Communication skills

3. Attendance and punctuality are extremely important in health care because:

   a.   You do not want the patients to be left alone for a long period of time

   b.   Your paycheck will be cut if you are late or absent

   c.   You want to leave on time

   d.   Another employee may be waiting to leave

4. The most effective method to study for a test is:

   a.   Studying at least a small amount every night

   b.   Cramming the night before the test

   c.   Skimming the material for important terms

   d.   Asking classmates for answers to your questions

5. When talking with an angry patient on the telephone, you should:

   a.   Tell them to calm down and listen to you

   b.   Stop talking

   c.   Let the patient verbalize his or her concern

   d.   Hang up the phone

6. A patient asks you about which laboratory she should go to. Your best answer would be:

   a.   "Don't go to the one on Main Street; they are too expensive."

   b.   "They are very nice at the one near the mall."

   c.   "Your doctor owns the one next door, so I would go there."

   d.   "Find out which laboratory accepts your insurance and is the most convenient for you."

Fill in the Blank

1. Your moral compass is known as _____.

2. Any statement that is offensive to you, regardless of how it was intended, is considered _____.

3. The process that scientists are using to alter a person's phenotype, or genetic makeup, to cure a disease or prevent a congenital condition in a newborn is known as _____.

Short Answer

1. **What characteristics would set you apart as a true professional?**

2. **When faced with an ethical decision, what questions should you ask to help make your decision?**

INTERNET RESOURCE		
Agency/Organization	Web Address	Resources/Functions
Are You a Professional	http://tipsforsuccess.org/professionalism.htm	Helpful tips for professional behavior
American Medical Association	http://ama-assn.org	Search "medical ethics" and follow the links to read AMA Code and articles
eHow.com	http://ehow.com/facts_7289412_professionalism-health-care.html	Facts about professionalism in health care
University of Georgia	http://coe.uga.edu/workethic/	Lessons in work ethics

PATIENT CONFIDENTIALITY 17

Learning Outcomes

17.1 Describe the components of the Health Insurance Portability and Accountability Act (HIPAA) laws

17.2 Apply HIPAA privacy and security mandates in the healthcare setting

17.3 Identify procedures for release of patient information

17.4 Identify individually identifiable health information

17.5 Discuss the importance of patient confidentiality

Competencies

CAAHEP

- Describe various types of content maintained in a patient's medical record. (CAAHEP V.C.6)
- Explore the issue of confidentiality as it applies to the medical assistant. (CAAHEP IX.C.2)
- Discuss the implications of HIPAA for the medical assistant in various medical settings. (CAAHEP IX.C.3)

ABHES

- Institute federal and state guidelines when releasing medical records of information. (ABHES 4.b)
- Comply with federal, state, and local health laws and regulations. (ABHES 4.f)
- Demonstrate professionalism by: (3) maintaining confidentiality at all times. (ABHES 11.b.(3))

Key Terms

abuse Billing for services that are medically unnecessary or unreasonably priced

covered entity Organizations with access to or need for personal health information, such as healthcare providers, health plans, and healthcare clearinghouses

emancipated minor A child who has been granted adult status by a court of law based on criteria such as joining the U.S. Armed Forces, becoming legally married, or demonstrating financial independence from his or her parents

fraud Intentional deception or misrepresentation for the purpose of financial gain

HIPAA Health Insurance Portability and Accountability Act, a federal law passed in 1996 to address health insurance issues related to job changes and the privacy of patients' health information

individually identifiable health information (IIHI) Information that can identify someone as a unique person, including name, date of birth, address, telephone number, or specific description of an illness or injury

Privacy Rule The federal law that protects a patient's IIHI

Your health information is your business. When you choose to share this information with your healthcare provider, you expect this information to remain private. Only those healthcare professionals who are directly involved with your care have a right to view your information and only to provide you with the best care possible.

In today's technological climate, many of our everyday activities are tracked, some without our knowledge. Your computer remembers sites that you visit, closed circuit cameras scan stores, and our financial institutions share information for credit ratings. Cases of identity theft occur as the result of unauthorized use of this information. One's ***individually identifiable health information (IIHI)*** should be exempt from this covert sharing. IIHI is any information that can identify you as an individual, such as your name, birth date, address, telephone number, or specific description of an illness or injury that is specific only to you. When all personally identifiable information is removed from your record so that you may not be associated with the information, the record is said to be "de-indentified," and it can be used in research or for statistical purposes. In the mid-1990s, there was much public concern that Americans were being denied health insurance when they changed jobs and that health information was being shared without regard to the patient's privacy. In 1996, Senators Edward Kennedy and Nancy Kassebaum introduced a bill into Congress to address health information and insurance known as H.R. 3103. The federal government passed the Health Insurance Portability and Accountability Act, commonly referred to as **HIPAA,** or Public Law 104-191, in September 1996. While the entire law is important and is reviewed in this chapter, the Privacy Law is most applicable to healthcare professionals.

Standard terminology was developed to ensure universal understanding when reading and interpreting all issues related to HIPAA. Those terms include:

- *Code set*: Any set of codes used to identify data elements of medical terms, physician codes for procedures and diagnoses, or medical concepts.
- *Healthcare clearinghouse:* A public or private company that processes medical information into a standard format that is acceptable for medical billing and processing.
- *Healthcare provider:* A provider of medical services or medical supplies.
- *Health information:* Oral or written information about a patient's diagnosis, treatment, prognosis, or supply use.
- *Health plan:* Programs that pay part or all of a patient's medical expenses based on a predetermined plan. These include private insurance companies and government programs such as Medicare and Medicaid.

HIPAA

There are four major components of the HIPAA law, which begins with the **portable insurance provision.** This component allows individuals who were continuously employed and insured for the previous 12 months to move to another job without lapse in insurance coverage or exclusion for preexisting conditions. New employees are provided with the same insurance benefits as those offered to current employees. Even if they have a preexisting condition, the law prevents these employees from being charged higher rates than any other employee. Should an employee lose his or her job, the employee is now able to convert the insurance to a private policy for a certain period. This provision offers some consolation to families who find themselves victims of the slow economy and decreasing job market.

Second, the law addresses fraud in health care. Increasing premiums often forced individuals into a managed care situation that limited their access to specific types of health care. Each insured person in the managed care program was assigned to a primary physician for basic care. Any special needs required a referral from the primary physician, who was also known as a "gatekeeper." This arrangement opened the door for double billing and increased costs associated with one medical encounter. This provision also put in place Medicare and Medicaid antifraud programs that expanded into the private insurance sector. **Fraud** is an intentional deception or misrepresentation to obtain financial gain, such as billing for a patient who did not visit the facility or billing for supplies that were not provided. **Abuse** is providing or billing for services that are not medically necessary or that are unreasonably priced. Before the law, unscrupulous healthcare entities billed for services long after the patient's death or inflated patients' bills beyond the services that the consumer received. Once the law passed, these providers were identified and prosecuted, with many serving jail time. The law sent a clear message to healthcare providers about illegal activities for financial gain.

The next provision rewards individuals who report healthcare fraud and abuse with civil immunity and often with monetary awards. The amount of money rewarded pales in comparison with the financial savings when offenders are stopped.

The final major provision of this law concerns patient files. The government was to establish unique identifier information for each physician, insurer, and patient. This effort would centralize and protect health information. In 2000, the government realized that the emergence of electronic health records may compromise the privacy of a patient's health information, and the government enacted the **Privacy Rule,** which specifically addressed the IIHI. The rule was revised in 2002 as the Administrative Simplification, and compliance was mandated by April 2003. The U.S. Department of Health and Human Services, Office for Civil Rights, is the government agency responsible for the direction of this federal law.

As individuals, the Privacy Rule provides rights concerning individuals' health information and addresses specifically who is allowed access to these personal health records. Before April 2003, individual state guidelines governed the release of records, and the rules varied from state to state. When the Privacy Rule went into effect, all states fell under the federal regulations concerning the release of medical information.

Flashpoint

There have been recent instances of healthcare workers losing their jobs and receiving jail time for accessing celebrities' records when the workers were not involved in the actual care of the patient.

Technology Adds Concerns

As electronic health records developed and outsourcing of medical record functions increased, the privacy of records became more of an issue. With increasing numbers of people having access to the records and health information available on the Web, the privacy of this information is more easily compromised. The advancements in technology are sometimes matched by the skills of hackers, making the security of health information an increasing concern. The Privacy Rule was ratified to keep the information secure at all costs.

Those required to follow the Privacy Rule are groups known as **covered entities,** those who have or need access to personal health information. Covered entities include health plans, healthcare providers, and healthcare clearinghouses. The health plans include, but are not limited to, health insurance carriers, health maintenance organizations (HMOs), group health insurance plans, and entitlement programs such as Medicare and Medicaid. Healthcare providers include all of those who provide care to consumers, such as hospitals, pharmacies, and physician offices, as well as those who transmit health information electronically to insurance companies or clearinghouses. A physician is a direct provider, and those that process the information are known as indirect providers. Healthcare clearinghouses receive and transmit nonstandard health information in the proper format for processing.

Flashpoint

The Privacy Rule does not mandate *how* a healthcare facility must protect personally identifiable health information, only that it *must.*

STOP, THINK, AND LEARN.
To determine who falls into the covered entity category, ask yourself these questions:

1. Does this entity provide, bill for, or receive payment for healthcare services?
2. Does this entity receive any HIPAA-sensitive information electronically?
3. Does this entity send any HIPAA-sensitive information electronically?

If you answered yes to any of these questions, this entity is a covered entity and is bound by all HIPAA rules.

Who Must Abide by the HIPAA?

There are other types of businesses that do not fall under the covered entity umbrella that are affected by the HIPAA. These are business associates who have a true need for information from the patient record. This includes attorneys, accountants, third-party claims administrators, and independent contractors who provide a specific service to healthcare facilities. A home medical transcriptionist is an example of an independent contractor.

The information governed by the Privacy Rule includes all entries in a medical record, regardless of who documents the information, any verbal transfer of information from the physician to other healthcare providers, information that is transmitted and stored by the insurance carrier, and billing information related to a patient's care.

There are entities with access to health information that do not have to abide by the Privacy Act. These include the employer, life insurer, workers compensation carriers, some law enforcement agencies, and automobile medical payment insurance. Many times, people voluntarily provide their health information to these entities in order to receive benefits. Examples include Internet self-help sites or public screenings for conditions such as diabetes, high blood pressure, and cholesterol.

It is the healthcare facility's responsibility to maintain physical security of patient information and establish limits as to who may view the information. The facility must also train all new employees on the privacy of the information and provide access on a "need to know" basis. A healthcare facility that uses a computer system maintained off-site must also ensure that the software agent has security in place to avoid the release of patient information, whether intentional or unintentional. A facility should have written policies and procedures indicating the security of information and levels of access for facility employees. Not everyone in the facility needs full access to the patient information. The security of the information can be accomplished with password protection scripts, computer screen guards, and secure record location.

 ### STOP, THINK, AND LEARN.

A radiology transport employee accessed a female patient's demographic information to get her telephone number to ask her out on a date.

As the patient, what would you do?
As the supervisor, how would you approach the employee?
As the employee, how would explain your actions?
How should the employee be punished?

The Privacy Rule gives patients unlimited access to view and receive copies of their health records on demand. Healthcare facilities must provide access within 30 days of the request. If you find a true error or omission in your record, you can ask that it be corrected or amended. You cannot, however, ask to have information removed simply because the information may be embarrassing or is no longer an issue. If you should need copies of your medical record, the facility must provide them, but they do have the right to charge a reasonable fee for the copies and postage if the copies are to be mailed. The information in the record is protected health information (PHI), which includes any information that can identify the patient personally and that is a written or electronic record of diagnoses, treatment, payment for services, or any other item that relates specifically to you. PHI also includes spoken words such as when a healthcare worker discusses your diagnosis or care within the hearing of those not directly involved in your care.

When a healthcare employee violates the HIPAA laws, there are consequences. The U.S. Department of Justice has established guidelines for who can be criminally liable under the HIPAA guidelines. Those who knowingly acquire or divulge any individually identifiable health information can face fines of up to $50,000 and possible prison time. If this information is acquired under false pretenses, the fines double and the person may face up to 5 years in prison. In a case where information is obtained and sold for commercial publication or personal gain, the fines increase to $250,000 and prison time increases up to a term of 10 years.

The American Recovery and Reinvestment Act of 2009 (ARRA) established a tiered system for HIPAA violations and penalties. The American Medical Association provides information for the member physicians on their website.

The Office of Civil Rights (OCR) is responsible for investigating all HIPAA violations as well as noncompliance by healthcare entities. The U.S. Department of Health and Human Services (DHHS) imposes penalties for such violations, and the Department of Justice (DOJ) imposes penalties for criminal violations. Table 17-1 outlines these penalties.

> *Flashpoint*
> It is disrespectful as well as illegal to tell friends and family about patients being treated in your healthcare facility.

Release of Information

When a record release is necessary, the patient must sign an authorization to do so. Patients who may legally sign their own release forms are competent adults, **emancipated minors,** pregnant women, military personnel regardless

TABLE 17-1

AARA PENALTIES FOR HIPAA VIOLATIONS

Civil Monetary Penalties (Department of Health and Human Services)	Criminal Monetary Penalties (Department of Justice)
Fines for the healthcare entity's known violations and willful violations range from $100 to $50,000 per violation with a $1.5 million maximum. No penalty will be enforced if the DHHS finds the violation was not intentional and corrected within 30 days of the discovery.	Those who intentionally violate the HIPAA standards can face up to 1 year in prison and face a $50,000 fine. If the violation involves false pretenses, the sentence can increase to 5 years and the fines to $100,000. In the event the information is used for intentional harm or profit, the prison time can increase to 10 years and the fines to $250,000.

Data from HIPAA Health Insurance Portability Accountability Act. American Medical Association Web site: http://ama-assn.org/ama/pub/physician-resources/solutions-managing-your-practice/coding-billing-insurance/hipaahealth-insurance-portability-accountability-act/hipaa-violations-enforcement.shtml. Accessed November 1, 2010.

of age, and a legal guardian or durable power of attorney for health care. An emancipated minor is allowed to conduct business or any other occupation on his or her own behalf or for his or her own account outside the influence of a parent or guardian. A durable power of attorney for health care is a legal document that authorizes an appointed person to be your healthcare agent (sometimes called an attorney-in-fact for health care, healthcare proxy, or surrogate) to make any necessary healthcare decisions for you and to see that physicians and other healthcare providers give you the type of care you wish to receive.

Custodial parents may sign for their children to release information. Authorization forms vary, but all include basic but thorough statements including the patient's name, birth date, medical record number, what information is to be released, to whom it is to be released, the purpose for release, the patient's signature, and the date signed. Each release should have an expiration date, and a new release is required for each request. The patient has the right to retract this release, in writing, if he or she chooses, but it does not apply to information already released. For all records that include information regarding HIV/AIDS, sexually transmitted diseases, alcohol and drug use and abuse, or mental health issues, the release form must contain specific wording to address the release of this information, meaning the patient knows the information is present in the record and he or she is willing to allow the release.

STOP, THINK, AND LEARN.

Did each of the following situations abide by the Privacy Rule?

1. A physician discusses an absent golf partner's test results with other members of their team while on a golf outing.
2. A laboratory calls a stat report to the physician's office and speaks with the nurse.
3. A nurse gives the oncoming shift a report of all patients' conditions in the private conference room on the nursing unit.
4. Two nurses discuss a pregnant friend over lunch at a local restaurant.
5. A mother is given details of her 21-year-old son's emergency room visit over the phone.

Prior to the Privacy Rule action, health information was routinely released for public interest. When a sports figure, celebrity, or other person of interest was injured or ill, the public was given probable diagnosis and regular updates on that person's condition. Since the Privacy Rule was enacted, only a general statement such as "stable condition" is released. These individuals have a right to protected health information just as everyone else does, and they can decide when and if information related to their accident or illness is released.

Your Health Information

Health information is your private information to be shared only with those involved in your care. If the need to share your health information arises, you can decide if the release is for an acceptable use. The facility should maintain and give you access to a record of when and with whom your information is shared. If you have reason to believe that your information has been compromised, there is a procedure for filing a complaint either with your healthcare provider or with the federal government.

Maintaining Confidentiality

Healthcare workers are obligated to maintain the confidentiality of their patients. This includes protecting both oral and written communication. When speaking with others about a patient, workers should ensure that other people in hallways, the cafeteria, elevators, stairwells, or restrooms cannot hear the conversation. To ensure this, restrict conversations regarding patients and their care to work areas only and not common areas of the facility. Avoid discussing patients with others at home, in public places, in social situations, or anywhere outside the facility.

Do not leave medical records in any area where unauthorized individuals may access them. Do not reveal any information found in the records without proper authorization and patient consent. If you are asked for patient information from someone and you are unsure of his or her right to the information, consult your supervisor.

Another important task in maintaining confidentiality as well as protecting patient privacy is to knock before entering any patient area and identify yourself. Tell the patient why you are in his or her room and what the patient may expect during your visit. Prior to performing any patient-related tasks, check the patient's armband against the medical record as well as ask the patient to tell you his or her name. This ensures that you do not call a patient by an incorrect name, which may jeopardize the confidentiality of another patient, and ensures that you are performing tasks and procedures on the correct patient.

Summary

Healthcare professionals have the duty to maintain strict confidentiality in the care of a patient, regardless of the situation. Always put yourself in the patient's position if you choose to divulge information. How would you feel if someone did the same to you?

Practice Exercises

Multiple Choice

1. Information found in your medical record concerning diagnoses, treatment, and outcomes is known as:

   a. HIPAA

   b. Individually important health information

   c. Private health information

   d. Protected health information

2. Which of the following is **not** a criterion for being an emancipated minor?

   a. Member of the armed forces

   b. Age 16 with a full-time job

   c. Has demonstrated financial independence from parents

   d. Legally married

3. Which senators introduced a bill in Congress to address health information and insurance?

   a. Kennedy and Kassebaum

   b. Graham and Ruddman

   c. Kennedy and Graham

   d. Kassebaum and Ruddman

4. A public or private company that processes medical information into a standard format that is acceptable for medical billing and processing is a:

   a. Covered entity.

   b. Clearinghouse

   c. Provider

   d. Third party

5. What entity investigates all HIPAA violations?

   a. OSHA

   b. CLIA

   c. FDA

   d. OCR

6. An intentional deception or misrepresentation to obtain financial gain is known as:

   a. Abuse

   b. Fraud

   c. Misfeasance

   d. Malfeasance

Fill in the Blank

1. It is the _____ responsibility to maintain physical security of patient information and establish limits as to who may view the information.

2. _____ may sign for their children to release information.

3. Each medical record release should have a(n) _____ and a new release is required for each request.

Short Answer

1. How can healthcare facilities protect a patient's information?

2. What is the definition of abuse as it relates to healthcare financing?

3. What are the four components of HIPAA?

INTERNET RESOURCES		
Agency/Organization	Web Address	Description
Privacy Rights Clearinghouse	http://privacyrights.org	Information about the privacy rules and sanctions
American Medical Association	http://ama-assn.org/ama/pub/ physician-resources/legal-topics/ regulatory-compliance-topics/ health-care-fraud-abuse.shtml	Cases of healthcare fraud and abuse
Health Information Privacy	http://hhs.gov/ocr/privacy/	Government Web site for all things HIPAA
HIPAA	http://hipaa.org/	HIPAA explanations

18 DOCUMENTATION

Key Terms

charting by exception The method of documenting patient care that requires a medical record entry only when a patient's response to treatment deviates from "normal"

continuity of care Documentation in the medical record that allows all healthcare personnel to provide ongoing, consistent care for the patient with each encounter

documentation Recording information about a patient's care for medical and legal purposes

electronic health record (EHR)

electronic medical record (EMR) Patient medical records that are stored in an electronic format

flow charts A format for documenting repeated medical information such as vital signs separate from the narrative summaries

medical record A file that contains the patient's demographic information and clinical data for past medical history, and current illnesses and treatments, including medications, vital signs, immunizations, and diagnostic studies

Learning Outcomes

18.1 State the importance of an accurate medical record

18.2 Recognize the importance of medical record confidentiality

18.3 Define the methods of documentation

18.4 Differentiate between subjective and objective information

18.5 Identify the ownership of the physical medical record and the information within

Competencies

CAAHEP

- Identify systems for organizing medical records. (CAAHEP V.C.5)
- Describe various types of content maintained in a patient's medical record. (CAAHEP V.C.6)
- Discuss principles of using electronic medical record. (EMR)(CAAHEP V.C.11)
- Identify types of records common to the healthcare setting. (CAAHEP V.C.12)

ABHES

- Prepare and maintain medical records. (ABHES 8.b)
- Identify and properly utilize office machines, computerized systems and medical software such as: (1) Efficiently maintain and understand different types of medical correspondence and medical reports; (2) Apply computer application skills using variety of different electronic programs including both practice management software and EMR software. (ABHES 7.b)

Documentation is an important issue in health care. The standard for a patient's medical record is "if it is not documented, it was not done." The ***medical record*** contains not only the patient's demographic information but also all of the clinical data for the patient's past medical history and current illnesses and treatments, including medications, vital signs, immunizations, and diagnostic studies. With a patient's first healthcare encounter, a baseline record is established from which physicians can monitor changes during the course of a treatment or the addition of medications. The information in a medical record is known as ***protected health information (PHI),*** information that is personally identifiable as belonging to the patient.

A medical record is both a medical and legal document, and it must be complete and accurate. The patient's medical record should reflect the care that is provided, the patient's compliance with any treatment, and any communications with the physician or the insurance company. Documentation should be factual, not a narrative involving unnecessary information. The patient should always be the focus of the entry, making the use of the pronoun "I" unnecessary. You should not try to speculate about any aspects of the patient's care or response to treatment. Simply state the facts without emotion or your opinion.

Patient Care Errors

In the event an error occurs with the patient, such as a wrong medication given or a treatment omitted, document what happened, not what should have happened. Make sure to follow your facility's guidelines for documenting patient care errors. Taking care of the patient should be your first priority, after which you should record the incident. Most facilities avoid the use of terms such as "error" or "inadvertent" in the medical record. In most facilities an "incident report" or "adverse occurrence" form may be used to document the error in its entirety. This form is not a part of the medical record and should not be referred to in the record. These forms are maintained by administration.

Ownership of the Medical Record

The permanent paper record becomes the physical property of the facility as does a computer system that houses electronic records, but the information belongs to the patient. A patient's medical record should be available to all healthcare providers involved in the patient's care. In a legal situation, you want the medical record to help you recall the details of the care you provided. You will care for many patients during your career, and it is impossible to remember them all in any detail. Should a patient and your facility become engaged in a legal situation, it may be a very long time before you may be called to testify. At that point, the patient's medical record will be your only reference. The record can be your best friend or your worst enemy in a court of law, based on how you documented the care you provided.

Documentation

The patient's medical record serves as written communication between you and the other members of the healthcare team as well as a legal account of the care provided to patients and their response to the care. The patient's medical record can provide legal protection to healthcare workers in the face of a lawsuit. The medical record also shows that the healthcare workers and facilities deliver care in compliance with government agencies and in a cost-effective manner. Medical documentation correctly reflecting the patient's care decreases denials from insurance companies and other third-party payers.

In a facility open all the time, you pass information from one shift to the next by documenting the events that took place during your shift. Changes in the patient's condition should be noted as well as medications given, treatments performed, and patient reactions. In a daily facility, your documentation will provide **continuity of care** for the next time the patient visits the office.

When you document, make sure that you state the facts and not your personal opinions. A direct quote from the patient may clarify a situation for others involved in his or her care. Table 18-1 indicates some examples of documentation. Decide which entry is the best choice for the patient record.

Key Terms—cont'd

polypharmacy The use of multiple medications by a patient treated by several physicians who each prescribe more than one medication

POMR A standardized documentation system called a problem-oriented medical record

progress note Continuous narrative summaries of the patient's care by physicians, nurses, and other healthcare professionals

protected health information (PHI) The information found in a medical record concerning diagnoses, treatment, and outcomes

SOAP How medical record documentation is done in the POMR, using subjective, objective, assessment, and plan criteria

TABLE 18-1

EXAMPLES OF DOCUMENTATION

Situation	Documentation	Good?	Documentation	Bad?
You find the patient on the floor in her room. She tells you that she just sat down for a minute to rest.	Patient found on floor. States she "sat down." Vital signs 98.7-88-22-134/78. No apparent injury. Patient assisted back to bed. Physician notified.		Patient fell out of bed. No broken bones. Informed patient that she would be restrained if she tried to get up again.	
A patient comes into your office for follow-up after being treated for a urinary tract infection. She says that she quit taking her antibiotics because they made her sick to her stomach, but she doesn't want you to tell the physician.	Vital signs 100.4-80-18-120/68. Patient says UTI is gone.		Vital signs 100.4-80-18-120/68. Follow-up visit for treatment of UTI with Septra. Patient discontinued medication after 3 days due to nausea. Denies UTI symptoms.	
The patient is hospitalized for an infected leg wound. The order is for dressing changes twice a day.	Dressing on R leg changed per protocol. Slight yellowish drainage noted on old dressing. Patient complains of slight itching at site. New dressing applied per protocol. Leg elevated as ordered.		Dressing changed X 2. No complaints.	
A new mother visits your office for her postpartum check. She tells you that she needs something to help her "nerves."	Vital signs 98.2-78-16-136/78. Patient wants prescription for nerve pills. She is depressed.		Vital signs 98.2-78-16-136/78. Patient appears anxious. States she needs "something to help her nerves."	

Methods of Documentation

In the 1980s, a form of acute care documentation known as **charting by exception** was developed in an effort to save nurses' time. The concept was that unless a patient's response to treatment deviated from "normal," there was no need to document in the record. It was believed that this would save the nurses' time, save space in the medical record, and make abnormal situations more obvious. Information was documented on **flow charts** and **progress notes** so that any deviations from normal stood out. Charting by exception was also designed to decrease the narrative aspect of written documentation and the number of entries in an electronic record. Some electronic health records have templates with built-in normal values that physicians and other healthcare providers can change with a simple click to note abnormal values or conditions.

STOP, THINK, AND LEARN.
What are your thoughts on charting by exception?
Would you be comfortable with such a system?
List three advantages and three disadvantages of charting by exception.
Who determines the definition of "normal"?

There will always be pros and cons for charting by exception. If healthcare providers are not comfortable with the system, they must let their facilities know this and the rationale for their discomfort. However, healthcare workers must always comply with their facilities' charting policies and procedures, even if they are not comfortable with them. Charting that does not follow facility policies and procedures can prove to be problematic should the chart go into legal proceedings.

The problem-oriented medical record **(POMR)** is a standardized documentation system that uses a master problem list and **SOAP** (subjective, objective, assessment, and plan) charting. The patient record begins with a comprehensive problem list based on a thorough patient assessment. Each problem or diagnosis is listed on the master problem list in the patient record. The list contains conditions that are active, inactive, temporary, and resolved and any potential problems. This list identifies the date of onset, action taken (treatment), the resolution, and the date of resolution. New problems may be added to the list as well as changes in treatment for active problems. The problem list serves as a quick check of the patient's history and treatment. Documentation in the POMR is done using the SOAP acronym: *s*ubjective is what the patient says; *o*bjective is what you observe; *a*ssessment is the overall impression of the patient's condition, and *p*lan is what treatment the patient needs. Using patient quotations in the subjective field is helpful to express the patient's own feelings without interjecting your own perceptions of the patient's complaint. The objective field is used to describe what you see from your observation of the patient, including the vital signs, laboratory or radiology reports, and examination of the patient by the provider. The assessment gives the provider's diagnosis based on the subjective and objective data, and the plan determines the diagnostics or treatment necessary. This method of documentation can be used in both paper and electronic record formats.

Narrative documentation may be the most common format for recording a patient's health information. Most physician office narrative records are kept in reverse chronological order, which means that the most recent encounters become the first documents. Acute care and long-term facilities use chronological order, meaning the beginning of the patient's care is at the beginning of the record. Most medical records are divided by discipline, such as laboratory reports, radiology reports, progress notes by the provider, nurse's notes, transcribed history and physical examination, operative reports, and any miscellaneous reports of the patient's care.

Learn and follow the system of documentation of your facility. Each healthcare facility decides what type of system works best, regardless of paper or electronic format.

Standards of Documentation

The patient's medical record serves as a communication tool among healthcare providers and a legal document because it is the official record of all care provided as well as the patient's response to care. Therefore, all entries in the patient's medical record must be thorough, legible, and professional. Table 18-2 demonstrates documentation do's and don'ts.

Figure 18-1 shows an example of how to correct a documentation error by drawing a line through the erroneous entry, writing the date and time and a brief explanation, signing the correction, and then writing the correct entry. Do not obliterate errors by erasing or using correction fluid or tape since the entry must remain legible.

Release of Information

The HIPAA laws discussed in Chapter 17 outline the **release of health information.** Only the patient can release the information in his or her medical record to other healthcare providers, insurance companies, or attorneys, except in the case of a worker's compensation claim or a subpoena. Custodial parents

TABLE 18-2
DOCUMENTATION DOS AND DON'TS

Documentation Do	Documentation Don't
Use black ink	Chart in pencil
Identify all documents with patient name and account number	Leave a blank line between the previous entry and later entries
Record an entry as soon after care is given as possible to prevent omission of important information	Go back at a later time to add information to a previous entry
Record data on the correct forms	Erase or use correction fluid or tape to get rid of errors
Write legibly and spell correctly	Chart in advance to providing care
Use only abbreviations and symbols approved by the facility	Make up new abbreviations, symbols, or terminology, or use any not approved by the facility
Sign and date all entries	Chart subjective opinions or assumptions
Include the military time in all entries	
Include appropriate credentials after signature (such as CMA, LPN, RN, etc.)	
Use correct medical terminology instead of lay terms and slang	
Accurately and objectively use standards of measurement to describe temperature, size, and amount (of fluids, drainage, medications, etc.)	
Indicate the patient's own words by using quotation marks	
Record data in a factual, accurate, nonjudgmental manner	
Identify any information added at a later time as a "late entry," with the current date and time indicated	

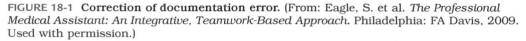

Date	
01/30/09: 9:15 a.m.	~~Pt c/o pain 7/10, in low back described as "sharp & intense."~~ ~~Administered 2 Vicoden per MD order~~ ~~————————————————— S. Gonzalez, CMA~~ Wrong chart. ————— S. Gonzalez, CMA, 0915, 01/30/09

FIGURE 18-1 **Correction of documentation error.** (From: Eagle, S. et al. *The Professional Medical Assistant: An Integrative, Teamwork-Based Approach.* Philadelphia: FA Davis, 2009. Used with permission.)

can request and release information on their children younger than 18 years, except in cases of emancipated minors, pregnancy, and those enlisted in the military. You always have a right to copies of your records if you need or want them. A healthcare facility has 30 days to provide you with copies of your records once you sign the release, and the facility can charge a "reasonable" fee for the copies, according to the HIPAA.

Certain situations require a special release of information authorization. Any patient record that contains information concerning the patient's HIV status or alcohol and drug use and abuse can be released only when the form states that the patient knows the information is contained in the record and authorizes its release.

Technology

In years past, records had to be shared by photocopying or transmittal by facsimile. This process often delayed treatment for the patient while physicians waited for the records. An ***electronic health record (EHR)*** or ***electronic medical record (EMR)*** streamlines the process of sharing a patient's medical information. In addition to reducing the amount of paper used, the electronic record saves time and increases the provider's access to the patient's medical information. The EHR allows all types of healthcare providers to develop interfaces for such processes as data sharing, quality management, decision algorithms, and outcome measurement. Information gathered through these programs provides knowledge for governmental agencies that study diseases, treatment, and prevention. Physician organizations, such as the American Medical Association, benefit from such information and provide the physician communities with the data. The more knowledgeable the physicians are about diseases, the better care patients receive. Such information also identifies quality issues in healthcare facilities and provides methods to improve the patient care. By using an electronic format, patient care can improve. There is less likelihood of errors and, as a result, there is a clearer and more accurate account of the patient's care. Duplication of diagnostic testing and treatment are avoided, and shared records can save the patient money and help prevent ***polypharmacy.*** Polypharmacy is the use of multiple medications by a patient and tends to be an issue in elderly patients who are treated by multiple physicians, each of whom may prescribe several medications. Because of EMRs, patients can be treated more effectively and make better decisions about their health care.

The initial government mandate was for all healthcare providers to convert to an electronic format by 2014. The conversion from paper to electronic record involves significant costs and training, which may impact the decision for some physicians and healthcare facilities. The economic stimulus package of 2009 provided $20 billion to promote the use of EHRs and other health information technologies in physician practices and other healthcare facilities in the United States.

In 2008, approximately 40% of physician offices began the process to institute a fully automated electronic format. This compares to only about 18% in 2001. The Harvard School of Public Health surveyed all members of the American Hospital Association in 2008 to determine the percentage of acute care facilities that initiated the conversion process. Of the 63% that responded to the survey, 1.5% had implemented a comprehensive EHR and an additional 7.6% had some form of basic EHR. The survey asked for specific reasons why the conversion had not started. Answers included the initial and maintenance costs, the resistance of physicians, and the lack of technology support, with costs being the most frequently cited reason. There are many different brands of EHR, but the concepts are similar and the interfaces will advance so that information can be shared between systems.

Security of **individually identifiable health information** (IIHI) is an issue that must be considered with the conversion to electronic formats and Internet storage of medical records. Many facilities are investigating the software packages to determine which provides superior information protection. Many physicians and patients remain skeptical of the privacy of health information with the emergence of hackers in today's society. There are companies that advertise a service that allows you, as a healthcare consumer, to store any health-related information that you want your healthcare providers to have access to on a company's secure Internet site. You choose the information and the entities that may have access. Access to your past medical history, immunization records, insurance information, and emergency contacts are especially helpful in emergency situations.

Summary

The patient medical record in any format is both a medical and legal document. Always remember: "If it isn't documented, it wasn't done."

Practice Exercises

Multiple Choice

1. The method of documenting patient care that requires a medical record entry only when a patient's response to treatment deviates from "normal" is called:

   a.   Charting with thought

   b.   Charting by exception

   c.   Charting by acceptance

   d.   Abnormal occurrence charting

2. Continuous narrative summaries of the patient's care by physicians, nurses, and other healthcare professionals are:

   a. Progress notes

   b. Flow charts

   c. Physician notes

   d. Discharge summaries

3. The permanent, physical medical record belongs to:

   a. The patient

   b. The healthcare facility

   c. The local hospital

   d. The physician's attorney

4. Records that document repeated information separate from narrative notes are:

   a. Operative notes

   b. Graphics

   c. Nurses notes

   d. Flow charts

5. Information that the patient tells you is listed as:

   a. Subjective

   b. Objective

   c. Assessment

   d. Notes

6. Who can release your medical records by signing an information release form?

   a. Your spouse

   b. Your children

   c. You

   d. Your parents

   e. All of the above

Fill in the Blank

1. A patient's medical record is both a _____ and _____ document.

2. When you document, make sure that you state the _____ and not your _____.

3. The initial government mandate was for all healthcare providers to convert to an electronic format by _____.

Short Answer

1. **What are the four components of SOAP charting?**

2. **How do you correct an error in a patient's medical record?**

3. **What are the advantages to using an electronic record format?**

INTERNET RESOURCES

Agency/Organization	Web Address	Resources/Functions
American Health Information Management Association	http://ahima.org	The official site for health information technicians and managers
U.S. Department of Health and Human Services	http://hhs.gov/ocr/privacy/	HIPAA and release of information statutes
Privacy Rights Clearinghouse	http://privacyrights.org/fs/ fs8-med.htm	Medical records privacy information
Centers for Disease Control and Prevention	http://cdc.gov/mmwr/preview/ mmwrhtml/m2e411a1.htm	Privacy Rules

5 Joining the Workforce

FINDING A JOB 19

Learning Outcomes

19.1 Define your career goals as a health-care professional

19.2 Describe how your clinical experience can be considered a job interview

19.3 Explain the importance of licensure, certification, or registration in your healthcare career

19.4 Determine the best type of résumé for your job search

19.5 Discuss the interview process

Competencies

CAAHEP

- Discuss licensure and certification as it applies to healthcare providers. (CAAHEP IX.C.5)
- List and discuss legal and illegal interview questions. (CAAHEP IX.C. 12)

ABHES

- Perform the essential requirements for employment such as résumé writing, effective interviewing, dressing professionally and following up appropriately. (ABHES 11.a)

Key Terms

application A form required by most employers to gather your basic information when you apply for a job with a company

budget A monthly statement of your salary and expenses

career services A division of a college that helps prepare students for graduation and entry into the workforce

certification Validation of the knowledge gained and skills learned in the educational process; conferred by the governing board of a profession

chronological résumé A summary of a job applicant's qualifications and experiences in order, with the most recent information listed first

Continued

School's out! When school is over, the "real world" begins. This can be an exciting yet scary time. It is an opportunity for reflection on what has been learned and accomplished in school and a time to prepare for the next step into a career. It is important to begin thinking about a job while you are still in school and to begin your job search with a plan. Taking the time to conduct an organized, well-planned job search can make the process less stressful and, it is hoped, more successful. In the event you decide after you graduate that a traditional healthcare career is not what you had envisioned or hoped for, you can use your education to become an informed healthcare consumer or a competent caregiver for a loved one.

Key Terms—cont'd

clinical experience A scheduled part of your education that allows you to gain work experience in the area of your studies in places such as hospitals, clinics, and physician offices

commute The distance you must travel to and from work each day

cover letter A letter of introduction that accompanies your résumé when applying for a job

expectations Characteristics you expect and ideals that you may have about a potential job or that potential employers may have about you

externship A volunteer clinical experience in a healthcare facility for medical students living outside the hospital

functional résumé A summary of a job applicant's skill sets, work abilities, and relevant career experience; this type of summary is best for applicants who have been out of the job market for some time or who have a history of many short-term jobs

job database Web sites Internet sites that provide information concerning available jobs in your area and adjacent areas, along with application instructions

licensure Validation of the knowledge and skills learned in the educational process; conferred by the governing board of a profession, it allows certain privileges while working in the healthcare arena

Determining Your Interests

While you are still in school, pay attention to any specific areas of study that you enjoy or one in which you excel. Think about the patient population that you prefer. Not all healthcare professionals can work with all types of patients. If you do not enjoy interaction with children, a pediatrics practice may not be the right job for you. If you prefer an exciting, constantly changing environment, you may consider an immediate care center or emergency room. Long-term care may be appropriate if you prefer getting to know your patients on a more personal level. If you can find your passion, you will have much more direction and motivation as you begin looking for a job after graduation. In addition, you will be more confident and successful doing something that you know you do well.

Use your instructors, externship opportunities, career services, and even your classmates to your advantage. They have experience and knowledge about the field, and you can learn a lot from them. Explore your options to decide what interests you most. You may not be able to determine your specific passion right away. It may even take a few years of work before you learn what you really love to do on the job, and that is acceptable. If you think you fall into this category, it is still important to stick to the guidelines of using your resources during school. Take the time to learn about the many opportunities available to you.

Gaining Experience

Every student should have a plan for life after graduation. As your graduation date approaches, you should gear up for your job search. Programs that offer *clinical experience* or *externships* may give you insight as to what setting you prefer. Volunteering is also an excellent way to learn about a facility and build career connections through networking. Keep in mind that you may not find your absolute passion, but you may find areas of health care that do not interest you at all. During your time in these clinical settings, keep your mind open as you may find an area not previously considered that does interest you.

If you do accept an externship or volunteer position, keep in mind that you are a guest of the facility and not an employee. This means that you should always be punctual and professionally dressed. Demonstrating initiative and a positive attitude can only benefit you in an externship situation. An externship provides you with a supportive environment in which to practice your clinical skills. Additionally, an externship can lead to potential employment or a great reference to share with another potential employer.

If your profession requires *licensure, certification,* or *registration,* determine when you will be ready to take the necessary examinations. If this process is not required, but suggested, it is always advisable to pursue the validation that comes with a license, certification, or registration. Most healthcare professions require it, and those that currently do not require it now may do so in the future. Taking an examination as soon as you graduate is preferable because you are still in the habit of studying, and all of your knowledge will be fresh in your mind.

Let's take a look at the certification process for the certified medical assistant (CMA). Although this credential is not legally required at the time this book was published, most employers seek out medical assistants with this credential because these individuals have demonstrated competency in educational knowledge and clinical and administrative skills.

A medical assistant earns the CMA credential by completing an accredited medical assisting program by the Commission on Accreditation of Allied Health Education Programs (CAAHEP) or by the Accreditation Bureau of Health Education Schools (ABHES) and passing an examination offered by the American Association of Medical Assistants (AAMA). After passing the examination, the new CMA is given a card demonstrating the credentials of certified medical assistant that may be presented to any potential employer across the country. The CMA must recertify credentials every 5 years by retaking the certification examination or by earning continuing education units (CEUs) by attending appropriate educational offerings.

Other healthcare professions require a similar process for licensure, credentialing, and registration that may also include a background check and fingerprinting, application to a state board, such as the state board of nursing, and payment to renew the license or credentials.

Companies that insure healthcare facilities and physicians will soon require professional validation for all employees.

Planning

When you are ready to begin your job search, it is important to have a plan. Winston Churchill said, "He who fails to plan is planning to fail." This holds true for your job search. You must answer specific questions as you prepare to enter the job market. The first question should be, "where do I want to live?" Many graduates choose to stay in the same city or town where they attended school whereas others want to explore job opportunities in other areas. Are you firmly rooted in your hometown, or does the possibility of moving to a new area seem exciting? Healthcare careers may be more plentiful in larger cities. Are you willing to **commute** to another city for the right job? If a commute is necessary, how far are you willing to drive each day to and from work? What time of day will you be on the road? Do you have reliable transportation? A job in a larger city may pay higher wages, but you must consider the cost of living may be higher as well. You should investigate housing costs in a new community and compare them to your current situation. Commutes and cost of living are expenses that you will need to include in your plan. When you are beginning your job search, determine what your priorities are and what you are willing to sacrifice.

How much money do you need to make? In some job postings, an employer lists the **salary range** for the position, and others do not. In your initial job search, be prepared that you may not receive as high a salary as you imagined, but also know that with time and experience, your salary will increase. When you go for an interview, be prepared for the prospective employer asking what salary you expect. Be careful that you do not price yourself out of their range, but do not undersell yourself. To prepare your salary expectation, you need to do some research. The U.S. Department of Labor Web site can give you an idea of salary ranges for all types of healthcare professionals in all areas of the

Key Terms—cont'd

nontraditional hours Work schedules that begin after the typical 9-to-5 job has ended, including evening and night hours as well as weekends and holidays

punctuality Arriving on time or slightly early for an interview or for work

recession A decline in economic trade and prosperity

reference A former employer that provides a summary of your work characteristics or a recommendation given by a former employer or instructor

registration A form of validation of your educational experiences from a regulatory agency associated with your profession

résumé A summary of a job applicant's skill sets, work abilities, and relevant career experience.

salary range Lowest to highest range of salaries for your healthcare profession; may vary according to location and benefit options

Continued

Flashpoint

A goal without a plan is just a dream.

country. Professional organization Web sites are also an effective way to determine average salaries for your profession.

You should determine what your living expenses are by creating a monthly **budget** for yourself, including the essentials such as housing, vehicle expenses, utilities, groceries, gas, and discretionary expenses such as entertainment. What amount do you need to make each month to cover these expenses? When comparing a potential salary against your expenses, remember that money is taken out of your paycheck for taxes and, in some cases, benefits. A human resources director can help you determine your net pay from a quoted salary.

Another consideration must then include your willingness to work evening or night shifts, weekends, and holidays. If you are required to work **nontraditional hours,** do you have needs such as child care that must be addressed? There are other healthcare facilities, such as physician or dental offices, that offer a routine schedule during typical business hours. Some larger healthcare facilities use creative staffing plans that may suit your needs. Before you commit to a position, make sure that you can work the required hours.

After you have determined the criteria for the job you wish to land, you have to pound the pavement to find the job. The Internet is an excellent job-search tool, as are local newspapers, the yellow pages, job fairs, healthcare career placement services, and healthcare trade magazines. Friends and family members can assist, too, by putting you in contact with people they know who may be able to help. When searching for a job, do not leave any stone unturned.

As discussed above, you may have discovered your passion during school, you may still be searching for it, or you may be equally as happy working in any area of the medical field. Your job search will be easier if you are open to working in any setting, but it is also important to try to pursue your passion if you have one. Research jobs in different settings and determine the pros and cons for each. Either way, try to remain open-minded during your search. If you do not find job opportunities in your preferred area, remember that you must begin somewhere.

Where you work in your first job will not necessarily determine the rest of your career. As long as you maintain your motivation and direction, the experience you gain in any job can help you achieve your future goals.

The Job Market

While the above questions are important, there is an outside influence that must be considered. You must base your expectations about what you find in your job search on the current state of the economy and resulting job market. In a good economy, you may have many jobs to choose from and be able to apply to those that appear to be the most exciting. You may even have multiple job offers and get to choose the job that is best for you. However, in a time of **recession** or a bad job market, you may find very few available jobs, rendering the questions above irrelevant. You may find only a few openings and be faced with competition from others hoping to land the same job. The job market can also vary from location to location. Remember that you have no control over the job market; you can only control how you handle it. Develop realistic **expectations** about your job search and be aware of the different experiences you may have in either a good or a bad job market. If the job market is good, be thankful and take advantage of the many opportunities available to you. If the market is

---

Flashpoint

Healthcare is a 24/7/365 business, and most facilities must staff around the clock.

Key Terms—cont'd

targeted résumé A summary that identifies the position desired and lists the applicant's specific experience and qualifications relevant to that job; ideal for applicants who know exactly what type of position they want

transcript A permanent record of all classes you have taken in your educational process, including class titles and the grades you earned.

work history A listing of your previous employers, job titles, and duties.

bad, be prepared to wait a little longer to find a job and know that you may have to make compromises.

Start your search with your school's **career services** department. In addition to job listings, they can provide assistance with the application process, your résumé, and your cover letter. Counselors and career advisors can offer insight into the job market and your search.

Like so many services today, many job postings are listed online. There are **job database Web sites** that allow you to organize your job search by location or position. It is a good idea to use broad search terms to return as many results as possible. Be aware of jobs that look like frauds, as many online postings are fraudulent. Never give out personal information in an online job application unless you have verified that the job and organization are legitimate. You can also use the job search function on the Web sites of specific hospitals or health organizations. Make sure to follow directions carefully in the online process; many places do not wish to receive phone calls or e-mails outside of the online application.

Applying for a Job

As you begin the application process, many of the applications require the same materials. Create a folder or notebook with all of your necessary materials. You can create a folder on your computer if you plan to apply online. If you begin with organized materials, you are able to apply to more jobs more easily. This folder might include copies of your **transcripts** from school, your **résumé** and **cover letter,** examination or certification results, a list of **references** and your **work history,** and other items listed as requirements in a job posting. While you may not have any healthcare work experience, many employers are looking to see that you have understanding of a work environment.

A résumé lists your contact information, education, qualifications, and work experience. Résumés should be specific. Most résumés should not be longer than one page and should appear organized and uncluttered, with strategic use of blank space to be visually appealing. Résumés should be printed on résumé-grade white paper using black ink. The use of colored paper or ink or paper with designs is unprofessional. All of the information found in the résumé should be accurate and easy for a potential employee to verify. Lying on a résumé is grounds for termination if discovered after the facility hires the applicant.

There are many types and styles of résumé, with the most common being the chronological résumé, the functional résumé, and the targeted résumé. A **chronological résumé** summarizes the applicants' qualifications and experiences in chronological order, with the most recent information listed first. The key areas are education and work experience. For new graduates, listing community involvement, volunteer experience, and professional affiliations can help expand a lean résumé (Fig. 19-1 is an example of a chronological résumé).

A **functional résumé** emphasizes skill sets, or groups of related work abilities, and describes the most valuable experiences of the applicant. This type of résumé is best for those applicants who have been out of the job market for some time or who have a history of many short-term jobs because a chronological listing of experiences is not necessary (Fig. 19-2 is an example of a functional résumé).

Flashpoint

A job will not likely come to find you. It takes effort on your part to find your right job.

Nicole Daniels
305 Apple Lane
Fruitdale, CT 06101

Home: (860) 123-3827
Cell: (861) 453-2345
E-mail: ndan@fruit.com

Education

2008 Certificate, Fruitdale Community College, Fruitdale, CT
Major: Medical Assisting

2005 Diploma, Fruitdale High School, Fruitdale, CT

Work Experience

6/06 – 6/08   Food server, Julio's Ristorante Italiano, Fruitdale, CT
                     Duties: waited tables, filled in for hostess and busser,
                     inventoried and ordered supplies, assisted with scheduling

8/04 – 5/06   Barista, Coffee Cupboard, Fruitdale, CT
                     Duties: made assorted coffee drinks, cashiered, weekend opener

Professional Affiliations

• American Assocation of Medical Assistants
• Connecticut Society of Medical Assistants
• Douglas County Chapter of Medical Assistants

Community Activities

• American Cancer Society volunteer
• Fruitdale Community Theater
• Fruitdale Middle School Volunteer Reading Tutor

References: Furnished upon request

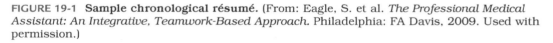

FIGURE 19-1 Sample chronological résumé. (From: Eagle, S. et al. *The Professional Medical Assistant: An Integrative, Teamwork-Based Approach.* Philadelphia: FA Davis, 2009. Used with permission.)

A **_targeted résumé_** identifies the position desired and summarizes the applicant's specific experiences and qualifications that are relevant to the job. This résumé is ideal for those who know exactly what position they want (Fig. 19-3 is an example of a targeted résumé).

Two essential components of the résumé are the cover letter and reference sheet. The cover letter highlights the applicant's best qualifications and requests a job interview. The cover letter, like the résumé, should be printed on résumé-quality white paper using black ink. The cover letter should demonstrate self-confidence and assertiveness without sounding arrogant or pushy. Be sure to carefully proofread your cover letter for any typos and employ the spell-check and grammar-check features on your computer to catch any errors in your letter. Have a friend or family member read your cover letter and résumé to ensure that there are no errors (Fig. 19-4 is a sample cover letter).

When developing your reference list, be sure to include only those people whom you have asked to use as a reference. Because the prospective employer

Karen Stephens
233 Apple Road
Fruitdale, CT 06101

Home: (860) 123-3344
Cell: (861) 453-6798
E-mail: bdbud@fruit.com

OBJECTIVE
To obtain a position as an administrative Medical Assistant

EDUCATION
2008 Certificate, Fruitdale Community College, Fruitdale, CT
Major: Medical Assisting

STRENGTHS AND ABILITIES
► Professional communication skills with clients in person and on the
  telephone
► Detail-oriented and organized
► Strong multi-tasking skills
► Double-entry bookkeeping
► Typing: 65 wpm

RELEVANT EXPERIENCE
► 2008   Medical Assisting Externship (160 hrs), Eastside Medical
                       Clinic Duties: prepared patients for examinations and
                       procedures, medication administration, phlebotomy, EKGs,
                       medical asepsis, WAIVE testing, data entry, reception,
                       appointment scheduling, filing, coding, inventoried and
                       ordered supplies
► 2006 – present   Receptionist, Fruitdale Family Dental Clinic
► 2000 – 2006   Homemaker
► 1995 – 2000   Stephens Chiropractic Center, Secretary/Bookkeeper

COMMUNITY ACTIVITIES
► American Red Cross volunteer
► Eastside Daycare Cooperative President
► Eastside Community Church Secretary

AFFILIATIONS
► Fruitdale Business and Professional Women's Organization
► Crested County Chapter of Medical Assistants
► Connecticut Society of Medical Assistants

FIGURE 19-2 **Sample functional résumé.** (From: Eagle, S. et al. *The Professional Medical Assistant: An Integrative, Teamwork-Based Approach.* Philadelphia: FA Davis, 2009. Used with permission.)

will most likely call the individuals listed on your reference sheet, you should include only those people who have agreed to provide a positive reference. Like the résumé, the reference list should be neatly typed on quality paper and provide accurate and complete contact information for the references.

When you apply for a job, make sure that you are providing the employer with accurate information. Most check your references, transcripts, and work history, so do not embellish this information. This is an official document, and telling the truth is essential. Your **application** is also your first impression with employers. Before they meet you, they see your résumé and cover letter and make note of how well you followed application directions. This can affect the likelihood of the employer contacting you for an interview, so make sure your application materials are professional. They must be neat and organized, with proper spelling and grammar, and be submitted on time.

```
                                               2321 Grant Road
                                                  Fruitdale, CT
                                                (860) 123-8976
    Brenda Williams                       bwill@anyserve.com


Objective:    Full-time Medical Assistant position in a primary care practice

Summary:      Seven years' experience in emergency and primary health care

Skills and Abilities
Administrative Skills
•   Reception and appointment scheduling
•   ICD-9-CM and CPT coding
Clinical Skills
•   First-aid and CPR
•   Phlebotomy
•   Electrocardiography
•   Medication administration
•   Preparation and assistance with sterile procedures
General Skills
•   Strong work ethic
•   Effective written and verbal communication ability
•   Detail-oriented, yet good at multitasking
•   Fluent in Spanish

Achievements
•   Helped organize new local chapter of AAMA
•   Organized and managed children's booth at local health fair
•   Taught first-aid course to seventh-grade students at summer camp
•   Earned CPR and CMA credential

Education
2008 – present    Fruitdale Community College, Fruitdale, CT
                  Major: Nursing
2003              Certificate, Fruitdale Community College, Fruitdale, CT
                  Major: Medical Assisting
2001              Certificate, Fruitdale Community College, Fruitdale, CT
                  Major: Emergency Medical Technician

Employment History
2006 – 2008       Fruitdale Family Medicine, Fruitdale, CT
                  Clinical Medical Assistant
2003 – 2006       Hartell Memorial Hospital, Blueville, CT
                  Administrative Medical Assistant
2001 – 2003       Gibbons Ambulance Service, Fruitdale, CT
                  Emergency Medical Technician

References: Furnished upon request
```

FIGURE 19-3 **Sample targeted résumé.** (From: Eagle, S. et al. *The Professional Medical Assistant: An Integrative, Teamwork-Based Approach.* Philadelphia: FA Davis, 2009. Used with permission.)

Interviewing

Even before you land your first interview, it is important to start practicing your answers to interview questions. Your career services office may be able to give you a list of common questions, or you may be able to find books of interview questions in the library or online. These practice questions help you to think about your interests, strengths, weaknesses, past experiences and challenges, and your future career goals. If your instructor does not offer practice interviews,

October 13, 2008

Brenda Williams
2321 Grant Road
Fruitdale, CT

Marcie Cross, Office Manager
1400 Peach Avenue
Fruitdale, CT 06101

Dear Ms. Cross,

I am interested in a position as a medical assistant for your family practice office. I have worked as a medical assistant for the past five years and very much enjoy helping people with their health care needs.

I am currently enrolled in the nursing program at FCC and am excited about a continuing career as a health care professional. I believe my varied experience and skills will enable me to be a versatile, valuable member of your health care team. As you can see from my enclosed resume, I have experience in clinical and administrative medical assisting. I would be happy to work in whatever capacity you may need. However, I would especially enjoy working in both areas if possible, as doing so will enable me to continue to develop and maintain my knowledge and skills in both areas.

Please call me at (860) 123-8976 so that we may schedule an interview and further discuss your needs and my qualifications. I can be contacted during the week after 3:00 p.m. and on weekends. I also have voicemail and respond to all messages promptly. I look forward to hearing from you.

Sincerely,

Brenda Williams

Brenda Williams, CMA (AAMA)

enclosure: resume

FIGURE 19-4 **Sample cover letter.** (From: Eagle, S. et al. *The Professional Medical Assistant: An Integrative, Teamwork-Based Approach.* Philadelphia: FA Davis, 2009. Used with permission.)

have a friend or classmate ask you the questions in random order so that you can practice answering questions aloud.

When you are called for an interview, you will likely not only be very excited but also nervous. If you have already started practicing your answers to interview questions, you are well on your way in your preparations for your interview. Keep practicing your questions and do any additional research on the employer that you may need to do. The more you know about the work they do, the more you have to talk about during the interview. You should also think about any questions that you might want to ask the employer during the interview. This shows that you are not only interested in the job but also engaging and thoughtful. Write these questions down and take them to the interview so that you will not forget to ask about details that may be important in making your decision. Keep your written questions in a folder or portfolio with your interview documents rather than on a scrap of paper.

STOP, THINK, AND LEARN.

Decide if you think the following questions are legal interview questions.

1. How old are you?
2. Where did you graduate from nursing school?
3. Do you have children?
4. Do you have any restrictions on your ability to travel?
5. When was your last physical examination?

It is important to choose a professional yet comfortable outfit for your interview. Not all job interviews require that you dress in a professional suit, and in most cases, business casual may be acceptable. Most prospective healthcare employers prefer that you not wear scrubs or uniforms to the interview. Make sure that any outfit you select is of relatively neutral color such as black, gray, navy, or brown and that you limit your accessories. Understated accessories, including neutral nail polish color and a natural hairstyle, are desirable. Less is more in this case. You want the interviewer to focus on your skills and intelligence and not a flashy outfit or extreme hairstyle. Healthcare is a specialized field, and appearance is important.

The night before your interview, be sure to have your materials prepared. If you need directions to the interview location, find and verify them. Give yourself some extra time to arrive at your interview so that you are on time. It is preferable to be early. This shows your *punctuality* and gives you a few minutes to relax and focus once you arrive.

Be prepared to meet with an interview committee rather than one person. Facilities are using committees in an effort to choose the person that fits best within the work area. Employees who may be working side by side with a new employee will have insight into a new employee that a human resources director may not have. An interview committee may be made up of various employees of the facility who have an interest in the new hire. As you go into your interview, take a deep breath and remain as calm as you can. Although the situation can be nerve-wracking, most interviewers are polite and accommodating, and they know you may be nervous. Be courteous, professional, and upbeat; it is essential that you project a good attitude during your interview. During an interview, the committee may take notes. This is standard procedure and necessary for them to remember each candidate once the interviews are completed. Try not to let this be a distraction to your train of thought.

As the interview progresses, listen closely to questions, and do not worry if you need a minute to develop thoughtful answers to the questions. Ask for clarification if you do not understand the question. If you speak too quickly and say something you do not mean, you may get flustered, and there may not be an opportunity to correct or explain your statement. The practice questions help you to avoid this interview pitfall. Near the end of the interview, the interviewer may ask whether you have any questions for him or her. It is possible that all of your questions are answered during the interview, but it is a good idea to ask at least one thoughtful question. Be prepared for a prospective employer to tell you that multiple interviews may be required. It is not uncommon for a potential employee to be called back to a second and third interview, especially is there is a large applicant pool. You should ask if further interviews

Flashpoint

An interview can be stressful. Wearing uncomfortable or ill-fitting clothes increases your stress level.

may be required, when a decision will be made, and if you will be notified regardless of the decision. Knowing when to expect a decision prevents needless concern. When your interview is over, make sure to offer a parting handshake and thank the interviewers for their time. A thank you letter sent within a day or two after the interview is a nice final touch and brings your name back up to your prospective employer who may have met with other interviewees in the meantime (Fig. 19-5 is a sample thank you letter). Be sure to keep the interviewers' information because, even if you do not get the job or you turn it down, you may want to network with the interviewers in the future. Interviewers may prove beneficial to your career in some other way.

STOP, THINK, AND LEARN.

Jane was interviewed by telephone for a job in a physician's office. She was hired and began work on Monday. When asked about her wrinkled scrubs, she says that she overslept. Jane sat at the nurse's station without participating in any patient care, stating, "I don't know how you do things here."

Do you think Jane will keep her job?
What would you do differently if you were Jane?

If you are offered the job at the end of the interview, it is best to ask when they need your answer. Most employers understand that you need to think about the offer or discuss it with your family, and they are willing to wait 24 to 48 hours for your response. If at the end of the interview you do not feel like

---

September 1, 2011

Ms. Cicley Jones
Nurse Manager
Groton Community Hospital
Groton, TX 55555

Dear Ms. Jones,

Thank you very much for taking the time to meet with me on the afternoon of August 30th, 2011. I am still very interested in the RN position with Groton Community Hospital, and I enjoyed learning more about your facility and its successes.

I feel that my professional demeanor, ability to work independently and lead others, and my upbeat nature will make a positive addition to your team. Additionally, as my references indicate, my clinical and patient communication skills are very solid.

I look forward to hearing from you in the near future. Thank you for your consideration.

Sincerely,

Nelly Nelson

Nelly Nelson

FIGURE 19-5 **Sample thank you note.**

the job is one that you want, you should ask that your name be removed from consideration for the position. This could prevent an awkward situation later if you are offered the job. Remain upbeat and show your gratitude for the opportunity to come in. While your interviewers have their notes on the things you said, they will likely remember your parting most clearly. Make sure to leave on a good note.

Summary

Do not wait until your education program is over to start thinking about where you would like to work. Evaluate all factors that will influence your decision for a potential job. Finding and landing the best job for you is always a boost to your morale. Once you get the job, make sure that your new employer knows they chose the right person.

Practice Exercises

Multiple Choice

1. A summary of a job applicant's skill sets, work abilities, and relevant career experience is a:

   a. Cover letter

   b. Reference

   c. Résumé

   d. Portfolio

2. A résumé that lists work experience in order, with the most recent information first, is:

   a. Targeted résumé

   b. Chronological résumé

   c. Functional résumé

   d. Experience résumé

3. When considering a position, you should evaluate which of the following?

   a. Salary

   b. Benefits

   c. Commute

   d. All of the above

4. During an interview, you do not understand the interviewer's question. You should:

   a. Ask for clarification

   b. Answer what you think you heard

   c. Excuse yourself to the restroom and regroup

   d. Tell them that you are a little hard of hearing and did not hear the question.

5. An excellent way to learn about a facility and build career connections through networking is:

   a. Calling the office daily to ask about activities going on

   b. Finding an employee and inviting them to dinner so that you can talk

   c. Volunteering at the facility

   d. Interviewing a patient of the facility to get his or her perspective

6. A comprehensive source of available jobs in your profession and preferred area is:

   a. Local newspaper

   b. Job database Web sites

   c. Bulletin boards in local businesses

   d. Fellow graduates

Fill in the Blank

1. Two important components of your résumé is the _____ and the _____.

2. A work shift that begins after 5:00 p.m. or on weekends is known as a _____ schedule.

3. Arriving on time or even a few minutes early for an interview shows _____.

Short Answer

1. **What questions are illegal during an interview?**

2. **What expenses must you consider when you are planning your monthly budget?**

3. **If you are offered a job after an interview, what is your best response?**

INTERNET RESOURCES

Agency/Organization	Web Address	Resources/Functions
Bureau of Labor Statistics	www.bls.gov	Job outlook, employment statistics, salary comparisons
About.com	http://jobsearch.about.com/od/interviewquestionsanswers/a/interviewquest.htm	Job search and interview tips
College Grad.com	http://collegegrad.com/jobsearch/Mastering-the-Interview/Fifty-Standard-Interview-Questions/	Interview questions
Job Interview Questions.org	http://jobinterviewquestions.org/	Resource for interview questions
Monster.com	www.monster.com	Job search Web site
Career Builder.com	www.careerbuilder.com	Job search Web site
Jobs.com	www.jobs.com	Job search Web site

SUCCEEDING IN YOUR JOB 20

Learning Outcomes

20.1 Identify characteristics of a successful employee

20.2 Recognize poor work ethics attributes

20.3 List characteristics of a positive attitude

20.4 Explain the advantages of networking

Competencies

CAAHEP

- Compare personal, professional and organization ethics. (CAAHEP X.C. 2)
- Identify the effect personal ethics may have on professional performance. (CAAHEP X.C. 5)

ABHES

- Demonstrate professionalism by: (1) Exhibiting dependability, punctuality, and a positive work ethic; (2) Exhibiting a positive attitude and a sense of responsibility; (5) Exhibiting initiative; (6) Adapting to change; (7) Expressing a responsible attitude; (8) Being courteous and diplomatic. (ABHES 11.b. 1, 2, 5, 6, 7, 8)

Key Terms

attitude An opinion or general feeling about something

backstabbing Talking maliciously about a coworker or friend to another coworker or friend to undermine that person or make yourself appear superior

cooperation Working together to achieve a common goal

gossip Statements or criticisms made to one person about another person that may be true, false, or based on rumors, but can be incriminating or hurtful

negativity Complaining about your working conditions or other aspects of your job and thus creating unnecessary tension in your relationship with coworkers

networking Communicating with other professionals to share ideas, information, and common interests so as to build relationships and enhance your reputation
Continued

Once you have successfully obtained a job in health care, you will want to keep it to gain experience and earn a salary. Will your first job always be your dream job? It is possible to get the job you have always wanted on your first attempt, but even if you do not get that perfect job, remember that any job worth doing is worth doing well. You want to succeed in your first job and all jobs thereafter because any prospective employers will contact your previous employers for a reference check. Chapter 16 discussed **professionalism,** which should be your top priority in a new job. This chapter expands on those traits that are necessary to be successful in a job.

There are rules to help you to excel in your new job. A positive **attitude** about your opportunity points you in the right direction. We all start out as the "new kid on the block," and from here we must prove that we are the right person for the job. Most employees will welcome you to the workplace and offer help in learning the routines. Do not be alarmed if some employees seem distant or unfriendly. Human nature occasionally causes people to feel threatened by new employees, which may trigger an attitude of being unapproachable. Make sure you are not displaying an attitude of overconfidence, which may escalate this type of reaction. Keep an open mind with these situations, and you may find that once you have proved to be a valuable employee, such attitudes will disappear. Be available and eager to learn from all employees.

In health care, being on time for your job—**punctuality**—is extremely important. In a facility that is open all the time, there is someone waiting for you to arrive so that he or she may go home. In a daily facility, there are tasks that must be completed before patients arrive. Arriving late may require you to play catch-up all day, which adds unnecessary stress to your job and may give the

Flashpoint

Attitudes are contagious. Is yours worth catching?

303

Key Terms—cont'd

professionalism Conducting yourself in a professional manner in terms of appearance, attitude, and energy

punctuality Arriving promptly and on time for a job or appointment

renewal A specific period in which you must gain an extension of your license, certificate, or registration through continuing education or completion of an examination

---

Flashpoint

Attitude is 10% what happens and 90% how you react.

Flashpoint

Every day may not be a good day, but there is something good in every day.

---

patients a feeling of being rushed. In addition to arriving at work on time, you should also be on time when you are returning from a break or from lunch. Being ready and available is a good trait to adopt. If you are going to be late for work or are unable to come in due to illness, let your employer know as soon as possible so that if a replacement is necessary, there is enough time to find someone. A "no call, no show" means that you have not notified your employer that you will not be in or will be late. This is a more serious event than being late or absent with notification, and the consequences are more significant.

 STOP, THINK, AND LEARN.
You are scheduled to leave at 7:15 p.m. At 7:00 p.m., your relief has not shown up for work. You have plans for 8:00 p.m. At 7:45 p.m., the relief has still not shown up for work. The supervisor asks you to stay until a replacement can be found. What do you do?

You should always complete an assignment before moving on to something else. As the day goes by, you may get busy and forget an important detail, such as ordering laboratory work or even giving a medication. Always complete your documentation when you are finished with a patient-care task. Details may become vague as you see other patients or complete other duties. The patient's medical record is a legal document and must be accurate and complete. Patients appreciate the fact that when you begin to care for them, they are your primary concern.

It should go without saying that you should always do your best work. Being unhappy with your job shows in your actions and by your inability to communicate effectively. Most employees or patients do not like being around negative people. The negative attitude can destroy the atmosphere in a healthcare facility. You do not want to stand out for the wrong reasons.

Complaining about your salary, your workload, or even something simple like the temperature in the building may cause other employees to avoid contact with you. This ***negativity*** can create unnecessary tension in the facility. Staying positive can mean remaining committed and focused in a stressful time; communicating in a calm, but friendly way; learning from mistakes and moving on; and taking the opportunity to encourage others when you have the chance. Every day may not be a great day at work, and you may not always feel like acting happy or cheerful, but if you can always maintain a positive attitude in spite of circumstances, bad days will be easier and good days will be even better.

Office ***gossip*** and ***backstabbing*** can be detrimental to the operations of any facility. Make a personal policy that you will not engage in such talk. You never know when you may be the subject of gossip yourself. If you steer clear of such "water cooler" talk, you can never be blamed for rumors that are spread about someone. Rumors and gossip can be hurtful. The golden rule certainly applies in this situation, and you earn your coworkers' trust by staying out of the gossip ring. If problems arise in the office with personnel or schedules, avoid the inclination to start criticizing the supervisor or company. You want to be remembered for your positive suggestions and willingness to help work on a solution rather than for being the one who adds to the trouble.

Keep current with the skills that your facility performs and be open to learning about new equipment that is purchased or procedures that are performed in your facility. Show that you are interested in your work by attending continuing education sessions when possible. If you are interested and the opportunity arises for you to further your education, talk with your employer to see if returning to school is a possibility. Some employers are willing to work with employees who want to better themselves, especially if an advanced education is beneficial to the facility. You must always maintain your licensure, certification, or registration in your field. The *renewal* process is determined by your professional organization, and if continuing education credits are necessary for renewal, ensure that you complete the requirements well before your expiration date. It is important that facilities hire and maintain a staff of certified, registered, or licensed personnel to provide the best possible care for patients. Companies that insure healthcare facilities also require validation of employees' professional credentials.

There may be times in your job that you are asked to take on additional responsibilities that you may not be familiar with or that you would rather not perform. Keep an open mind if this happens. Do not allow an employer to use you, but do try to accommodate the needs of the facility when possible. It is not a good idea to immediately ask for an increase in pay for an increase in job duties. *Cooperation* is essential in today's economic state, and some facilities are not able to replace employees. Employers will notice your willingness to help out in such a situation.

STOP, THINK, AND LEARN.

Today is your birthday and you are excited to be going out for dinner with family and friends. A coworker has become involved in a tense patient/family situation. Her other duties are being neglected while she cares for the patient. You notice that she keeps looking at her desk, and you notice the amount of work. She has not always helped you when you were behind. Do you help her out by assuming some of her tasks? Do you ask someone else to help her? Do you say nothing and leave?

Many times employees are tempted by today's technology. Cellular telephones are unnecessary during your working hours. Texting and calls can be a distraction from your primary goal of patient care. Your family should have the emergency contact number for the facility if a need to reach you during working hours arises. Using office computers for social networking is not acceptable in most facilities. When you are being paid to perform a job, using these technologies is technically stealing from your employer.

Do not be known as the office know-it-all. While you may be really good at your job, there may be others whose work habits and skills are equal to or better than your own. It is fine to accept compliments on your work, but when others are involved with that work, be sure to include them. If you are given credit for a task that you did not perform, give the credit to the right person. You do not want to stand out to your employer for the wrong reasons.

Networking is an important part of succeeding in a job. Building relationships with other healthcare professionals and facilities allows you to share ideas and knowledge that can build your reputation in the event you need to look for another job opportunity. A professional network also provides contacts in the healthcare field for educational opportunities. Occasionally, the perfect job will come to you through a network, so you will want to keep your résumé current by regularly updating it. Always be open to the idea of a new job if the opportunity presents itself, but before leaving your current job make sure that the move is beneficial. Take the time to compare job responsibilities, salary, work hours, and benefits. Do your homework before submitting your resignation and accepting the other job. Do not advertise the fact that you are job hunting, even if you are unhappy in your current position. Do not use work time to search job sites or make contact with facilities in your network. When you are at work, be at work, and perform your duties to the best of your ability. Remember that a prospective employer will call your current employer for a reference. If you decide to take another job, give your employer a minimum of 2 weeks' notice (but preferably 1 month) so that a replacement can be hired before you leave. Do not leave your current job before you have a new one. Set up a time with your employer to communicate personally that you will be leaving your current job. You should write a letter of resignation to bring with you to the meeting, but never give the letter to the employer without also talking with the employer. Tell your employer before you tell any of your coworkers. You do not want the news to get to the employer before you have had a chance to explain your reasons for leaving. Be honest with your employer if there are problems in the office that are causing you to leave. If there are unsolved issues, bringing them to the attention of the employer may prevent a revolving door of employees in the future.

In an economic downturn, there are not enough jobs for the people who are searching. A person who is a valuable employee who gives an honest day's work is more likely to keep his or her job if the employer has to reduce the number of staff members. If it appears that your job may be in jeopardy, try to negotiate with your employer to work fewer hours, take a temporary decrease in pay, or offer to work as an independent contractor who does not require benefits. These options may convince your employer to keep you until the economic situation improves. If you do get laid off or fired from a job, leave in a professional manner, and do not leave showing an angry attitude because you never know where and when you may meet your supervisors and coworkers again. Box 20-1 demonstrates the top reasons healthcare employees are fired.

Flashpoint

"Successful people are always looking for opportunities to help others. Unsuccessful people are always asking, 'What's in it for me?'"—Brian Tracy

Box 20-1 Top Reasons Why Healthcare Workers Get Fired

- Missing too much work
- Unprofessional behavior and attitude
- Dishonesty/stealing
- Lying on a résumé
- Doing job slowly with too many errors
- Conducting personal business during work hours
- Inability to work well with others
- Facility downsize/purchase by another company
- Drug and alcohol use/failed drug test

Summary

Your goal should always be to prove that you are a valuable team member capable of providing quality patient care even in the face of an increasing workload or changing workplace conditions.

Practice Exercises

Multiple Choice

1. Your top priority in a new job should be:

   a. Getting to work early every day

   b. Bringing refreshments on the first day

   c. Professionalism

   d. Negativity

2. Working together to accomplish a common goal is the definition of:

   a. Cooperation

   b. Attitude

   c. Aptitude

   d. Productivity

3. A "no-call, no-show" means that you have:

   a. Notified your supervisor that you are not coming to work

   b. Taken a vacation day

   c. Did not call your supervisor and did not show up for work

   d. Did not let the office know that you were going to be late

4. You can show your supervisor that you are truly interested in your job by:

   a. Being punctual

   b. Taking initiative

   c. Sharpening your skills through continuing education

   d. All of the above

5. A professional network can:

   a. Help with your license renewal

   b. Provide contacts in the healthcare field to help you with continuing education

   c. Supplement your salary

   d. Provide health insurance coverage

Fill in the Blank

1. Office _____ and _____ can be detrimental to the operations of the healthcare facility.

2. You should give your employer a minimum of _____ prior to leaving your job.

Short Answer

1. **Why is it important to finish one task before you move on to the next?**

2. **How do you handle the situation when your supervisor asks you to take on additional responsibility or tasks that you are not familiar with?**

INTERNET RESOURCES		
Agency/Organization	Web Address	Resources/Functions
Mayo Clinic, Adult Health	http://mayoclinic.com/health/job-satisfaction/WL00051	Tips for job satisfaction
Mayo Clinic	http://mayoclinic.com/health/shift-work/AN01616	Tips for sleeping when working the night shift
The Riley Guide	http://rileyguide.com/	Insight into the many aspects of job satisfaction
Quintessential Careers	http://quintcareers.com/first_days_working.html	Tips for succeeding in your job

CENTERS FOR DISEASE CONTROL AND PREVENTION GROWTH CHARTS

Birth to 36 months: Boys
Length-for-age and Weight-for-age percentiles

NAME _____

RECORD # _____

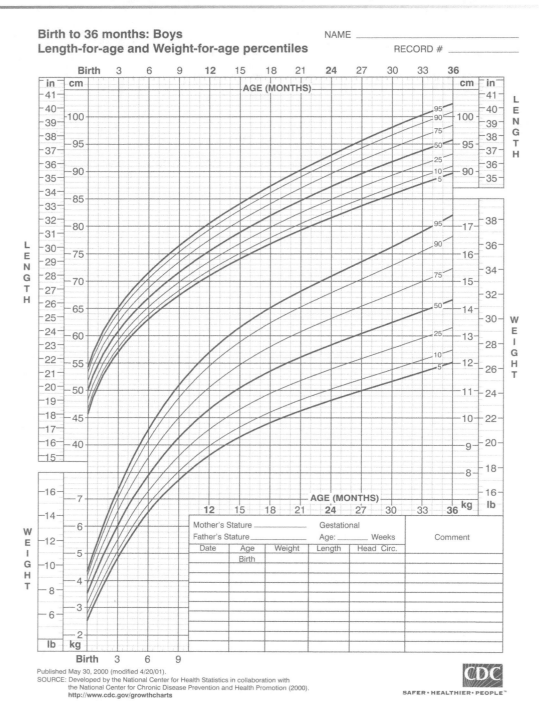

Published May 30, 2000 (modified 4/20/01).
SOURCE: Developed by the National Center for Health Statistics in collaboration with
the National Center for Chronic Disease Prevention and Health Promotion (2000).
http://www.cdc.gov/growthcharts

CDC
SAFER · HEALTHIER · PEOPLE™

Birth to 36 months: Girls
Length-for-age and Weight-for-age percentiles

NAME _____

RECORD # _____

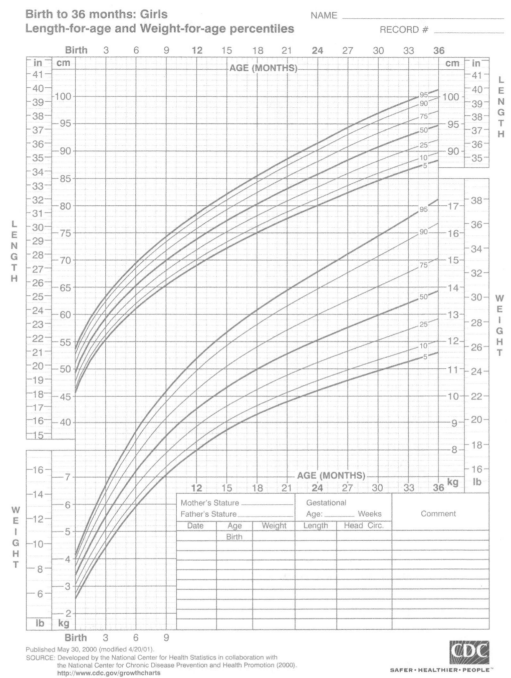

Published May 30, 2000 (modified 4/20/01).
SOURCE: Developed by the National Center for Health Statistics in collaboration with
the National Center for Chronic Disease Prevention and Health Promotion (2000).
http://www.cdc.gov/growthcharts

CDC
SAFER · HEALTHIER · PEOPLE™

INFECTION CONTROL TRAINING AND COMPETENCY DOCUMENTS

**EXPOSURE CONTROL PLAN FOR BLOOD AND AIRBORNE PATHOGENS
TRAINING DOCUMENTATION FORM**

NAME_____

Purpose of Training: ☐ Initial Training ☐ Annual Refresher

Date of Training:_____

Training Summary

The above-indicated participant received instruction on the following topics:

1. OSHA Standard CFR 1910.
2. Epidemiology, signs and symptoms of bloodborne diseases.
3. Modes of transmission.
4. Technical institution exposure control plan for blood and air-borne pathogens.
5. Identifying tasks that may involve exposure to blood or O.P.I.M.
6. Workplace practices and equipment used to prevent/minimize potential exposure.
7. Personal protective equipment: types, selection of appropriate type, proper use, location, storage, removal, handling, decontamination, and disposal.
8. Hepatitis B vaccination.
9. Emergency first aid and contact person for exposures.
10. Procedures to be followed after an exposure.
11. Postexposure evaluation and follow-up.
12. Labels and sign requirements.
13. Mode of transmission, pathogenesis, signs and symptoms of TB.
14. Diagnosis and assessment of TB.
15. Potential for occupational exposure to TB, practices to prevent exposure.

16. PPD testing, test results, and positive TB status (treatment, active disease vs. latent infection, reinfection, BCG vaccination, and false-positive status).
17. Drug therapy for active TB.
18. Preventive therapy for latent infection status.
19. Risk of TB in HIV seropositive or AIDS patients and other immunosuppressive diseases/conditions.
20. Medical evaluation postexposure and PPD conversion.
21. Confidentiality secondary to assessment and treatment of faculty or students who develop TB disease, HIV seropositive status, or AIDS.
22. Voluntary duty reassignment options.

Signature of Instructor

_____   Date _____

Competency Checklist

**Infection Control Procedures
Hand Washing**

Student Name:_____

Instructor:_____

Specific Task: Hand washing is a task that must be performed before and after each patient contact, after using the restroom, and after handling contaminated objects. The aseptic hand wash must be completed within 3 minutes. The student will gather all materials prior to beginning.

Equipment/Supplies: Water, liquid soap, clean paper towels, proper trash receptacle.

Safety/Standard Precautions: Student must be aware of water/soap spills. Note allergies to soap or latex.

Standard of Performance: Student must follow proper sequence and complete the task within 3 minutes. Student may be given a maximum of five (5) points for each step in the procedure, or the instructor may simply give a satisfactory or unsatisfactory grade for the procedure. Failure to properly complete all steps may result in a failing grade. The instructor will determine how many times a student may attempt the procedure.

Conditions of Performance:

TASK/PERFORMANCE STEP	S	U
1. Gather equipment and supplies (5)		
2. Remove all jewelry from hands (5)		
3. Obtain paper towels to turn faucet on. Adjust water temperature to moderately warm. Dispose of the paper towels. (5)		
4. Wet both hands and apply soap to obtain a significant lather. (5)		
5. Work the lather into hands including palmar surface, back, and between all fingers. Rub vigorously. (5)		
6. If necessary, use a nailbrush or orange stick to remove dirt from around and under fingernails and cuticles. (5)		
7. With hands in a downward position, rinse thoroughly. (5)		
8. Using a paper towel, blot and dry hands completely. Discard paper towel. Using another clean paper towel, turn faucet off. (5)		

Successful Completion ☐ Yes ☐ No   Number of attempts _____

Comments:_____

Instructor Initials _____   Date:_____

Competency Checklist

Infection Control Procedures
Personal Protective Equipment

Student Name:_____

Instructor:_____

Specific Task: Personal protective equipment (PPE) is important to your protection when working in healthcare situations that may involve exposure to blood and body fluids. Learning the correct way to don and remove PPEs to prevent contamination is a skill that all healthcare workers need. The student will gather all materials prior to beginning.

Equipment/Supplies: Nonpermeable gown, gloves, mask, goggles, shoe covers, head cover.

Safety/Standard Precautions: Note allergies to latex.

Standard of Performance: Student must follow proper sequence and complete the task within 3 minutes. Student may be given a maximum of five (5) points for each step in the procedure, or the instructor may simply give a satisfactory or unsatisfactory grade for the procedure. Failure to properly complete all steps may result in a failing grade. The instructor will determine how many times a student may attempt the procedure.

Conditions of Performance:

TASK/PERFORMANCE STEP	S	U
1. Gather equipment and supplies. (5)		
2. Perform medical aseptic hand wash. (5)		
3. Don the nonpermeable gown and secure. (5)		
4. Don head covers and shoe covers. (5)		
5. Apply mask to face and secure ties or elastic band. Bend nosepiece to fit bridge. (5)		
6. Apply gloves. (5)		
7. Remove PPE without contaminating clothes or skin. (5)		
8. Properly dispose of PPE in biohazard container. (5)		

Successful Completion ☐ Yes ☐ No   Number of attempts _____

Comments:_____

Instructor Initials _____   Date:_____

C HEPATITIS B VACCINE DECLINATION STATEMENT

Student Name: _____

I understand that due to my occupational duties, and the potential exposure to blood or other potentially infectious body materials, I may be at risk of acquiring hepatitis B virus (HBV) infection. I have been advised to complete the hepatitis B vaccination series. However, I decline hepatitis B vaccination at this time. I understand that by declining this vaccine, I continue to be at risk of acquiring hepatitis B, a serious disease. If in the future, I continue to have occupational training exposure to blood or other potentially infectious body materials and I want to be vaccinated with hepatitis B vaccine, I can receive the vaccination series at no cost.

_____

Signature of Student   Date

_____

Signature of Instructor   Date

HEALTHCARE PERSONNEL VACCINATION RECOMMENDATIONS

Healthcare Personnel Vaccination Recommendations

Vaccine	Recommendations in brief
Hepatitis B	Give 3-dose series (dose #1 now, #2 in 1 month, #3 approximately 5 months after #2). Give IM. Obtain anti-HBs serologic testing 1–2 months after dose #3.
Influenza	Give 1 dose of influenza vaccine annually. Give inactivated injectable influenza vaccine intramuscularly or live attenuated influenza vaccine (LAIV) intranasally.
MMR	For healthcare personnel (HCP) born in 1957 or later without serologic evidence of immunity or prior vaccination, give 2 doses of MMR, 4 weeks apart. For HCP born prior to 1957, see below. Give SC.
Varicella (chickenpox)	For HCP who have no serologic proof of immunity, prior vaccination, or history of varicella disease, give 2 doses of varicella vaccine, 4 weeks apart. Give SC.
Tetanus, diphtheria, pertussis	Give a one-time dose of Tdap as soon as feasible to all HCP who have not received Tdap previously. Give Td boosters every 10 years thereafter. Give IM.
Meningococcal	Give 1 dose to microbiologists who are routinely exposed to isolates of *N. meningitidis*. Give IM or SC.

Hepatitis A, typhoid, and polio vaccines are not routinely recommended for HCP who may have on-the-job exposure to fecal material.

Hepatitis B

Healthcare personnel (HCP) who perform tasks that may involve exposure to blood or body fluids should receive a 3-dose series of hepatitis B vaccine at 0-, 1-, and 6-month intervals. Test for hepatitis B surface antibody (anti-HBs) to document immunity 1–2 months after dose #3.

• If anti-HBs is at least 10 mIU/mL (positive), the patient is immune. No further serologic testing or vaccination is recommended.

• If anti-HBs is less than 10 mIU/mL (negative), the patient is unprotected from hepatitis B virus (HBV) infection; revaccinate with a 3-dose series. Retest anti-HBs 1–2 months after dose #3.

– If anti-HBs is positive, the patient is immune. No further testing or vaccination is recommended.

– If anti-HBs is negative after 6 doses of vaccine, patient is a non-responder.

For non-responders: HCP who are non-responders should be considered susceptible to HBV and should be counseled regarding precautions to prevent HBV infection and the need to obtain HBIG prophylaxis for any known or probable parenteral exposure to hepatitis B surface antigen (HBsAg)-positive blood.[1] It is also possible that non-responders are persons who are HBsAg positive. Testing should be considered. HCP found to be HBsAg positive should be counseled and medically evaluated.

Note: Anti-HBs testing is not recommended routinely for previously vaccinated HCP who were not tested 1–2 months after their original vaccine series. These HCP should be tested for anti-HBs when they have an exposure to blood or body fluids. If found to be anti-HBs negative, the HCP should be treated as if susceptible.[1]

Influenza

All HCP, including physicians, nurses, paramedics, emergency medical technicians, employees of nursing homes and chronic care facilities, students in these professions, and volunteers, should receive annual vaccination against influenza. Live attenuated influenza vaccine (LAIV) may only be given to non-pregnant healthy HCP age 49 years and younger. Inactivated injectable influenza vaccine (TIV) is preferred over LAIV for HCP who are in close contact with severely immunosuppressed persons (e.g., stem cell transplant patients) when patients require protective isolation.

Measles, Mumps, Rubella (MMR)

HCP who work in medical facilities should be immune to measles, mumps, and rubella.

• HCP born in 1957 or later can be considered immune to measles, mumps, or rubella only if they have documentation of (a) laboratory confirmation of disease or immunity (HCP who have an "indeterminate" or "equivocal" level of immunity upon testing should be considered nonimmune) or (b) appropriate vaccination against measles, mumps, and rubella (i.e., 2 doses of live measles and mumps vaccines given on or after the first birthday, separated by 28 days or more, and at least 1 dose of live rubella vaccine).

• Although birth before 1957 generally is considered acceptable evidence of measles, mumps, and rubella immunity, healthcare facilities should consider recommending 2 doses of MMR vaccine routinely to unvaccinated HCP born before 1957 who do not have laboratory evidence of disease or immunity to measles, mumps, and/or rubella. For these same HCP who do not have evidence of immunity, healthcare facilities should recommend 2 doses of MMR vaccine during an outbreak of measles or mumps and 1 dose during an outbreak of rubella.

Varicella

It is recommended that all HCP be immune to varicella. Evidence of immunity in HCP includes documentation of 2 doses of varicella vaccine given at least 28 days apart, history of varicella or herpes zoster based on physician diagnosis, laboratory evidence of immunity, or laboratory confirmation of disease.

Tetanus/Diphtheria/Pertussis (Td/Tdap)

All HCPs who have not or are unsure if they have previously received a dose of Tdap should receive a one-time dose of Tdap as soon as feasible, without regard to the interval since the previous dose of Td. Then, they should receive Td boosters every 10 years thereafter.

Meningococcal

Vaccination is recommended for microbiologists who are routinely exposed to isolates of *N. meningitidis*. Use of MCV4 is preferred for persons younger than age 56 years; give IM. Use MPSV4 only if there is a permanent contraindication or precaution to MCV4. Use of MPSV4 (not MCV4) is recommended for HCP older than age 55; give SC.

References

1. See Table 3 in "Updated U.S. Public Health Service Guidelines for the Management of Occupational Exposures to HBV, HCV, and HIV and Recommendations for Postexposure Prophylaxis," *MMWR*, June 29, 2001, Vol. 50, RR-11.

For additional specific ACIP recommendations, refer to the official ACIP statements published in *MMWR*. To obtain copies, visit CDC's website at www.cdc.gov/vaccines/pubs/ACIP-list.htm; or visit the Immunization Action Coalition (IAC) website at www.immunize.org/acip.

Adapted from the Michigan Department of Community Health

Technical content reviewed by the Centers for Disease Control and Prevention. March 2011.

www.immunize.org/catg.d/p2017.pdf • Item #P2017 (3/11)

Immunization Action Coalition • 1573 Selby Ave. • St. Paul, MN 55104 • (651) 647-9009 • www.immunize.org • www.vaccineinformation.org

RECOMMENDED IMMUNIZATION SCHEDULES

Please note that the following recommendations were developed by the Advisory Committee on Immunization Practices and borrowed from the Centers for Disease Control and Prevention (www.cdc.gov/vaccines/recs/acip).

Recommended Immunization Schedule for Persons Through 6 Years— United States, 2012 (for those who fall behind or start late, see the catch-up schedule)

Vaccine Age	Birth	1 month	2 months	4 months	6 months	9 months	12 months	15 months	18 months	19–23 months	2–3 years	4–6 years
Hepatitis B[1]	Hep B	HepB					HepB					
Rotavirus[2]			RV	RV	RV [2]							
Diphtheria, tetanus, pertussis[3]			DTaP	DTaP	DTaP		see footnote [3]	DTaP				DTaP
Haemophilus influenzae type b[4]			Hib	Hib	Hib [4]		Hib					
Pneumococcal[5]			PCV	PCV	PCV		PCV					PPSV
Inactivated poliovirus[6]			IPV	IPV		IPV						IPV
Influenza[7]						Influenza (Yearly)						
Measles, mumps, rubella[8]							MMR		see footnote [8]			MMR
Varicella[9]							Varicella		see footnote [9]			Varicella
Hepatitis A[10]							Dose 1 [10]			HepA Series		
Meningococcal[11]							MCV4 — see footnote [11]					

Range of recommended ages for all children	Range of recommended ages for certain high-risk groups	Range of recommended ages for all children and certain high-risk groups

This schedule includes recommendations in effect as of December 23, 2011. Any dose not administered at the recommended age should be administered at a subsequent visit, when indicated and feasible. The use of a combination vaccine generally is preferred over separate injections of its equivalent component vaccines. Vaccination providers should consult the relevant Advisory Committee on Immunization Practices (ACIP) statement for detailed recommendations, available online at http://cdc.gov/vaccines/pubs/acip-list.htm. Clinically significant adverse events that follow vaccination should be reported to the Vaccine Adverse Event Reporting System (VAERS) online (http://vaers .hhs.gov) or by telephone (800-822-7967).

1. **Hepatitis B (HepB) vaccine** (Minimum age: birth)

At birth:

- Administer monovalent HepB vaccine to all newborns before hospital discharge.
- For infants born to hepatitis B surface antigen (HBsAg)–positive mothers, administer HepB vaccine and 0.5 mL of hepatitis B immune globulin (HBIG) within 12 hours of birth. These infants should be tested for HBsAg and antibody to HBsAg (anti-HBs) 1 to 2 months after receiving the last dose of the series.

- If mother's HBsAg status is unknown, within 12 hours of birth administer HepB vaccine for infants weighing ≥2000 g and HepB vaccine plus HBIG for infants weighing <2000 g. Determine mother's HBsAg status as soon as possible and, if she is HBsAg-positive, administer HBIG for infants weighing ≥2000 g (no later than age 1 week).

Doses after the birth dose:

- The second dose should be administered at age 1 to 2 months. Monovalent HepB vaccine should be used for doses administered before age 6 weeks.
- Administration of a total of 4 doses of HepB vaccine is permissible when a combination vaccine containing HepB is administered after the birth dose.
- Infants who did not receive a birth dose should receive 3 doses of a HepB-containing vaccine starting as soon as feasible
- The minimum interval between dose 1 and dose 2 is 4 weeks, and between dose 2 and 3 is 8 weeks. The final (third or fourth) dose in the HepB vaccine series should be administered no earlier than age 24 weeks and at least 16 weeks after the first dose.

2. **Rotavirus (RV) vaccines** (Minimum age: 6 weeks for both RV-1 [Rotarix] and RV-5 [Rota Teq])
   - The maximum age for the first dose in the series is 14 weeks, 6 days; and 8 months, 0 days for the final dose in the series. Vaccination should not be initiated for infants age 15 weeks, 0 days or older.
   - If RV-1 (Rotarix) is administered at ages 2 and 4 months, a dose at 6 months is not indicated.

3. **Diphtheria and tetanus toxoids and acellular pertussis (DTaP) vaccine** (Minimum age: 6 weeks)
   - The fourth dose may be administered as early as age 12 months, provided at least 6 months have elapsed since the third dose.

4. *Haemophilus influenzae* **type b (Hib) conjugate vaccine** (Minimum age: 6 weeks)
   - If PRP-OMP (PedvaxHIB or Comvax [HepB-Hib]) is administered at ages 2 and 4 months, a dose at age 6 months is not indicated.
   - Hiberix should be used only for the booster (final) dose in children age 12 months through 4 years.

5. **Pneumococcal vaccines** (Minimum age: 6 weeks for pneumococcal conjugate vaccine [PCV]; 2 years for pneumococcal polysaccharide vaccine [PPSV])
   - Administer 1 dose of PCV to all healthy children age 24 through 59 months who are not completely vaccinated for their age.
   - For children who have received an age-appropriate series of 7-valent PCV (PCV7), a single supplemental dose of 13-valent PCV (PCV13) is recommended for:
     - All children age 14 through 59 months
     - Children age 60 through 71 months with underlying medical conditions
   - Administer PPSV at least 8 weeks after last dose of PCV to children age 2 years or older with certain underlying medical conditions, including a cochlear implant. See *MMWR* 2010:59 (No. RR-11), at http://cdc.gov/mmwr/pdf/rr/rr5911.pdf

6. **Inactivated poliovirus vaccine (IPV)** (Minimum age: 6 weeks)
   - If 4 or more doses are administered before age 4 years, an additional dose should be administered at age 4 through 6 years.

- The final dose in the series should be administered on or after the fourth birthday and at least 6 months after the previous dose.

7. **Influenza vaccines** (Minimum age: 6 months for trivalent inactivated influenza vaccine [TIV]; 2 years for live attenuated influenza vaccine [LAIV])
   - For most healthy children age 2 years and older, either LAIV or TIV may be used. However, LAIV should not be administered to some children, including (1) children with asthma, (2) children 2 through 4 years who had wheezing in the past 12 months, or (3) children who have any other underlying medical conditions that predispose them to influenza complications. For all other contraindications to use of LAIV, see *MMWR* 2010;59 (No. RR-8), at http://cdc.gov/mmwr/pdf/rr/rr5908.pdf
   - For children age 6 months through 8 years:
     - For the 2011–12 season, administer 2 doses (separated by at least 4 weeks) to those who did not receive at least 1 dose of the 2010–11 vaccine. Those who received at least 1 dose of the 2010–11 vaccine require 1 dose for the 2011–12 season.
     - For the 2012–13 season, follow dosing guidelines in the 2012 ACIP influenza vaccine recommendations.

8. **Measles, mumps, and rubella (MMR) vaccine** (Minimum age: 12 months)
   - The second dose may be administered before age 4 years, provided at least 4 weeks have elapsed since the first dose.
   - Administer MMR vaccine to infants age 6 through 11 months who are traveling internationally. These children should be revaccinated with 2 doses of MMR vaccine, the first at age 12 through 15 months and at least 4 weeks after the previous dose, and the second at age 4 through 6 years.

9. **Varicella (VAR) vaccine** (Minimum age: 12 months)
   - The second dose may be administered before age 4 years, provided at least 3 months have elapsed since the first dose.
   - For children age 12 months through 12 years, the recommended minimum interval between doses is 3 months. However, if the second dose was administered at least 4 weeks after the first dose, it can be accepted as valid.

10. **Hepatitis A (HepA) vaccine** (Minimum age: 12 months)
    - Administer the second (final) dose 6 to18 months after the first.
    - Unvaccinated children 24 months and older at high risk should be vaccinated. See *MMWR* 2006;55 (No. RR-7), at http://cdc.gov/mmwr/pdf/rr/rr5507.pdf
    - A 2-dose HepA vaccine series is recommended for anyone age 24 months and older, previously unvaccinated, for whom immunity against hepatitis A virus infection is desired.

11. **Meningococcal conjugate vaccines, quadrivalent (MCV4)** (Minimum age: 9 months for Menactra [MCV4-D], 2 years for Menveo [MCV4-CRM])
    - For children age 9 through 23 months (1) with persistent complement component deficiency; (2) who are residents of or travelers to countries with hyperendemic or epidemic disease; or (3) who are present during outbreaks caused by a vaccine serogroup, administer 2 primary doses of MCV4-D, ideally at ages 9 months and 12 months or at least 8 weeks apart.
    - For children age 24 months and older with (1) persistent complement component deficiency who have not been previously vaccinated; or

(2) anatomic/functional asplenia, administer 2 primary doses of either MCV4 at least 8 weeks apart.

- For children with anatomic/functional asplenia, if MCV4-D (Menactra) is used, administer at a minimum age of 2 years and at least 4 weeks after completion of all PCV doses.
- See *MMWR* 2011;60:72–6, at http://cdc.gov/mmwr/pdf/wk/mm6003.pdf; Vaccines for Children Program resolution No. 6/11-1, at http://cdc.gov/vaccines/programs/vfc/downloads/resolutions/06-11mening-mcv.pdf; and *MMWR* 2011;60:1391–2, at http://cdc.gov/mmwr/pdf/wk/mm6040.pdf for further guidance, including revaccination guidelines.
- This schedule is approved by the Advisory Committee on Immunization Practices (http://cdc.gov/vaccines/recs/acip), the American Academy of Pediatrics (http://aap.org), and the American Academy of Family Physicians (http://aafp.org).

Recommended Immunization Schedule for Persons Age 7 Through 18 Years—United States, 2012 (for those who fall behind or start late, see the schedule and the catch-up schedule)

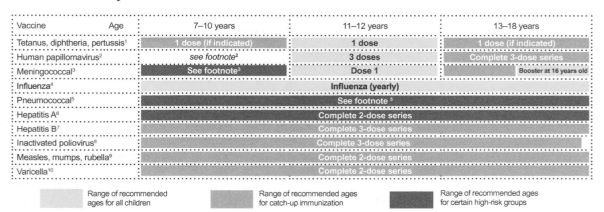

This schedule includes recommendations in effect as of December 23, 2011. Any dose not administered at the recommended age should be administered at a subsequent visit, when indicated and feasible. The use of a combination vaccine generally is preferred over separate injections of its equivalent component vaccines. Vaccination providers should consult the relevant Advisory Committee on Immunization Practices (ACIP) statement for detailed recommendations, available at http://cdc.gov/vaccines/pubs/acip-list.htm. Clinically significant adverse events that follow vaccination should be reported to the Vaccine Adverse Event Reporting System (VAERS) online (http://vaers.hhs.gov) or by telephone (800-822-7967).

1. **Tetanus and diphtheria toxoids and acellular pertussis (TDaP) vaccine** (Minimum age: 10 years for Boostrix and 11 years for Adacel)
   - Persons age 11 through 18 years who have not received TDaP vaccine should receive a dose followed by tetanus and diphtheria toxoids (Td) booster doses every 10 years thereafter.
   - TDaP vaccine should be substituted for a single dose of Td in the catch-up series for children age 7 through 10 years. Refer to the catch-up schedule if additional doses of tetanus and diphtheria toxoid–containing vaccine are needed.

- TDaP vaccine can be administered regardless of the interval since the last tetanus and diphtheria toxoid–containing vaccine.

2. **Human papillomavirus (HPV) vaccines (HPV4 [Gardasil] and HPV2 [Cervarix])** (Minimum age: 9 years)
   - Either HPV4 or HPV2 is recommended in a 3-dose series for females age 11 or 12 years. HPV4 is recommended in a 3-dose series for males age 11 or 12 years.
   - The vaccine series can be started beginning at age 9 years.
   - Administer the second dose 1 to 2 months after the first dose and the third dose 6 months after the first dose (at least 24 weeks after the first dose).
   - See *MMWR* 2010;59:626–32, at http://cdc.gov/mmwr/pdf/wk/mm5920.pdf

3. **Meningococcal conjugate vaccines, quadrivalent (MCV4)**
   - Administer MCV4 at age 11 through 12 years with a booster dose at age 16 years.
   - Administer MCV4 at age 13 through 18 years if patient is not previously vaccinated.
   - If the first dose is administered at age 13 through 15 years, a booster dose should be administered at age 16 through 18 years with a minimum interval of at least 8 weeks after the preceding dose.
   - If the first dose is administered at age 16 years or older, a booster dose is not needed.
   - Administer 2 primary doses at least 8 weeks apart to previously unvaccinated persons with persistent complement component deficiency or anatomic/functional asplenia, and 1 dose every 5 years thereafter.
   - Adolescents age 11 through 18 years with human immunodeficiency virus (HIV) infection should receive a 2-dose primary series of MCV4 at least 8 weeks apart.
   - See *MMWR* 2011;60:72–76, at http://cdc.gov/mmwr/pdf/wk/mm6003.pdf; and Vaccines for Children Program resolution No. 6/11-1, at http://cdc.gov/vaccines/programs/vfc/downloads/resolutions/06-11mening-mcv.pdf for further guidelines.

4. **Influenza vaccines (trivalent inactivated influenza vaccine [TIV] and live attenuated influenza vaccine [LAIV])**
   - For most healthy nonpregnant persons, either LAIV or TIV may be used, except LAIV should not be used for some persons, including those with asthma or any other underlying medical conditions that predispose them to influenza complications. For all other contraindications to use of LAIV, see *MMWR* 2010;59 (No.RR-8), at http://cdc.gov/mmwr/pdf/rr/rr5908.pdf
   - Administer 1 dose to persons age 9 years and older.
   - For children age 6 months through 8 years:
   - For the 2011–12 season, administer 2 doses (separated by at least 4 weeks) to those who did not receive at least 1 dose of the 2010–11 vaccine. Those who received at least 1 dose of the 2010–11 vaccine require 1 dose for the 2011–12 season.
   - For the 2012–13 season, follow dosing guidelines in the 2012 ACIP influenza vaccine recommendations.

5. **Pneumococcal vaccines (pneumococcal conjugate vaccine [PCV] and pneumococcal polysaccharide vaccine [PPSV])**
   - A single dose of PCV may be administered to children age 6 through 18 years who have anatomic/functional asplenia, HIV infection or other immunocompromising condition, cochlear implant, or cerebral spinal

fluid leak. See *MMWR* 2010:59 (No. RR-11), at http://cdc.gov/mmwr/pdf/rr/rr5911.pdf

- Administer PPSV at least 8 weeks after the last dose of PCV to children age 2 years or older with certain underlying medical conditions, including a cochlear implant. A single revaccination should be administered after 5 years to children with anatomic/functional asplenia or an immunocompromising condition.

6. **Hepatitis A (HepA) vaccine**
   - HepA vaccine is recommended for children older than 23 months who live in areas where vaccination programs target older children, who are at increased risk for infection, or for whom immunity against hepatitis A virus infection is desired. See *MMWR* 2006;55 (No. RR-7), at http://cdc.gov/mmwr/pdf/rr/rr5507.pdf
   - Administer 2 doses at least 6 months apart to unvaccinated persons.

7. **Hepatitis B (HepB) vaccine**
   - Administer the 3-dose series to those not previously vaccinated.
   - For those with incomplete vaccination, follow the catch-up recommendations.
   - A 2-dose series (doses separated by at least 4 months) of adult formulation Recombivax HB is licensed for use in children age 11 through 15 years.

8. **Inactivated poliovirus vaccine (IPV)**
   - The final dose in the series should be administered at least 6 months after the previous dose.
   - If both OPV and IPV were administered as part of a series, a total of 4 doses should be administered, regardless of the child's current age.
   - IPV is not routinely recommended for U.S. residents age 18 years or older.

9. **Measles, mumps, and rubella (MMR) vaccine**
   - The minimum interval between the 2 doses of MMR vaccine is 4 weeks.

10. **Varicella (VAR) vaccine**
    - For persons without evidence of immunity (see *MMWR* 2007;56 [No. RR-4], at http://cdc.gov/mmwr/pdf/rr/rr5604.pdf), administer 2 doses if not previously vaccinated or the second dose if only 1 dose has been administered.
    - For persons age 7 through 12 years, the recommended minimum interval between doses is 3 months. However, if the second dose was administered at least 4 weeks after the first dose, it can be accepted as valid.
    - For persons age 13 years and older, the minimum interval between doses is 4 weeks.
    - This schedule is approved by the Advisory Committee on Immunization Practices (http://cdc.gov/vaccines/recs/acip), the American Academy of Pediatrics (http://aap.org), and the American Academy of Family Physicians (http://aafp.org).

Catch-Up Immunization Schedule for Persons Age 4 Months Through 18 Years Who Start Late or Who Are More Than 1 Month Behind—United States, 2012

See the catch-up schedule and minimum intervals between doses for children whose vaccinations have been delayed. A vaccine series does not need to be restarted, regardless of the time that has elapsed between doses. Use the section appropriate for the child's age. **Always use this table in conjunction with the accompanying childhood and adolescent immunization schedules and their respective footnotes.**

Vaccine	Minimum Age for Dose 1	Minimum Interval Between Doses			
		Dose 1 to dose 2	Dose 2 to dose 3	Dose 3 to dose 4	Dose 4 to dose 5
Persons aged 4 months through 6 years					
Hepatitis B	Birth	4 weeks	8 weeks and at least 16 weeks after first dose; minimum age for the final dose is 24 weeks		
Rotavirus[1]	6 weeks	4 weeks	4 weeks[1]		
Diphtheria, tetanus, pertussis[2]	6 weeks	4 weeks	4 weeks	6 months	6 months[2]
Haemophilus influenzae type b[3]	6 weeks	4 weeks if first dose administered at younger than age 12 months / 8 weeks (as final dose) if first dose administered at age 12–14 months / No further doses needed if first dose administered at age 15 months or older	4 weeks[3] if current age is younger than 12 months / 8 weeks (as final dose)[3] if current age is 12 months or older and first dose administered at younger than age 12 months and second dose administered at younger than 15 months / No further doses needed if previous dose administered at age 15 months or older	8 weeks (as final dose) This dose only necessary for children age 12 months through 59 months who received 3 doses before age 12 months	
Pneumococcal[4]	6 weeks	4 weeks if first dose administered at younger than age 12 months / 8 weeks (as final dose for healthy children) if first dose administered at age 12 months or older or current age 24 through 59 months / No further doses needed for healthy children if first dose administered at age 24 months or older	4 weeks if current age is younger than 12 months / 8 weeks (as final dose for healthy children) if current age is 12 months or older / No further doses needed for healthy children if previous dose administered at age 24 months or older	8 weeks (as final dose) This dose only necessary for children age 12 months through 59 months who received 3 doses before age 12 months or for children at high risk who received 3 doses at any age	
Inactivated poliovirus[5]	6 weeks	4 weeks	4 weeks	6 months[5] minimum age 4 years for final dose	
Meningococcal[6]	9 months	8 weeks[6]			
Measles, mumps, rubella[7]	12 months	4 weeks			
Varicella[8]	12 months	3 months			
Hepatitis A	12 months	6 months			
Persons aged 7 through 18 years					
Tetanus, diphtheria/tetanus, diphtheria, pertussis[9]	7 years[9]	4 weeks	4 weeks if first dose administered at younger than age 12 months / 6 months if first dose administered at age 12 months or older	6 months if first dose administered at younger than age 12 months	
Human papillomavirus[10]	9 years	Routine dosing intervals are recommended[10]			
Hepatitis A	12 months	6 months			
Hepatitis B	Birth	4 weeks	8 weeks (and at least 16 weeks after first dose)		
Inactivated poliovirus[5]	6 weeks	4 weeks	4 weeks[5]	6 months[5]	
Meningococcal[6]	9 months	8 weeks[6]			
Measles, mumps, rubella[7]	12 months	4 weeks			
Varicella[8]	12 months	3 months if person is younger than age 13 years / 4 weeks if person is aged 13 years or older			

1. **Rotavirus (RV) vaccines (RV-1 [Rotarix] and RV-5 [Rota Teq])**
   - The maximum age for the first dose in the series is 14 weeks, 6 days; and 8 months, 0 days for the final dose in the series. Vaccination should not be initiated for infants age 15 weeks, 0 days or older.
   - If RV-1 was administered for the first and second doses, a third dose is not indicated.

2. **Diphtheria and tetanus toxoids and acellular pertussis (DTaP) vaccine**
   - The fifth dose is not necessary if the fourth dose was administered at age 4 years or older.

3. *Haemophilus influenzae* **type b (Hib) conjugate vaccine**
   - Hib vaccine should be considered for unvaccinated persons age 5 years or older who have sickle cell disease, leukemia, human immunodeficiency virus (HIV) infection, or anatomic/functional asplenia.
   - If the first 2 doses were PRP-OMP (PedvaxHIB or Comvax) and were administered at age 11 months or younger, the third (and final) dose should be administered at age 12 through 15 months and at least 8 weeks after the second dose.
   - If the first dose was administered at age 7 through 11 months, administer the second dose at least 4 weeks later, and a final dose at age 12 through 15 months.

4. **Pneumococcal vaccines** (Minimum age: 6 weeks for pneumococcal conjugate vaccine [PCV]; 2 years for pneumococcal polysaccharide vaccine [PPSV])
   - For children age 24 through 71 months with underlying medical conditions, administer 1 dose of PCV if 3 doses of PCV were received previously, or administer 2 doses of PCV at least 8 weeks apart if fewer than 3 doses of PCV were received previously.
   - A single dose of PCV may be administered to certain children age 6 through 18 years with underlying medical conditions. See age-specific schedules for details.
   - Administer PPSV to children age 2 years or older with certain underlying medical conditions. See *MMWR* 2010:59 (No. RR-11), at http://cdc.gov/mmwr/pdf/rr/rr5911.pdf

5. **Inactivated poliovirus vaccine (IPV)**
   - A fourth dose is not necessary if the third dose was administered at age 4 years or older and at least 6 months after the previous dose.
   - In the first 6 months of life, minimum age and minimum intervals are only recommended if the person is at risk for imminent exposure to circulating poliovirus (i.e., travel to a polio-endemic region or during an outbreak).
   - IPV is not routinely recommended for U.S. residents age 18 years or older.

6. **Meningococcal conjugate vaccines, quadrivalent (MCV4)** (Minimum age: 9 months for Menactra [MCV4-D]; 2 years for Menveo [MCV4-CRM])
   - See "Recommended immunization schedule for persons age 0 through 6 years" "Recommended immunization schedule for persons age 7 through 18 years" for further guidance.

7. **Measles, mumps, and rubella (MMR) vaccine**
   - Administer the second dose routinely at age 4 through 6 years.

8. **Varicella (VAR) vaccine**
   - Administer the second dose routinely at age 4 through 6 years. If the second dose was administered at least 4 weeks after the first dose, it can be accepted as valid.

9. **Tetanus and diphtheria toxoids (Td) and tetanus and diphtheria toxoids and acellular pertussis (TDaP) vaccines**
   - For children age 7 through 10 years who are not fully immunized with the childhood DTaP vaccine series, TDaP vaccine should be substituted for a single dose of Td vaccine in the catch-up series; if additional doses are needed, use Td vaccine. For these children, an adolescent TDaP vaccine dose should not be given.
   - An inadvertent dose of DTaP vaccine administered to children age 7 through 10 years can count as part of the catch-up series. This dose can count as the adolescent TDaP dose, or the child can later receive a TDaP booster dose at age 11 to 12 years.

10. **Human papillomavirus (HPV) vaccines (HPV4 [Gardasil] and HPV2 [Cervarix])**
    - Administer the vaccine series to females (either HPV2 or HPV4) and males (HPV4) at age 13 through 18 years if patient is not previously vaccinated.
    - Use recommended routine dosing intervals for vaccine series catch-up; see "Recommended immunization schedule for persons age 7 through 18 years".
    - Clinically significant adverse events that follow vaccination should be reported to the Vaccine Adverse Event Reporting System (VAERS) online (http://vaers.hhs.gov) or by telephone (800-822-7967). Suspected cases of vaccine-preventable diseases should be reported to the state or local health department. Additional information, including precautions and contraindications for vaccination, is available from CDC online (http://cdc.gov/vaccines) or by telephone (800-CDC-INFO [800-232-4636]).

GLOSSARY

A

Abduction: A directional medical term that indicates movement away from the center of the body.

Abuse: Billing for services that are medically unnecessary or unreasonably priced.

Acquired immunodeficiency syndrome (AIDS): A disease caused by the human immunodeficiency virus, which destroys a person's immune system, opening the way for opportunistic infections.

Adduction: A directional medical term that indicates movement toward the center of the body.

Adenosine triphosphate (ATP): The body's energy source.

Adipose: Fatty tissue found below the skin.

Adjective suffix: A suffix that changes the meaning of a medical term to one that describes the body organ. Example: gastr/ + -ic becomes "gastric," meaning "pertaining to the stomach."

Administrative: The portion of the medical record that provides demographic and insurance information and is maintained by clerical healthcare workers.

Afebrile: Without fever.

Afferent: Impulses moving from the nerve receptors to the central nervous system.

Airborne: Passage of germs through the air by cough or sneeze.

Algorithm: Detailed treatment scenarios developed based on best practices and used with the patient's profile to determine an "if/then" plan of care.

Allergic reaction: Signs and symptoms such as itching, hives, nausea, or difficulty breathing that may indicate the patient cannot tolerate a medication.

Amphiarthrosis: A joint that exhibits only slight movement. Example: pubic symphysis.

Anatomical position: Standing straight, facing forward, arms at the side and palms facing forward.

Anatomy: The study of the body structure.

Aneroid: A device that uses air pressure to measure a patient's blood pressure.

Antecubital space: The portion of the forearm commonly known as the bend of the elbow.

Antibiotic: Medication that destroys most bacterial organisms.

Antibiotic-resistant organism: An organism that cannot be destroyed by antibiotic medications.

Antigen: A protein found on the red blood cell that recognizes a foreign or incompatible cell.

Apical: The bottom-most area of the heart where the heartbeat can be heard.

Apothecary system: The least used and oldest of the three systems used in drug calculations.

Appearance: The way someone looks or seems to other people.

Application: A form that must be completed to give potential employers information about your qualifications for the job.

Arabic numerals: Traditional numbering system that is used every day.

Artery: An elastic vessel that carries oxygenated blood to the cells.

Asclepion: An ancient Greek healing temple used by those who believed in the supernatural treatment of diseases.

Aseptic: Clean, without infection.

Aspiration: Inhaling liquids or other foreign materials into the lungs.

Atom: The smallest unit of matter.

ATP: Adenosine triphosphate; the energy produced by the body to facilitate metabolism.

Attendance: Arriving at the scheduled place at the scheduled time.

Attenuated: A term used to describe a disease-causing organism that has been weakened and used in a vaccine to protect against that disease.

Attitude: A general feeling or opinion. A characteristic of your manner and disposition. An attitude can be positive, negative, or indifferent.

Auditory tube: Also called the eustachian tube, the tube that connects the nasopharynx with the middle ear to equalize pressure on both sides of the eardrum.

Auscultation: The act of listening to body sounds. Typically done with a stethoscope to hear both normal and abnormal sounds.

Autogenous: Self-generation of a disease. Example: scratching an infected lesion and transferring the infection to another portion of the body.

Avatar: A newly emerging virtual reality that can simulate a disease process and provide computer-based algorithms and an if/then plan of care.

Axon: The long process that extends from the nerve cell body to transmit impulses to the next nerve cell.

B

Backstabbing: Talking maliciously about a coworker or friend to another coworker or friend to undermine that person or make yourself appear superior.

Bacterium (bacteria): A single-celled organism that is capable of causing disease.

Bioethics: Ethical or moral implications of medical research using newer technologies.

Biohazard: An object that is contaminated with blood or body fluids.

Birth order: The ordinal position that a child is born into a family. Research suggests that birth order may have some effect on development.

Blackwell, Elizabeth (1821–1910): The first female to qualify as a physician in the United States.

Bloodborne pathogens: Blood or body fluids that are potentially infectious.

Body mechanics: The way in which the body moves and maintains balance while making the most efficient use of all its parts.

Bradycardia: A very slow heart rate; less than 60 beats per minute.

Broad spectrum: A medication that covers a wide range of bacterial organisms.

Broad-spectrum antibiotics: Antibiotics that kill a wide range of bacteria, are relatively inexpensive, and nontoxic.

Budget: A personal evaluation of finances that determine income and expenses.

C

Calorie: The unit of energy gained from food that, if not used, is converted to adipose tissue.

CA-MRSA: Community-associated methicillin-resistant *Staphylococcus aureus*. A strain of MRSA that affects a community, usually surrounding athletic venues and players.

Capillaries: Blood vessels that connect arteries and veins.

Career services: A division of the college that helps prepare students for graduation and entry into the workforce.

Catheterization: Insertion of a catheter into a body cavity, such as a urinary catheter in the bladder.

CDC: Centers for Disease Control and Prevention. A governmental agency that closely monitors and prevents the outbreak of disease, implements prevention strategies, and maintains national health statistics.

Cell: The basic unit of life. A cell is capable of all processes necessary to life.

Centigrade: The system of temperature measurement used in health care; also known as Celsius.

Central line: An intravenous line that is inserted into the thoracic portion of the vena cava for delivery of concentrated or long-term medication or intravenous fluids.

Cephalocaudal: A term used describe an infant's pattern of growth from head to toe.

Cerebellum: The smaller portion of the brain that is located posterior to the cerebrum and is responsible for body positioning and balance.

Cerebrum: The larger portion of the brain that provides processing of stimuli that control movement, sensation, intellect, and emotion.

Certification: A validation of a healthcare worker's education and successful completion of a capstone examination administered by the accrediting agency for that profession. Example: Certified Medical Assistant (CMA).

Character: The qualities that make you unique, including your morals and actions.

Charting by exception: The method of documenting patient care that requires an entry only when a change occurs in the patient or the treatment.

Chickenpox: A highly contagious viral illness caused by the varicella virus, which produces flu-like symptoms followed by a rash that progresses to blister lesions.

CHIP: Children's Health Insurance Program. A joint federal and state program that provides insurance coverage for children and pregnant women who do not qualify for Medicaid but are unable to afford insurance.

Chlamydia: The most commonly reported sexually transmitted disease; may cause damage to the female reproductive system.

Choroid: The middle layer of the eye that contains the blood vessels and pigments.

Chronological résumé: A summary of a job applicant's qualifications and experiences in order, with the most recent information listed first.

Circadian rhythm: A 24-hour human clock that is synchronized with the normal light of day and dark of night.

Clean: 1. Free of all infectious organisms. 2. Infections that do not involve the respiratory, gastrointestinal, or genitourinary systems.

Clean-contaminated: Surgical procedures that enter the respiratory, gastrointestinal, or genitourinary systems with no obvious lapses in sterile technique.

CLIA: Clinical Laboratory Improvement Amendments. An agency of the federal government that regulates all laboratory testing on the human body.

Clinical: Providing hands-on care for the patient in a healthcare facility.

Clinical experience: A scheduled part of your education that allows you to gain work experience in the area of your studies. Examples include hospitals, clinics, and physician offices.

Closed drainage system: A drainage system that does not have a continuous opening, such as a Foley catheter system.

Colonized: A group of foreign organisms that has settled into a body area without causing disease.

Combining form: A letter or combination of letters that joins the parts of a medical term together.

Combining vowel: A vowel that helps to join prefixes, word roots, and suffixes into a medical term. The most common combining vowel is *o*.

Communicable: The term used to describe a disease that is transmissible between humans.

Communication: The art of conversation and actions by which thoughts and ideas are exchanged. The exchange of information by written, spoken, or nonverbal means.

Commute: The amount of travel time that you must drive or take public transportation to your job.

Compromised immune system: A weakened immune system as the result of a disease process or medication.

Cones: A photoreceptor for clear color vision in bright light.

Conscientious objection: A personal disagreement on moral or ethical grounds to refuse participation in a procedure or practice.

Contagious: The state in which a person can transmit a disease to another person.

Contaminated: Surgical procedures that include gross spillage from the gastrointestinal tract, entry into the biliary or urinary systems when there is infected bile or urine, and major breaks in sterile technique.

Continuity of care: Documentation in the medical record that allows all healthcare personnel to provide continuous care for the patient with each encounter.

Controlled substances: Medications that have the potential for use and abuse. There are five classifications of controlled substances based on the abuse potential.

Cooperation: Working together to achieve a common goal.

Copay: A payment set by the insurance company that a patient must pay at the time of service at the physician's office or pharmacy.

Cornea: The outer layer of the eye where light rays first pass through.

Cover letter: A professional letter that introduces an applicant to a prospective employer and precedes the résumé.

Covered entity: Organizations with access or need for personal health insurance, such as healthcare providers, health plans, and healthcare clearinghouses.

Credentialed: Having successfully completed a certification or licensure examination, a healthcare professional may use the appropriate initials following his or her signature to identify a professional affiliation.

Cross-contamination: Spreading germs by reusing dirty equipment or supplies, and not washing the hands between caring for patients.

Cultural competency: Functioning within the framework of cultural needs, beliefs, and behaviors both as an individual and as a healthcare organization.

Cultural knowledge: The concepts that you know and understand about other cultures and their beliefs, behaviors, and customs.

Culture: The normal practices of a specific population that guide all decisions and actions, learned from the elders and passed to younger generations.

Culture and sensitivity test: A test done to identify the infecting bacteria and the antibiotic that will sufficiently destroy the organism.

Current medications: A list of all medications that the patient is currently taking. Includes dosage and schedule of all medications.

Custom: The actions of a specified individual or group in a given situation.

Cyanosis: A bluish discoloration of the skin, usually indicating a lack of oxygen.

D

DEA: Drug Enforcement Agency. The federal agency that oversees the distribution and regulation of controlled substances.

Decimal: Used to define parts of numbers expressed in units of ten. They represent the number of tenths, hundredths, thousandths, and so forth that are available.

Declination statement: A form that may be signed by a healthcare professional that states his or her objection to receiving a particular immunization. Example: the hepatitis B series.

Deductible: A preset amount that the patient must pay each year prior to the insurance company's payment.

Defensiveness: A barrier to effective communication in which a person feels he or she must protect his or her personal views and opinions.

Demographics: The patient's full name, date of birth, social security number, current address, telephone numbers, e-mail address, insurance information, and emergency contact information.

Dendrite: The short branching processes that receive information and carry it to the cell body.

Denver Developmental Screening Test: A standardized platform to measure a child's development.

Dependability: Being able to be counted on or trusted to complete a task.

Dermis: The second layer of skin that contains nerves, blood vessels, and glands.

Development: An increase in the functionality of a child's physical, mental, and emotional abilities.

DHHS: Department of Health and Human Services. The federal governmental agency that protects the health of Americans and provides health services to those who cannot care for themselves.

Diarthrosis: A joint that exhibits free movement within a fluid-filled capsule.

Diastolic: The bottom number of a blood pressure reading, which indicates the blood pressure during relaxation of the heart.

Direct contact: Transmission of disease through touching an infected source, the result of improper or lack of hand washing.

Directly observed therapy: A type of therapy that reminds patients to take their medication by meeting with a healthcare professional daily or several times per week.

Disinfectant: A chemical solution that kills pathogenic organisms but does not sterilize.

Diversity: The understanding that there will always be patients and other healthcare workers with ideas and beliefs that differ from yours.

DNA: Deoxyribonucleic acid. The chemical substance that contains each person's specific genetic characteristics.

Documentation: Recording information about a patient's care for medical and legal purposes.

Droplet: The aerosol produced with a cough or sneeze.

E

E. coli: *Escherichia coli.* A normal flora organism in the gastrointestinal system, but the primary cause of urinary tract infections.

-ectomy: Suffix to indicate "removal of."

Efferent: The motor pathway that sends impulses back to the body after interpretation by the CNS.

Effort (respiratory): The amount of energy that a patient must exert to breathe.

Electronic health record (EHR): Patient health record that is maintained in an electronic format that can be accessed by Internet regardless of patient location.

Electronic medical record (EMR): Patient health record that is maintained in an electronic format that can be accessed by Internet regardless of patient location.

Emancipated minor: A child who has been granted adult status by a court of law based on criteria such as joining the U.S. Armed Forces, a legal marriage, or by demonstration of financial independence from his or her parents.

Emergency medical services: A network of police, fire, rescue, and ambulance services used to care for and transport patients in emergency situations to the nearest healthcare facility for treatment.

Endemic: A slow but steady progression of a particular disease.

Endocrine gland: A gland of the endocrine system that secretes the product directly into the blood. Example: pancreas.

Engineering control: Equipment, when used correctly, helps minimize exposure to potentially infectious materials.

EPA: Environmental Protection Agency. A governmental agency that studies the effects of the environment on diseases and protects us from pollutants in the air, soil, and water.

Epidemic: An outbreak of a disease that affects a large group of people in a geographic region or defined population group.

Epidermis: The outer layer of the skin.

Epstein-Barr virus: The organism that causes infectious mononucleosis.

Ergonomics: The correct placement of furniture and equipment, training in required muscle movements, efforts to avoid repetitive motions, and an awareness of the environment to prevent injuries.

Erythrocyte: A red blood cell that carries oxygen to the tissues of the body.

Estimating: The process used to approximate the result of a calculation to detect any possible errors.

Ethics: A person's moral compass that allows them to make the best decision.

Ethnicity: Identity associated with nationality, religion, or other cultural systems of a larger group.

Eversion: A directional medical term that indicates turning outward.

Exocrine gland: A gland that secretes the product directly to the outside of the body. Example: sweat gland.

Expectations: Characteristics you anticipate and ideals that you may have about a potential job or that potential employers may have about you.

Extension: A directional medical term that indicates pushing outward.

Externship: A clinical experience in a healthcare facility based on your educational qualifications.

F

Fahrenheit: The system of temperature measurement more familiar to people living in the United States.

Failure to thrive: An infant who is consistently below the predicted height and weight of the standardized growth charts.

Family history: A thorough investigation of the patient's family history of diseases. Includes, but is not limited to, grandparents and their descendents.

FDA: Food and Drug Administration. The governmental agency that is responsible for the safety of all cosmetics, food, medications, medical devices, vaccines, and even cellular telephones and other radiation-emitting devices.

Febrile: With fever.

Fetal alcohol syndrome: A documented condition of infants born to mothers who consumed alcohol during pregnancy, including delayed growth and development, decreased muscle tone, poor coordination, and significant functional impairments.

Fifth disease: The common name for erythema infectiosum, a common childhood virus that causes a "slapped cheek" rash. Caused by the human parvovirus B19.

Flexion: A directional medical term that indicates pulling inward.

Flow charts: A format for documenting repeated medical information such as vital signs separate from the narrative summaries.

Fraction: A method of expressing numbers that represents part of a whole. The numerator is the top number, which represents actual number of parts of a whole, and the denominator is the bottom number, which signifies how many parts it takes to make a whole.

Fraud: Intentional deception or misrepresentation to obtain financial gain.

Functional résumé: A summary of a job applicant's skill sets, work abilities, and relevant career experience; this type of summary is best for applicants who have been out of the job market for some time or who have a history of many short-term jobs.

Fungus: A classification of organisms that typically cause diseases of the skin, hair, and nails. Example: yeasts and molds.

G

Galen of Pergamom (129–199/217): A Roman philosopher and physician who is best known for his extensive observation and investigation, which led to today's modern research techniques.

Gamete: The sex cell that contains half of the adult genetic material. Example: the egg or the sperm.

General hospital: A general hospital encompasses services to meet the healthcare needs of the community, including emergency services, intensive care, surgery, maternity and newborn care, and some basic psychiatric care.

Generalization: Ideas based on trends in specific population groups.

Genetics: The branch of biology that deals with heredity.

Germ: A generic term that describes organisms that might cause disease.

German measles: The common name for rubella, a form of 3-day measles caused by a virus. This disease can cause birth defects if contracted by a woman in her first trimester of pregnancy.

Gonorrhea: A sexually transmitted bacterial disease.

Gossip: Statements made to a person about another person that may be true or false but can be incriminating or hurtful.

Gram-negative: The staining properties of bacterial organisms. A gram-negative organism does not retain the stain applied in the Gram stain process. These organisms appear pink or red under the microscope.

Gram-positive: The staining properties of bacterial organisms. A gram-positive organism retains the stain applied in the Gram stain process. These organisms appear purple under the microscope.

Gram staining: The division of bacteria into two large groups–gram-positive or gram-negative–based on the bacteria's cell wall.

Group: Members of a specific population that each have individual goals and tasks.

Group policy: An insurance policy that covers all employees of a business. An employer may pay a portion of the premium as a benefit to the employee.

Growth: A measurable increase in physical size.

H

Half-life: The amount of time that the body takes to metabolize or eliminate one-half of a medication dosage.

Hand washing: Cleaning your hands with soap, water, and friction for a minimum of 20 seconds.

Healthcare-associated infection (HAI): An infection that a patient develops within 48–72 hours of admission to a healthcare facility that was not present or incubating on admission.

Height: The measurement of the person's stature or length from the feet to the top of the head.

Hematopoiesis: The formation and production of blood cells.

Hepatitis: A viral illness that affects the liver. There are currently five forms of the disease, each transmitted by a specific mechanism.

Heredity: The passage of certain characteristics from parent to the child through DNA.

Herpes simplex virus (HSV): A virus that causes infections of the skin and mucous membranes.

Hierarchy of needs: A theory of Abraham Maslow that states humans must pass through a series of developmental stages to become a fully functional adult.

HIPAA: Health Insurance Portability and Accountability Act.

Hippocrates (circa 460–370 BC): An early Greek physician, known as the "father of Western medicine," Hippocrates believed that the body should be treated as a whole with the healing process of fresh air, good food, rest, and above all, cleanliness.

Hippocratic oath: A pledge in which a new doctor swears to uphold a number of professional ethical standards, a promise that can be boiled down to "harm not."

Holistic: A method of using the patient's physical, social, and psychological needs in the treatment of disease.

Homeostasis: The body's ability to maintain a stable internal environment regardless of external changes.

Hospital: A facility that provides care on a short-term basis for those in need of treatment of diseases or surgical procedures.

Hospitalist: A physician who chooses to practice exclusively in the hospital environment treating the patients of local physicians.

Household system: A system of measurement commonly used in U.S. households that also has applications in heath care, including volume, length, and weight.

HSV-1: The form of HSV that causes infections in the oral cavity; fever blisters.

HSV-2: The form of HSV that causes infections in the genital tract.

Human immunodeficiency virus (HIV): A virus that attacks the immune system and destroys the white blood cells necessary to fight diseases.

Human papillomavirus (HPV): A sexually transmitted virus with over 40 different strains causing genital skin infections and cancers; genital warts.

Hypertension: Consistently elevated blood pressure readings over a defined period of time.

Hypotension: Blood pressure readings that are significantly below the American Heart Association's "normal" range.

Hypothalamus: The portion of the brain that is responsible for maintaining homeostasis.

I

if/then: Through a series of questions and best practices, a treatment plan can be established. Example: If the patient has a fever above 102, then order a CBC (complete blood count).

IIHI: Individually identifiable health information. Information that can identify a person as an individual, such as name, birth date, address, telephone number, or social security number.

Immunity: A person's ability to ward off bacterial and viral illnesses.

Immunization: An injection that may provide immunity to certain diseases.

Improper fraction: A fraction that has a numerator that is larger than its denominator.

Incubation period: The period of time in which an organism invades the body and symptoms of the disease appear.

Indirect contact: Transmission of disease through an improperly cleaned or contaminated piece of equipment.

Individual policy: An insurance policy that an individual must purchase independently.

Infected or dirty: Procedures for major traumatic injuries, excess leakage from the gastrointestinal tract into the wound, and significant breaks in sterile technique. Also, patients with a known wound or other infection.

Infectious waste: Any item or product that has the potential to transmit disease, such as linens, sharps, or trash.

Influenza: An acute viral respiratory illness that can affect adults and children in varying degrees of severity.

Initiative: Taking the responsibility to make a decision or act without having to be instructed to do so.

Insertion: The moveable point of attachment for a muscle.

Inspection: Observation of the patient to note changes in skin color, swelling, or respiratory and other signs of distress.

Insurance: A policy purchased by a group or individual that covers medical expenses. A premium is paid monthly to maintain coverage.

Internship: A clinical experience in a healthcare facility based on one's educational qualifications.

Interstitial: Between the cells. Example: Interstitial fluid, the fluid found between the cells.

Intravenous immunoglobulin (IVIG): A newer form of treatment for necrotizing fasciitis which involved a direct intravenous injection of immunoglobulin, a protein found in blood plasma.

Inversion: A medical term that indicates turning inward.

Iris: The colored portion of the eye, which includes the pupil, or opening in the center. The iris controls the size of the pupil based on the availability of light.

Irregularly irregular: A pulse rate that is irregular in pattern and rate.

-itis: Suffix to indicate "inflammation."

J

Job database Web sites: Internet sites that provide information concerning available jobs in your area and adjacent areas with instructions for application.

L

Language barriers: The lack of ability to communicate through the spoken word due to different languages.

Legal documents: Documents, including medical records, that are admissible in a court of law.

Leukocyte: White blood cells that are responsible for immunity and fighting infections in the body.

Licensure: Validation of knowledge and skills learned in the educational process. Licensure is conferred by the governing board of a profession and allows certain privileges while working in the healthcare arena. Successful completion of an examination that validates an individual's education and knowledge in a particular field. Example: physician.

Ligament: A band of connective tissues that joins bone to bone.

Lumen: The center or opening of a structure such as a blood vessel.

Lymphocyte: A specialized type of white blood cell.

M

Managed care: A program of care that helps to control the rising costs of health care by focusing on quality care at reduced costs by using a primary care physician as the gatekeeper for a patient's care.

Material safety data sheet (MSDS): A compilation of material from the manufacturer describing in detail the make-up of a substance, with the requirements for proper care, handling, storage, and first aid, and the known health risks. This printed information must be made available to employees.

Math anxiety: A situation in which learners react to math so strongly that their ability to memorize, concentrate, and pay attention is negatively impacted.

Measles: A viral illness that produces respiratory symptoms and a spotty rash.

Medical history: The patient's history of diseases, medications, and surgical procedures.

Medical record: A complete and accurate account of all patient visits to the facility. Records may be paper or electronic.

Medicare: A government health insurance plan for citizens over age 65 and others under age 65 with certain disabilities.

Meiosis: The reproductive process of the sex cells.

Meninges: The three layers of membranes that surround the brain and spinal cord. In order from inner to outer, the layers are pia, arachnoid, and dura.

Meningitis: Inflammation of the membranes surrounding the brain and spinal cords. Bacterial meningitis is contagious and often fatal. Viral meningitis is less common and has few lasting effects.

Menstruation: The sloughing of the endometrium if an egg is not fertilized. The cycle occurs every 28 days.

Mensuration: The act or process of measuring.

Metabolism: The chemical processes that take place in the body to maintain life.

Metric system: A measurement system based on units of 10.

Microorganism: A microscopic living organism too small to be seen with the unaided eye.

Micturition: The act of urinating.

Military time: Time based on a 24-hour day, meaning that the 12th hour represents 12 noon and the 24th hour represents 12 midnight.

mm Hg: Millimeters of mercury. The unit of pressure measurement used in blood pressure readings.

MMR: The vaccine that provides immunity to measles, mumps, and rubella.

Molecule: A particle made of at least two atoms that, when arranged in a orderly fashion, build cells.

Mononucleosis: An infectious disease caused by the Epstein-Barr virus.

MRSA: Methicillin-resistant *Staphylococcus aureus*, a highly resistant strain of *Staphylococcus* that does not respond to treatment with most antibiotics.

Mumps: A viral illness that presents with respiratory symptoms and swelling of the parotid glands.

Mutation: A change in the DNA sequence of a gene. Mutations can cause an organism to become resistant to medications.

N

National Fire Protection Agency (NFPA): An international nonprofit organization that develops and publishes consensus codes to minimize the effects of fire and other risks.

National Health Service: A service in Great Britain that provides health care to all residents at little to no cost through taxation.

Necrotizing fasciitis: "Flesh-eating bacteria." A devastating disease caused by group A *Streptococcus* bacteria that can destroy the skin and fascia.

Negativity: Lacking any positive qualities or feelings.

Networking: Communicating with members of your profession to share ideas, information, and common interests.

Neuron: A nerve cell.

Neurotransmitter: A chemical substance that allows for transmission of a nerve impulse across the synapse or junction of two neurons.

Nightingale, Florence (1820–1910): The highly respected pioneer in nursing whose work laid many of today's nursing foundations.

NIH: National Institutes of Health. A governmental agency that provides detailed research and documented studies of today's most devastating diseases.

Nomenclature: Method of naming.

Nontraditional hours: Hours that begin after the traditional 9-to-5 job has ended, including evening and night hours as well as weekend and holiday hours.

Nonverbal clues: Signs that may indicate the patient is uncomfortable with a question or does not understand what you are asking.

Normal flora: Bacteria that reside on and in the human body that perform useful and essential tasks to help the body function. Under normal conditions, these bacteria do not cause disease.

Nosocomial: A term once used to describe a healthcare-associated infection (HAI).

Nurse practitioner (NP): A master's degree–prepared registered nurse who has been trained to diagnose and manage the most common diseases. The NP is licensed by the state in which he/she practices.

Nutrition: The ability of the body to take in food and use it for normal body functions.

O

Obstetrical history: A woman's history of all pregnancies with outcomes and reproductive status.

-ology: Suffix to indicate "the study of."

-otomy: Suffix to indicate "create an opening."

Open drainage system: A drainage system that has a continuous opening.

OPIM: Other potentially infectious materials. Body fluids other than blood or those contaminated with blood.

Orchitis: Inflammation of the testicles as a possible complication of the mumps.

Organization: Having a plan to accomplish daily tasks in an orderly and complete fashion.

Origin: The stationary point of an attachment for a muscle.

OSHA: Occupational Safety and Health Administration. An agency of the federal government that protects all workers in all industries by setting standards, providing education, and encouraging continuous improvement in work practices.

Osteoclast: The cells that allow for calcium reabsorption.

Osteocyte: Mature bone cells.

Ova: A human egg.

Ovaries: Small, almond-shaped reproductive organs found in the female pelvis.

P

Palpation: Using the fingertips to lightly press on the patient's body to determine the size of a mass or the amount of tenderness in a certain part of the body.

Papillae: Small projections found on the tongue that absorb flavors.

Parasite: A group of microorganisms that live their entire life cycle in or on the human body.

Parasympathetic: The division of the autonomic nervous system that calms the body after an emergency situation.

PASS: Pull, aim, squeeze, sweep. Acronym that describes proper steps in the use of a fire extinguisher.

Pathogen: A germ that is capable of causing disease.

Patient interview: The initial contact with the patient to determine medical history, current medications, and chief complaint.

Penicillin: The world's first antibiotic, discovered in 1928, that paved the way for modern antibiotic therapy.

Percentage: A number that expresses either a whole (100%) or part of a whole (for example, 25%).

Percussion: A method of tapping with the fingers over body organs to determine size, fluid collection, or gas accumulation.

Peristalsis: The muscular contractions of the digestive tract that moves food through for absorption.

Personal sensitivity: Being fully aware of your own feelings and reactions.

Personality: A person's social and moral characteristics.

PHI: Protected health information. The information found in a medical record concerning diagnoses, treatment, and outcomes.

Physical assessment: The patient interview, review of systems, and physical examination.

Physical examination: The process of using the four techniques of inspection, auscultation, palpation, and percussion to evaluate a patient's health status and determine a diagnosis.

Physician's assistant: A healthcare professional that is licensed to provide treatment for medical conditions as determined by the supervising physician. Many PAs are given autonomy by the physician in caring for the patient.

Physiology: The study of the function of the body.

Platelets: Blood cells that are responsible for the clotting process of blood.

Polypharmacy: A situation that occurs when patients use multiple physicians to get multiple prescriptions, often for the same medications.

POMR: Problem-oriented medical record.

Portal of entry: The orifice of the body through which a pathogen may enter.

Portal of exit: The orifice of the body through which a pathogen will exit.

PPE: Personal protective equipment. Gowns, gloves, masks/face shields, head/shoe covers provided to employees for protection against blood and body fluid contamination.

Prefix: The beginning portion of a medical term that is used to describe a process, number, or location.

Prejudice: An unfavorable opinion or feeling formed beforehand or without knowledge, thought, or reason and having a negative effect on health care.

Premium: A monthly payment for insurance coverage.

Prenatal care: Necessary care during pregnancy to help assure a healthy outcome of delivery.

Privacy Rule: The government-sponsored law that protects IIHI.

Productivity: The ability to accomplish a set amount of work within a specified time.

Professionalism: Conducting yourself in a professional manner with your appearance, attitude, and energy.

Progress notes: Continuous narrative summaries of the patient's care by physicians, nurses, and other healthcare professionals.

Pronation: A directional medical term that indicates turning the body part over.

Proportion: The equality and relationship between two ratios.

Proof of vaccinations: The permanent record that documents all immunizations that a person has received.

Proximodistal: Development that begins in the midline of the body and extends outward.

Pulse: The heart rate per minute.

Pulse oximetry: The measurement of the oxygen content in arterial blood. Measured with a spectrophotoelectric instrument applied to the skin.

Punctuality: The art of being on time for your job or an appointment.

Punnett square: A diagram used to see all the possible combinations of genotypes two parents can pass on to their offspring.

Pupil: The opening in the iris of the eye that allows light into the eye.

Q

Quality control: The process that ensures that every healthcare facility has sufficient sterile supplies for procedures and sterilization capabilities for major equipment.

R

RACE: Rescue, activate, contain, extinguish. Acronym used to remember steps in a fire emergency.

Rash: A reddened, possibly raised lesion that appears on the skin as the result of some viral diseases.

Rate: How many times a patient breathes or the number of heart beats per minute. Also used with descriptors of regular or irregular.

Ratio: The relationship between one value and number as compared to another like value.

Recertification: A renewal of a professional licensure, certification, or registration as required by the accrediting affiliation.

Recession: A period of time in which the economic outlook declines, typically with a drop in the stock market, increased unemployment, and a decline in the housing market.

Reciprocal: A fraction that is inverted, or turned upside down.

Reference: An employer, previous employer, instructor, or personal friend who will provide information on your character and job qualifications.

Registration: A form of validation of your educational experiences from a regulatory agency associated with your profession.

Religious beliefs: Believing in and showing devotion or reverence for a deity or deities.

Renewal: A specific period of time in which you must gain an extension of your license, certificate, or registration through continuing education or completion of an exam.

Repetitive motion injuries (RMI): Injuries that are generally based on the overuse of one part of the body and generate undue stress on tendons, nerves, or joints while causing inflammation; also called cumulative trauma injuries.

Reservoir: A place in which microorganisms reside, including plants, soil, and the human body.

Resistance: 1. The ability of an organism to withstand the effects of a medication that would normally destroy it. 2. The ability of the body to defend itself against diseases after exposure.

Resistant organism: An organism that cannot be destroyed by antibiotic medications.

Respect: A feeling of admiration for another person or his or her thoughts and ideas.

Respiration: The cycle of one inhalation and one exhalation.

Responsibility: Accepting a task or being accountable for an action or idea.

Résumé: A summary of your personal information, education, and work experiences that is presented to a potential employer in consideration for a job.

Retina: The innermost portion of the eye that contains the photoreceptors.

Review of systems (ROS): A portion of the patient assessment that includes questions about each body system. Notes are made if a symptom may need further investigation.

Rhythm: A measurement of an occurrence such as respiration or pulse to determine the interval between each.

Rods: The photoreceptors for dim light vision and peripheral vision.

Roman numerals: An ancient numbering system consisting of seven key numbers represented by capital letters; still used in health care for medications, solutions, and ordering systems.

Rounding numbers: Changing a number to the nearest whole, tenth, hundredth, or thousandth, depending on the original number and your final product.

Rubella: A form of 3-day measles, often called German measles.

Rubeola: Often called "red measles," a viral illness that produces a rash that begins around the hairline and behind the ears, then progresses toward the feet.

S

Salary range: A monetary range that includes the lowest and highest potential salary that a job pays based on the applicant's education and experience.

Sclera: The white covering of the eye.

Sebaceous gland: An exocrine gland that secretes sebum, an oily substance that lubricates and protects the skin and hair.

Self-confidence: Your ability to believe in yourself and your ability to succeed.

Sharps: Any piece of equipment with a sharp surface that can penetrate the skin. Example: needles and scalpels.

Shingles: The result of the varicella-zoster virus that lays dormant in the body until the adult years. Causes a painful, blister-like rash along the pathway of one nerve.

SOAP: Subjective, objective, assessment, and plan format of medical record entries.

Social history: The patient's marital status, occupation, sexual habits, use of alcohol and tobacco, or other recreational drugs.

Sphygmomanometer: An instrument used to measure blood pressure using an inflatable cuff wrapped around the patient's arm and a pressure gauge.

Stereotyping: The assumption that all persons in a certain culture believe and act on identical standards.

Sterile: Free of all microorganisms.

Strength: The ability to exert pressure.

Subscriber: A person who buys insurance coverage for himself or herself and family members.

Suffix: The end of a medical term that further defines the condition, procedure, or disease.

Superbug: Another term for a resistant organism; one that will not respond to most antibiotics.

Supination: A directional term that indicates turning a body part upward.

Surgical site infection (SSI): An acquired infection of an operative wound. One of the most common healthcare-acquired infections.

Sympathetic: The division of the autonomic nervous system that speeds up vital body functions during an emergency situation.

Synapse: The space between two nerve cells.

Synarthrosis: A joint that exhibits no movement. Example: the cranial sutures.

Syphilis: A bacterial sexually transmitted disease that develops in three phases from acute to latent.

Systolic: The top number of a blood pressure reading that indicates the pressure during contraction of the heart.

T

Tachycardia: A rapid heart rate, usually over 100 beats per minute.

"Take Three" challenge: A CDC challenge for the prevention of influenza. Take a flu shot; take everyday precautions; and take antiviral medications when ordered by the physician.

Targeted résumé: A summary that identifies the position desired and lists the applicant's specific experience and qualifications relevant to that job; ideal for applicants who know exactly what type of position they want.

Team: A group of individuals who may work individually toward one specific goal.

Team building: Activities that allow a team to bond as members and develop techniques to be successful in their goal.

Teamwork: The act of individuals working together to accomplish a unified goal.

Temporal artery thermometer: An electronic thermometer that uses infrared technology to measure the temperature in a major artery.

Tendon: A band of connective tissue that joins muscles to bones.

Testes: The male reproductive organs.

Tissues: Cells with similar structure and function.

Transcripts: A permanent record of all classes that you have taken in your educational process, including class titles and grades earned.

Transcultural health care: The knowledge and attitudes required to provide quality care to patients from different cultural, ethnic, and racial backgrounds.

Trauma center: A unit within a hospital that specializes in the care of catastrophic physical events. Trauma centers are designated by the state.

Triage systems: Guidelines used to assess patients' conditions and determine where they should be sent and what treatments should be administered.

Tuberculosis: A bacterial infection that typically attacks the lungs by destroying the healthy tissue and creating holes in the lungs.

Tympanic thermometer: An electronic thermometer that uses infrared technology to measure the temperature at the tympanic membrane (eardrum).

U

Universal precautions: The guidelines developed by the CDC in 1987 specific to health care that say that blood and body fluids could contain transmissible infectious organisms.

Ureter: The tube that drains urine from the kidney to the bladder.

Urethra: The tube that drains urine from the bladder to the outside of the body.

Urinary tract infection (UTI): An infection of any part of the urinary system, including the urethra, bladder, ureters, or kidneys.

Utilization management: The process used to determine if the future services used by the patient in terms of medical services and procedures, facilities, and practitioners are necessary, appropriate, and the most cost-effective.

Utilization review: A process used to review medical treatment already received by the patient to evaluate if the medical services were appropriate and cost-effective.

V

Vaccine: A solution containing a killed or attenuated (weakened) form of a pathogen given as an injection to provide immunity against the pathogen.

Vancomycin: An older generation of antibiotic that is effective against MRSA in some situations.

Varicella-zoster virus: The virus that causes chickenpox or shingles.

Vector-borne: The transmission of a disease from one host to another, usually through the bite of an insect.

Vein: A blood vessel that transports blood back to the heart.

Vena cava: The largest vein that drains all of the circulating blood from the body back into the heart.

Ventilator: A machine that provides assistance in breathing for patients unable to breathe independently.

Virus: A submicroscopic organism that is unable to replicate without a host cell and is capable of causing disease. It invades a cell and uses the cell's activity to survive.

Vital signs: The patient's temperature, pulse rate, respiratory rate, and blood pressure. Sometimes includes height and weight.

VRE: Vancomycin-resistant *Enterococcus*. Like MRSA, an enterococcal infection that is resistant to vancomycin.

W

Weight: The heaviness of the body usually stated in pounds or kilograms.

Whistle-blower: Someone who reports safety issues in the workplace with no fear of retribution.

Whole numbers: Traditional numbers that do not contain fractions or decimals and that are used in counting.

Word root: The foundation of a medical term. Denotes the body part, organ system, or process.

Work history: A portion of your resume that contains all of your previous jobs, how long you worked, and what your duties were.

Work practice control: The physical acts of hand washing, wearing PPEs, proper disposal of sharps and biohazardous material to prevent the spread of infectious organisms.

Z

Zero out: Calibrating or adjusting the scales to 0 pounds prior to measuring a patient's weight.

Zygote: The reproductive cell with the full adult genetic complement formed by the joining together of the egg and the sperm.

INDEX

Note: Page numbers followed by "f" refer to figures (illustrations); page numbers followed by "t" refer to tables.